Children
Without Homes

Children Without Homes

An Examination of Public Responsibility to Children in Out-of-Home Care

This study was conducted by Jane Knitzer, Mary Lee Allen and Brenda McGowan. Dr. Knitzer participated in all phases of the project from its inception in 1975. Ms. Allen joined the project in 1976, and is primarily responsible for analysis of the federal role. Dr. McGowan, a member of the Children's Defense Fund staff from 1974 to 1976, participated in the conceptualization of the study and data collection. The final report was written by Jane Knitzer and Mary Lee Allen.

Children's Defense Fund
Washington, D.C.

Inquiries concerning the report should be addressed to the Children's Defense Fund, 1520 New Hampshire Avenue, N.W., Washington, D.C. 20036.

362.73
K74
c.

Copyright © 1978 by Children's Defense Fund.
All rights reserved.
No part of this publication may be reproduced, stored in a retrieval system, or transmitted in any form or by any means, electronic, mechanical, photocopy, recording, or otherwise, without prior written permission from the publisher.
Library of Congress Catalog Card Number: 78-74230
Printed in the United States of America
Designed by Marilyn Worseldine

To Justine Wise Polier who has, with unfailing vision and persistence, initiated countless advocacy efforts on behalf of children and inspired succeeding generations of advocates to do the same.

Contents

Foreword ix
Preface xiii
Acknowledgments xv

Introduction and Overview 1
No One's Children 1
The CDF Study 3
Highlights of Our Findings 5
What Can Be Done? 10
How the Report is Organized 12

Part I. Defining the Problem

1. Families Don't Count: Severing Family Ties 15
Separating Children from Families 15
Reducing Family Ties After Placement 22
When Out-of-Home Care Ends: Is There Any Family? 25
What Can Be Done? 34

2. Children Don't Count: Patterns of Public Neglect 37
What Public Neglect Looks Like 37
The Reasons for Public Neglect 42
Special Burdens of Minority Children 49
Local Efforts Can Work 54
What Can Be Done? 55

3. Children Placed Out of State: Public Neglect Compounded 57
How Many Children Are Out of State? 58
Which Children Are Sent Out of State? 61
The Inadequacy of Regulatory Efforts 66
What Can Be Done? 74

Part II. State and Federal Responsibility

4. The Role of the State: Assessing Responsibility 77
The State's Responsibility 77
The CDF Findings 78
What Can Be Done? 100

5. The Federal Role: In Search of a Viable Federal Policy 105
Major Federal Programs: An Overview 106
The CDF Findings 123
What Can Be Done? 140

Part III. Effecting Change

6. Programs That Work: Varied Approaches 153
Direct Service Programs for Families and Children 153
Administrative and Judicial Protections 160
Advocacy Groups 165

7. Advocacy for Children Without Homes: Strategies for Change 169
Case Advocacy 169
Class Advocacy 170
Responding to Excuses 178
Action at the National Level 179

Appendices

A. The Study Methodology — 182

B. Status of Audits of the AFDC Foster Care Program by the HEW Audit Agency — 184

C. Findings from the CDF Survey of County Child Welfare and Probation Offices — 185

D. Policy Statement on Parental Visiting — 192

E. Statutory Provisions for Counsel in Neglect and Termination Proceedings — 195

F. Citations to State Adoption Subsidy Statutes — 210

G. Adoption Exchanges — 211

H. Interstate Placements — 216

I. Interstate Placements Reported by Child Welfare Administrators in 1976 — 221

J. Selected Demographic Characteristics of Seven Study States — 222

K. Number of Children in Out-of-Home Placement — 224

L. Description of Statutory Provisions for Foster Care Reviews — 228

M. Administrative Structure of State Agencies Responsible for Children in Out-of-Home Care as of 1976 in the Study States — 252

N. Organization of Child Welfare Services in the Study States as of 1976 — 254

O. 1975-1976 Adoption Data for the Study States — 256

P. Federal Programs Affecting Children Without Homes — 258

Q. AFDC Foster Care Program Expenditures for Fiscal Year 1976, and June 1976 Program Recipients — 276

R. Medicaid Eligibility Coverage of Financially Needy Children Under 21 — 278

S. Contacts Concerning Innovative Efforts Discussed in Chapter 6 — 280

Photographs: The photographs in this book are for illustrative purposes only. There is no direct relationship between any particular person and the text. *Credits:* Iris Rothman, pp. 4, 25, 59, 81, 112, 115, 118, 129, 139, 141, 143, 168, 173. Janie Eisenberg, pp. 20, 34, 76, 119, 121, 134, 152. J. Wayne Higgs, pp. 48, 127, 162. Marilyn Worseldine, pp. 70, 125. William Lohr, p. 9. Leslie Cooper, p. 36. Michael A. Woodlon, p. 43. Janet Dinsmore, p. 47. Roland L. Freeman, p. 67. Ted Webersinn, p. 101. Joan Larson, p. 155. Suzanne Rhodes, p. 174. Other photographs courtesy of Administration for Children, Youth and Families, U.S. Department of Health, Education and Welfare; President's Committee on Mental Retardation; and U.S. Commission on Civil Rights. Photographs by J. Wayne Higgs courtesy of Law Enforcement Assistance Administration, U.S. Department of Justice.

Foreword

It is a safe assumption that, at predictable intervals, a dramatic story about some particular homeless, neglected or abused child who has suffered hardship or damage at the hands of an insensitive bureaucracy will be spread upon the front page of a newspaper with an otherwise dull crop of news. These stories range from that of a child torn from his mother's loving arms for seemingly trivial or irrelevant reasons, to that of a child who has reached a hospital badly beaten by a parent. In the first instance the cry is "Why can't the government leave them alone?" and in the second, "Why didn't the government do something?" But between these bouts of outraged societal conscience, little is done to strengthen the public child welfare responsibility and the agencies charged with giving it reality. They are left to try to function in a limbo of neglect: underfunded, little appreciated, and generally misunderstood.

Every public function runs the risk of bureaucratic lassitude and failure of performance. Dedication, imagination and zeal do not thrive readily in the thicket of governmental procedure. But where child welfare is concerned there is double jeopardy. On the one hand, the child already damaged by parental failure or handicap is further endangered by the failure or inadequacy of the back-up public agency. On the other hand, the agency falters because of the absence of public understanding and support. The outrage felt at the plight of a particular child is rarely translated into support for the child welfare service program charged with his protection.

Child welfare is the function that derives from the unique and extended dependency of the human child on adult care and nurture. Normally this care is provided by the child's family: in the first instance by his parents—preferably both but in our time frequently by a lone mother. In the second instance there may be a widening circle of secondary family care: grandparents, uncles and aunts, cousins or even neighbors. This outer circle is common in tribal or subsistence agricultural societies. But in our own society—urban, mobile, and fragmented—the larger family is scattered and the child is increasingly dependent on his own parents or parent. Thus, as in so many other areas, the back-up function has been assumed by organized societal institutions, both governmental and voluntary, with ultimate authority assigned to the courts. Where parental responsibility is lacking or in dispute, the authority of a family court may be necessary. But the responsibility for shoring up or providing substitutes for that parental care rests with child welfare.

The role of the child welfare agency is little understood even though the social disorganization that creates it is widely deplored. In the days before antibiotics and other miracles of modern medicine reduced premature death and before social security reduced economic dependency when a parent died, most people directed their philanthropic impulses toward aiding orphans and orphanages. But today the full orphan or the destitute half-orphan is a relative rarity. Instead, we are overwhelmed by family breakdown, illegitimacy, desertion, or the incapacity of an ill or over-burdened single mother. And we are overwhelmed with related problems of truancy, runaways, juvenile delinquency, alienation and other products of failed child nurturance. People deplore the outcome of neglect but they ignore or reject the agency charged by society for its mitigation.

Few even understand the difference between the need for protection of a child in a particularly vulnerable home situation and the economic relief needed by an impoverished family with children. The latter may be a strong and supportive family in every respect except income; the former may be the child of an economically privileged family unable to function for other reasons. It is ironical that, while the economic relief program of AFDC (Aid to Families with Dependent Children)—unpopular though it may be—spent over ten billion dollars in 1976, the Child Welfare Services Program received only $50.5 million in federal funds (out of a previously authorized sum of $266 million).

This lack of understanding and support for the child welfare service function has had another predictable result: fragmentation. The separate parts have tended to overshadow the whole. Thus, as public outrage responded to awareness of one part, the physical abuse of children by their parents, a new program of federal grants was authorized to deal with "Child Abuse and Neglect." Similarly with runaway children, teen-age pregnancies, day care, juvenile delinquency prevention, and others. Even certain of the primary care aspects of child welfare services, including foster care for children needing temporary care away from their own homes and adoptive placement for children without families, have tended to overshadow the preventive and protective service matrix from which they draw their lifeblood. It is little wonder that a demoralized service tends to jog listlessly along accustomed paths until a fresh outcry breaks the conspiracy of silence and indifference surrounding their difficult and sensitive task.

It is fortunate for these supremely vulnerable children that a number of recent studies and legislative initiatives have begun to break through the wall of isolation that has obscured their plight. Outstanding among the studies is this one, *Children Without Homes*, undertaken by Dr. Jane Knitzer, Mary Lee Allen and Dr. Brenda McGowan for the Children's Defense Fund. It is outstanding in its successful wedding of scholarship in the gathering and analysis of factual material with the graphic interpretation of what these facts mean to real children.

The facts and drama of *Children Without Homes* all contribute to single theme: that when the government assumes responsibility for children, it owes them the kind and degree of nurture children require for their development. This, as the report documents, it is tragically failing to do in myriad ways. Children require, before all else, the sense that they belong to reliable and loving adults who will care for their needs, emotional as well as physical. Yet repeatedly, it is demonstrated, families are permitted to fall apart, parents to throw in the sponge—when an investment of supportive services and aids would have given them the strength and security to function as parents. Children require stability, most particularly an inner assurance that caring adults will remain firmly in their lives. Yet children removed from their own homes are repeatedly moved from foster home to foster home or institution while little is done to strengthen their ties to their own families. Many, who might with skillful strengthening of the home situation return to their own homes, remain in the limbo of "placement" until they are grown. Some, in fact many, are sent to institutions far from their own homes even in distant states, and are there forgotten. No one seems to know or care where they are: they are not visited, rescued or even recorded. Except for the heavy fees paid by the sending state with help from the federal assistance program, they are effectively abandoned.

The irony of this whole sad picture lies in its departure from our typical American addiction to cost-benefit economy. It would obviously serve the welfare of the children better to strengthen their own homes or free them for adoption if that proved impossible. But it would also be infinitely cheaper for the taxpayer. Study after study confirms simple common sense on this score. This being true, one is driven to ask why do we persist in such destructive and counter-productive practices?

Last year Congress initiated a number of moves to strengthen the basic child welfare sevices program by incorporating procedural protections against the overuse of foster care, and by instituting financial subsidy for some adoptions that would begin to turn this situation around. That legislation did not pass and child welfare must now be given priority in the next session of Congress. Yet whatever happens in terms of federal financial aid and leadership, the continuing problem remains primarily at the state and community level. People need to understand and enthusiastically support an adequate and caring child welfare service and related programs. This report should be widely read and studied to this end, not only by policy makers but also by all devoted and informed advocates for children.

Elizabeth Wickenden
Consultant on Social Policy

Preface

This is the seventh Children's Defense Fund report on major problems facing large numbers of American children: problems which cry out for immediate public response and remediation.

In 1975, we decided to examine the numerous problems facing the hundreds of thousands of children at risk of being placed or already placed out of their own homes. We wanted to determine how well publicly supported child care agencies were carrying out their mandated responsibilities to these children and their families; how effective existing laws covering out-of-home placements were; where local, state and federal policies and practices fail to meet the needs of these children and families; and what can be done about it. CDF staff visited seven states, talked with over 200 people, and read many, many pages of reports and public documents describing federal and state policies.

What we have found and detail in this report is a national disgrace—a pattern of institutional abuse and neglect of our most vulnerable children that cannot wait one more day for correction. The daily plight of these children, often left family-less, makes a mockery of our professed belief in family, our concern for our young, and for the cost-effective use of taxpayers' money.

Remedies to help this group of children must be comprehensive. They must involve all levels of government and address all the systems having responsibility for these children—child welfare, juvenile justice, mental health, mental retardation and special education. At the federal level there is a pressing need for strong leadership and legislative reform. Particularly crucial is the passage of child welfare legislation which would: erase federal fiscal incentives to keep children in out-of-home care; increase funds for preventive and restorative services; strengthen protections for children and families; and ensure children permanent families.

At local and state levels there is much to be done as well. Advocates and citizens must seek a redirection of those policies and practices which result in children being victimized by public neglect. They must work to see that services are strengthened, that reviews are meaningful, and that meeting the needs of this group of children and families becomes a political priority.

Our report is a first step. It defines the problems, and lays out some steps for advocates to take. The Children's Defense Fund is committed to making the needed changes — but we need your help.

Marian Wright Edelman
Director, Children's Defense Fund

Acknowledgments

Many people in many different places have made this report possible. But there are also a number of individuals without whose efforts this report would simply not exist, and who should be thanked individually.

Don Rademacher participated in the early stages of the report as co-director and shared with us his broad experience with the juvenile justice system. Carol Furst and Kathleen Reynolds made site visits to several states, bringing back insightful observations concerning the problems and needs. Ms. Furst also conducted and assisted in the analysis of surveys of children placed out of state. Carol Larson, Karen Milner, and Ellen Segal helped in the difficult task of trying to understand the state statutes. Paul Smith and Shannon Ferguson, of the CDF staff, enabled us to make sense out of the not always sensible statistical information we gathered from the counties. And to Burstelle Simmons and Luba Lynch we are deeply grateful for patience and fortitude in typing the many versions of the report. We are also grateful to the many CDF staff members who provided information and encouragement, and particularly to Janet Dinsmore for her editorial assistance. A special thank you to the Edna McConnell Clark Foundation without whose generous support this report would not have been possible.

We must also express our appreciation to officials, professionals, parents and others around the country who took the time to share with us information, both the good and the bad, about what really happens to children without homes. Our thanks too to numerous staff at the federal level who shared program information with us.

And above all, deep gratitude is due to Justine Wise Polier and Elizabeth Wickenden who helped us conceptualize the report, critiqued it often, and throughout the long process, encouraged us to speak out on behalf of children without homes.

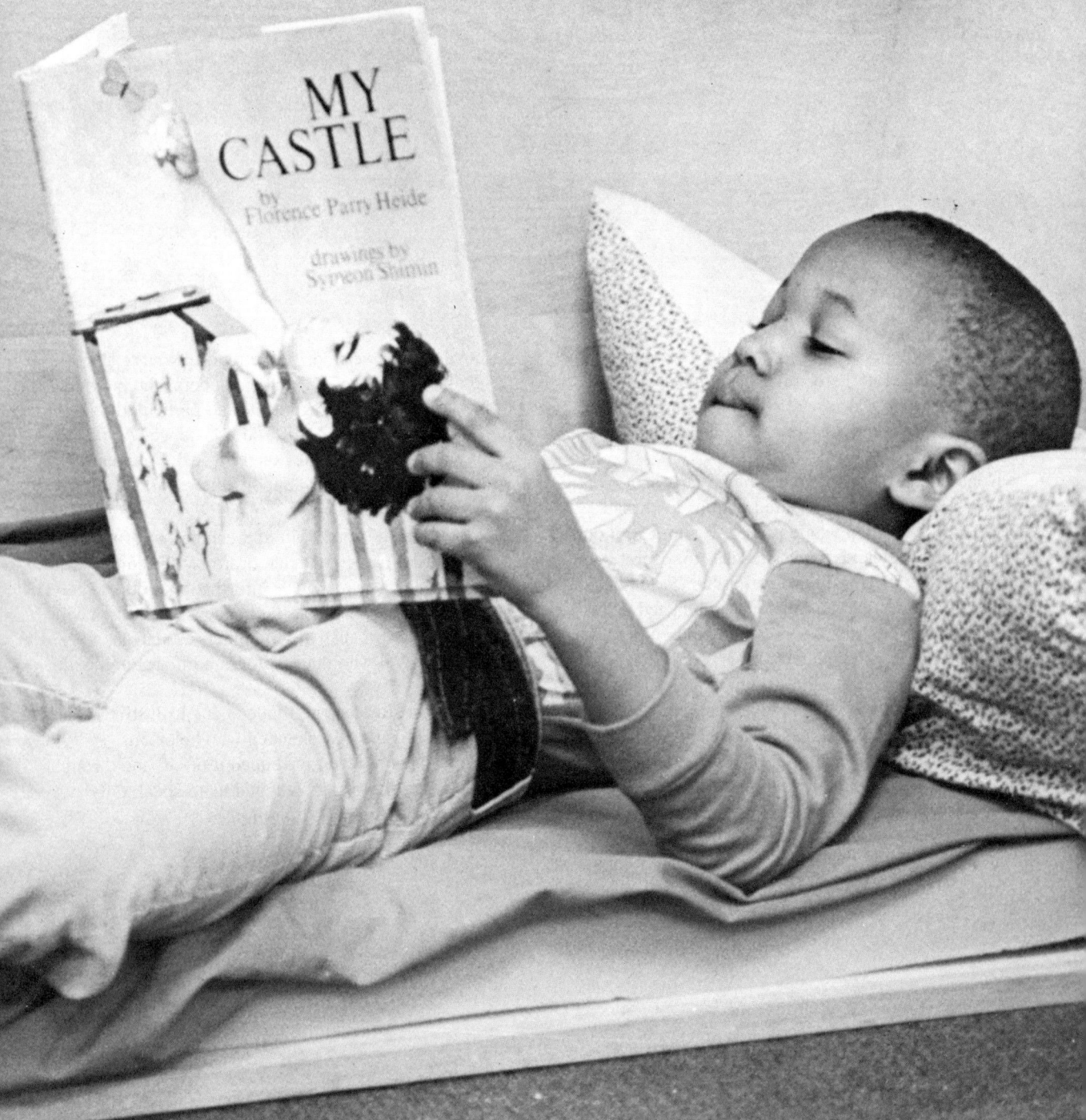

Introduction and Overview

"Hey, anybody who wants to read this, I am a nine-year-old boy. I have a mommy, but she doesn't live with me. She comes to see me sometimes. I live in a shelter. The place I'm living my mommy says is better than living with her, but I don't think so. It's kind of lonely living here. I don't get much mail. Please write to me because its lonely here."

A note found in a laundromat in a southern state, Spring 1978.

Almost everyone agrees that families are vital to the healthy development of children. Professionals and researchers confirm the conventional wisdom: children need to feel wanted and accepted, they need continuity in their relationships with biological or psychological parents; they need guidance to cope with the demands of growing up; and they need to have some sense that there is a regular, dependable quality to the world.[1]

---

[1] See, for example, E. Erikson, *Identity: Youth and Crisis* (New York: W. W. Norton and Company, 1968), Joint Commission on Mental Health for Children, *Crisis In Child Mental Health: Challenge for the 1970's* (New York: Harper & Row, 1969), and Advisory Committee On Child Development, *Toward a National Policy for Children and Families* (Washington, D.C.: Assembly of Behavioral and Social Sciences, National Research Council, National Academy of Sciences, 1976).

No One's Children

The majority of American children grow up secure in their own families. Over 500,000 children do not. These are children who, for a variety of appropriate and inappropriate reasons, are removed from their homes and made the responsibility of public child care systems. Sometimes they lack families. Sometimes their families don't care. Too often they are children whose families have been wrongly written off by the responsible public child care systems as too poor, too sick, or too inadequate to bring up children. Public agency decisions have been made on the children's behalf, but they have little to do with individual circumstance or need. The result is that many of these children grow up without the psychological roots vital to their security. They are no one's children.

The children without homes are a heterogeneous group. Some are infants; many more are preadolescents and adolescents. Some have special needs stemming from physical or emotional handicaps; others have been involved with the juvenile court; some have families in which pressures to cope were too great and their parents requested the children be removed from home; and some have abusive or neglectful parents. Typical among them are Timmy, Terri, Cindy, and Alvin.

Timmy is one and a half years old. He is an abused child who was born deaf. His home for the last 15 months has been a hospital ward in a large city. No one charged with his responsibility can find a foster home for him, although he no longer needs hospital care and his mother does not want him back.

Terri is an alert, warm, engaging eight-year-old who is beginning to show signs of learning difficulties and aggressiveness. Terri is entering her third school and her fourth foster home in four years. She has not seen her own parents in four years but no one is making plans for her to ensure she has a permanent family.

Cindy is a seven-year-old retarded child whose mother made numerous unsuccessful attempts to enroll her in the public school system in the southern rural community where they live. Cindy could already do many things for herself. Yet the school system argued it had no services for her, offered no alternatives and told her mother to keep Cindy at home. Cindy and her mother were receiving public assistance but the local welfare officials did nothing to help Cindy's mother insist the schools provide an appropriate education. Instead, they wanted to place Cindy in a state institution for the mentally retarded. When Cindy's mother refused, the local department formally charged her with neglect. The Court upheld the charge and ordered that Cindy be placed in the state institution.

Alvin is 15. He rarely attends school and has a history of troubled behavior. Alvin has been away from home for seven years. Three years ago, he tried to run away from his foster home to his own home. He was brought to court and declared a status offender—a child in need of supervision. He was then sent to a school 3,000 miles away from his home state. No one visits him there, and his mother, despite requests, cannot get reports on his progress. She cannot find the caseworker assigned to Alvin, and her letters to the out-of-state facility have not been answered.

No one knows exactly how many children are in placement out of their own homes, or of those, how many are completely cut off from their own families. Piecing together the scattered data, we estimate that public child care systems are responsible for one-half to three-quarters of a million children in out-of-home placement.[2]

Five major child care systems have responsibility for children without homes: child welfare, juvenile justice, mental health, mental retardation, and special education.[3] These systems place the children, pay for their care, and make crucial decisions about what happens to them. The children live in foster homes, group homes, residential treatment centers, special schools, and child care institutions.[4] Sometimes they live in hospitals and nursing homes for long periods of time, not because they are sick but for lack of any other place to go.

The majority of the children in out-of-home care, regardless of age, special need, or family circumstance,

---

[2]On the basis of a 1975 CDF survey of children out of their homes in a random sample of 140 counties, CDF projected nationally that there were over 448,000 children in out-of-home care who are the responsibility of public child welfare agencies. This figure does not include children who are the responsibility of probation, mental health, mental retardation or special education systems. For an explanation of the basis for our projection, see Appendix A.

Data collection efforts relevant to children out of their homes, as we show in later chapters, are grossly inadequate. For example, no federal agency knows how many children are indeed in out-of-home care. Various surveys, however, do give some indication. According to 1970 Census data, there were approximately 2.5 million children under 18 years of age who were living with neither parent; 1.6 million were in homes with relatives, 434,000 in households in which they were not related to the head, 247,000 in institutions and another 160,000 in group quarters other than institutions. U.S. Bureau of the Census, Census of Population: 1970, *Subject Reports, Persons by Family Characteristics*, Final Report PC(2)-4B (Washington, D.C.: U.S. Government Printing Office, 1973), Table 1. Although it is not possible to know the proportion of children in these various settings who were in the care of public agencies, it is likely that many of them would fit our definition of children without homes.

Other survey data from studies of individual child care systems also suggest that our estimate of over one-half to three-quarters of a million children is realistic. Preliminary findings from a recently completed national survey of a sample of over 9,000 children served by public social services departments in the United States indicate that in March 1977, social services were provided to 1.8 million children, 28 percent of whom, or over half a million children, were in foster care. See A. Shyne and A. Schroeder, *National Study of Social Services to Children and Their Families–Overview* (Washington, D.C.: Children's Bureau, Office of Human Development Services, Administration for Children, Youth and Families, HEW, 1978), pp. 8-9. The 1975 Annual Juvenile Detention and Correctional Facility Census reported that there were approximately 47,000 juveniles in public juvenile detention centers, training schools and other correctional facilities, and an additional 27,000 in private juvenile custody facilities, over 80 percent of whom were in long-term care facilities. U.S. Department of Justice, Law Enforcement Assistance Administration, National Criminal Justice Information and Statistics Service, *Children in Custody: Advance Report on the Juvenile Detention and Correctional Facility Census of 1975* (Washington, D.C.: U.S. Government Printing Office, 1977), pp. 18-19.

[3]For the purpose of this report, we use the term "system" to refer to each of the particular public bureaucracies that has responsibility for the out-of-home placement and care of children. When we refer to the "systems" collectively, we speak of child care systems.

[4]Rigorous definitions of what constitutes these different types of settings are lacking. In general, foster homes serve up to six children, group homes between 6 and 15, sometimes up to 25, and institutions 25 or more. The term "institution" is often used to refer to both residential treatment centers and custodial child care institutions and is used that way in our report, except where we specifically discuss one or the other.

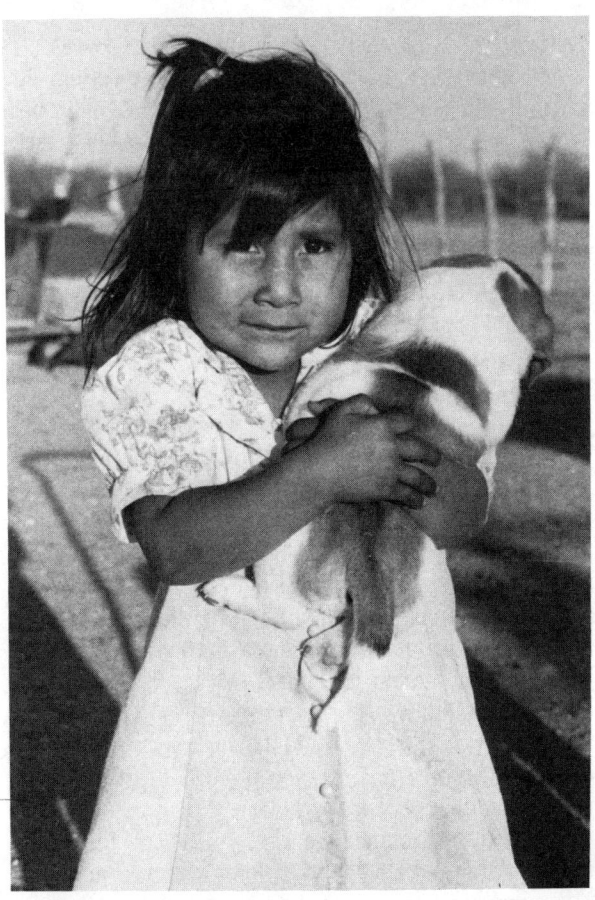

The CDF Study

In 1975, the Children's Defense Fund (CDF) decided to examine the problem of children at risk of placement or already placed out of their own homes.[6] We sought to determine how well public child care agencies were carrying out mandated responsibilities to these children and their families; how effective existing laws covering out-of-home placements were; where local, state and federal policies and practices fail to meet the needs of the children and families; and what can be done about it.

We looked at all of the public systems responsible for children out of their homes.[7] However, since the majority of children out of their homes become the responsibility of the child welfare system, we examined its role most carefully. We identified eight basic questions needing answers.

The Questions

1. To what extent do public systems take account of a child's need for a family? What are the legal and psychological dilemmas in sorting out public and parental responsibility for these children?

2. Which public policies and practices are most harmful to children without homes?

3. What is the state's initial and continuing responsibility to children at risk of removal from their homes or

are the responsibility of the child welfare system;[5] a smaller number become the responsibility of the other child care systems. Theoretically, each system responds to children with different needs: e.g., children involved in status offenses fall under the jurisdiction of the juvenile justice system; children with emotional difficulties are cared for by systems for the mentally ill. In practice, however, the needs of the children entering different systems are interchangeable. And some of the children become the responsibility of no one system, but are shuttled from one to the other.

---

[5]Many of the terms used in speaking of children at risk of placement or in out-of-home care have multiple meanings. For example, "child welfare" has at least two meanings. In its broadest sense, it refers to a general social concern with the well-being of children. In this sense, all public systems with responsibility for children are concerned with child welfare. In its second meaning, child welfare refers to a particular body of professional practices, services and regulations pertaining to the placement of children in out-of-home care and to the protection of children at risk of such placement. Historically, child welfare has been particularly concerned with those children who are vulnerable as a result of family problems, and do not themselves have severe handicapping conditions.

[6]By "children" we mean persons who are minors consistent with the particular state definition. Thus, we include both younger children and adolescent youth.

[7]Few studies have looked across child care systems to identify patterns of equal and unequal treatment to similar types of children, who happen, often by chance, to be the responsibility of different systems.

Examinations of the child welfare system, however, have repeatedly shown that once in foster care, children are likely to remain for long periods and that the foster care system does not provide "temporary" but rather long-term care for children away from their families. See, for example, D. Fanshel and E. B. Shinn, *Children in Foster Care: A Longitudinal Investigation* (New York: Columbia University Press, 1978); B. Ferleger and M. J. Cotter, eds., *Children, Families and Foster Care, New Insights from Research in New York City* (New York: Community Council of Greater New York, 1976); R. Geiser, *The Illusion of Caring* (Boston: Beacon Press, 1973); H. Maas and R. Engler, *Children in Need of Parents* (New York: Columbia University Press, 1959); R. Mnookin, "Foster Care -- In Whose Best Interest?" *Harvard Educational Review* 43 (November 1973): 599-638; and S. M. Vasaly, *Foster Care in Five States: A Synthesis and Analysis of Studies from Arizona, California, Iowa, Massachusetts and Vermont* (Washington, D.C.: Social Research Group, George Washington University, 1976).

To a much lesser extent there have also been examinations of other systems caring for children out of their homes. These have focused primarily on what happens to the children within each system. See, for example, R. C. Sarri and R. D. Vinter, *Time Out: A National Study of Juvenile Correctional Programs* (Michigan: National Assessment of Juvenile Corrections, University of Michigan, 1976); Task Force on Children Out of School, *Suffer the Children: Politics of Mental Health in Massachusetts* (Boston: Task Force on Children Out of School, 1972).

in placement? What should it be? How adequately does a group of representative states actually meet its responsibility to these children?

4. What is the role of the federal government in exercising leadership and in assisting states to carry out their responsibility to children at risk of removal or in placement?

5. What informational gaps impede effective change on behalf of children without homes?

6. What types of existing programs are responsive to the needs of children at risk of or already in placement, as well as their families?

7. What specific legislative or administrative changes are required of the states and federal government to end policies and practices that are destructive for large numbers of children?

8. What can advocates do to improve conditions for children without homes?

How We Conducted The Study

CDF gathered answers to these eight questions in four ways. First, we sent a two-page questionnaire to both child welfare and probation offices in a stratified random sample of 140 counties: 27 with populations over 300,000, 113 with populations under 300,000. We requested basic information about the children placed in out-of-home care—age, sex, race, type of placement, length of stay in care, number of moves, and legal status—to determine what is known about the children by the agencies directly responsible for them. We also requested information about specific placement-related policies.

Second, we studied seven states in depth: Arizona, California, Massachusetts, New Jersey, Ohio, South Carolina, and South Dakota. These states reflect different geographic regions, different patterns of urban and rural concentration, different proportions of minority populations and different minority groups, different per capita incomes, and different social service structures.

In each state, our purpose was to understand the policies and responsibilities of the various child care systems, and to examine how they work in practice at the local level. We sought to build a profile of the state and to identify areas of strength and weakness regarding policies and practices affecting individual children without homes. We sought, too, to determine which forms of public neglect and abuse cut across states and child care systems, and what factors contribute to these abuses.

We spent two to four weeks in each state meeting with state officials responsible for the children, interested citizen advocates, lawyers and legislators. We also visited three or four counties in each state to talk with staff who daily must make hard decisions about the strengths of families, which children must be placed out of their homes, and where they are placed. This gave us a first-hand sense of the constraints and problems those "on the firing line" experience. In addition, we reviewed statistical data, advocates' reports and relevant national information.

Third, we undertook a special survey in the 50 states and the District of Columbia of children placed in residential facilities in states other than their own. Because children in out-of-state placements are cut off from their families and the view of state officials by geographic distance and jurisdictional boundaries, we wanted to know how much officials in the sending states knew about what happens to these children.

Finally, we conducted a detailed analysis of federal policies, including relevant legislation, regulations, funding patterns, research and demonstration grants, and the administrative organization of federal programs affecting children at risk of placement or in out-of-home care. We also examined the extent of federal leadership and innovation in relation to children without homes.

A summary of our major findings follows.

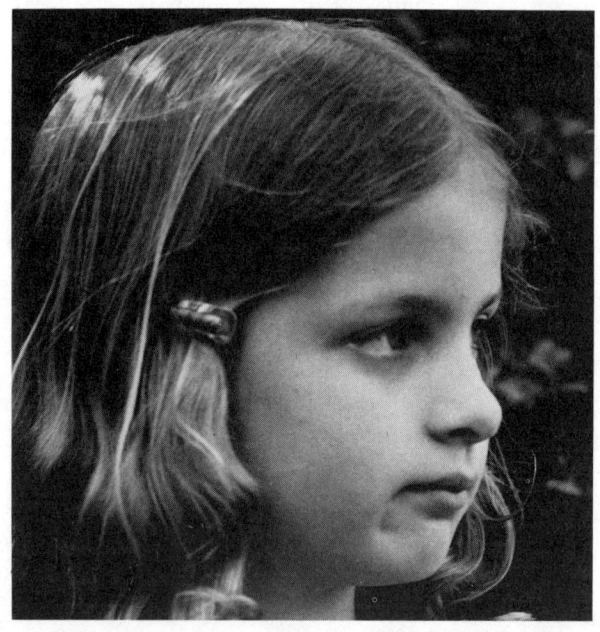

Highlights of Our Findings

Families Don't Count

At every point in the placement process children and their natural families are isolated from one another by the action and inaction of those with official responsibility. Pro-family rhetoric notwithstanding, a pervasive, implicit anti-family bias often shapes decisions about children at risk of removal or in out-of-home care.

When the Child is Placed

- The initial separation of child and family is often by default. Few alternatives such as homemakers, day care,[8] specialized day treatment, alternative housing and other supportive services are available. Removing a child from home is often the easiest course. Funds for removal are available; adequate funds for alternatives are not.

- Sometimes, in order to get appropriate educational or social services for handicapped children, parents are told they must place their children in out-of-home care. Sometimes, they are even told they must give up legal custody of their children.

- When it is necessary to place a child out of the home, little thought typically is given to placement with familiar relatives. Sometimes states do not pay foster care rates to relatives, although they will to strangers. Yet without such assistance, relatives often cannot care for the children. This means that even when willing relatives are available, a child is likely to be totally uprooted and placed with strangers.

When the Child is in Out-Of-Home Care

- Typically, parents are not explicitly encouraged to maintain contact with their children. Sometimes they are actively discouraged from doing so. Only one-half of the reporting counties in our child welfare survey had specific written policies about parent-child visitation. One county reported it permitted such visits only on special occasions, such as the child's birthday. Another permitted visiting only in the courtroom, hardly a setting designed to put either the child or parent at ease.

---

[8]While day care services theoretically can have a significant role in relieving stress on families, public policy in general has limited eligibility for publicly supported day care to children of working parents. Only a very small proportion of day care funds has been used for day care to prevent out-of-home placements.

- Parents who want to maintain close contact with a child in placement get little help from local or state officials. Funds to pay transportation costs for visits are limited even though children are often placed long distances from their families. Parents are not routinely informed about the progress children are making. Sometimes they are not even informed when their children are moved. All this serves to reduce psychological ties and lessen the likelihood of reunification.

- While the child is in out-of-home care, parents generally get little help with the problems that led to the removal. Funds for services that would enable the family to be reunited are seldom available.

When Ties with the Natural Family are Broken

- There is far too little concern for the child's right to a family when initially removed from his or her own home, often before other alternatives are tried. Yet it is a tragic irony that once parental ties have been severed, either as a consequence of parental abandonment or the action or inaction of public systems, legal termination of parental rights is rare. Regardless of the reality of the child's current situation or needs, there is widespread reluctance to initiate proceedings to terminate the rights of biological parents.

- For children who should have parental rights terminated or who have had parental rights terminated, efforts to ensure new permanent homes are often not vigorous enough. Adoption efforts are hampered by fiscal barriers, inadequate funds for subsidized adoptions or legal fees, as well as deeply embedded views that certain children—minority children, older children, and children with special medical needs—are "hard to place," and thus "unadoptable."

Children Don't Count

Children placed out of their homes are not only likely to be cut off from families, but also abandoned psychologically and sometimes literally by the public systems that assume responsibility for them. They are, in effect, children in double jeopardy.

- In every county we visited, those who work directly with children report great pressures: impossibly large caseloads, excessive and meaningless paperwork, no time to get to know children for whom they make decisions, no time to visit families, and no training to deal with complex family problems.

- Children remain in care for long periods of time, often moving from place to place, without the chance to experience stable caring from any adult. In our survey, 13 percent of the children had been out of their own homes for over four years, and an additional 20 percent for over six years. In all, 52 percent had been in out-of-home care for two or more years. Moreover, the responding survey counties reported that 18 percent of the children in out-of-home care had been moved more than three times.

Children in institutional or group home settings rather than foster home care appear to be particularly vulnerable to public neglect and various forms of institutional abuse. Mechanisms for ensuring that these children are appropriately placed and receive quality care are ineffective or nonexistent.

- Sixty-four of the 140 county child welfare offices in our survey reported having written policies requiring caseworker-child contact. But while 46 percent of the counties reporting required such contact if a child was in a foster home, only 30 percent required contact if a child was in a group home; 25 percent if the child was in an institution; and only 12 percent if a child was in out-of-state placement. In other words, the further away the child was from a family context, the less caseworker-child contact was required.

- Too many children are in institutions. In each of the seven study states, public officials openly acknowledged that children who did not belong in institutions were placed there. On the other hand, children who do need institutional care or care in residential treatment facilities may not get it. Children with special needs, for instance, are frequently placed in institutions with no appropriate programs or specialized services.

- Despite immense public concern about familial abuse, no state CDF staff visited had set up mechanisms, nor issued guidelines to monitor and eliminate the institutional abuse of children. Such abuse takes many forms: the unmonitored, excessive use of seclusion or drug therapies, severe behavioral restrictions, or harsh physical punishment. Despite evidence that abuse of children in institutions and other group settings is widespread, no state studied had a licensing statute spelling out specific sanctions for institutional abuse.

- Children are sent far distances from their own communities, sometimes within the same state, but often out of state. Out-of-state placement virtually ensures that there will be no contact with family or caseworker. Nationally, we estimate over 10,000 children are placed out of state at any one time.

The Failure of State Responsibility

States are often neglectful parents—sometimes even abusive ones—failing to meet their ongoing obligations to individual children at risk of or in placement. Public systems lack the capacity to ensure coordinated program planning and service delivery. Compliance with even weak laws and regulations is inadequate. We found evidence of such failures in each of the study states.

State statutory protections for children and families facing placement were inadequate.

- Statutory criteria in the seven study states for the court's removal of a child from home were often vague and did not require that alternatives be tried in non-emergency situations.[9] Counsel was not uniformly provided at all points in the placement process.

- None of the child welfare statutes in the study states explicitly required that consideration be given to placing a child with willing relatives as opposed to strangers; that a child be placed in the least restrictive setting; or that a child be placed in his or her own community unless there was specific evidence that to do so would be harmful to the child.

- Only one study state (South Carolina), at the time of our visit, exercised its continuing responsibility to individual children in out-of-home care. It requires by statute a periodic review of the children, conducted independently of the public child welfare agency responsible for the care of the children.

- Only three study states (Ohio, South Dakota, and Massachusetts) made it possible for minors at risk of voluntary psychiatric hospitalization to have access to counsel prior to hospitalization.

Efforts to provide permanence for children were limited.

- No study state had placed emphasis in its statute or policy on reunification efforts to ensure, whenever appropriate, that children and natural families were reunited.[10]

- South Carolina was the only study state which, as a matter of state policy, had taken a strong stand in

---
[9]There is such a requirement in two of California's 58 counties as a result of experimental time-limited legislation. See Chapter 4.
[10]The California legislation cited in footnote 9 refers specifically to reunification efforts.

regard to a child's right to permanence. The state had created an Office of Child Advocacy within the Governor's Office to act as advocate and ombudsman for children in foster care and to ensure that their right to permanence was protected.

- All seven study states provided for subsidized adoptions, but only two gave *priority* to foster parents for the adoption of children they had cared for for long periods of time. Most study states failed to provide adequate funding for their subsidy programs.

Efforts by the state to ensure that children out of their homes received quality services were lacking.

- Licensing, which theoretically constitutes a core component of the state's efforts to protect children, was ineffective. Even in Massachusetts and California, the two study states that had recently substantially modified licensing procedures and regulations, licensing efforts were still beset with enforcement failures, and the licensing process was isolated from other placement activities. The same isolation pervaded program reviews.

- No study state had developed explicit procedures for monitoring purchase-of-service agreements and ensuring that private providers met agreed-upon performance standards.

The administrative structure of children's services was varied and complex, but bore little relationship to the quality of services.

- Fragmentation of children's services was widespread. Only three study states had sought administrative solutions, either through offices for children (Massachusetts and South Dakota), or through liaison staff across systems (New Jersey). Yet in each state we found "exchangeable children," who, with the same needs, were the responsibility of different systems.

- State oversight of local practice was inadequate regardless of whether child welfare services were administered by the state or by local jurisdictions, with the state in a supervisory role. No local child welfare office that we visited reported receiving any substantive in-service training from the state child welfare agency. Staff did receive training in how to fill out forms.

Shockingly little was known about the status of children in placement. No study state monitored the treatment of minority children for evidence of discrimination.

- Based on CDF's survey of child welfare and probation offices in 140 counties, the lack of information about children out of their homes, even in their own counties, was appalling. Responding child welfare officials could not provide data on the race of 54 percent of the children reported to be in out-of-home care; on the age of 49 percent of the children; on the length of time in care for 53 percent of the children; on the number of moves for 87 percent of the children; and on the legal status for 73 percent. Probation officials did no better. Fifty-nine percent could not identify the race of the children reported in out-of-home placement; 66 percent could not report age; and 42 percent could not identify the types of facilities in which the youths were placed.

- Only two of the seven study states were even attempting to gather statewide data within the child welfare system, and only one across systems. No study state had systematic accurate information concerning the numbers of children and families receiving services to prevent placement, what services they received, or how effective such services were. No state could routinely and systematically identify those children who move in and out of placements, or trace the pathways of children moving from one system to another.

- No study state was monitoring the treatment of minority children. We found evidence of unequal treatment of Indian children in both study states with large Indian populations, Arizona and South Dakota. In general, data about minority children were inadequate, but information available suggested minority children were even more susceptible than other children to the failures of the child-placing systems.

Efforts to give parents, children and foster parents an opportunity to voice complaints or problems were almost nonexistent.

- Massachusetts was the only study state that had created within the Office for Children a mechanism for individual parents, children, foster parents, providers, and others to register complaints about services or seek resolution of difficult situations. Families in New Jersey had access to the Office of the Public Advocate empowered to engage in case and class advocacy in a variety of areas. No other study state had specific mechanisms for redressing procedural wrongs or service inequities and inadequacies, other than through normal legal processes, or in several instances, through ombudsman programs within institutions.

The Failure of Federal Leadership and Policy

There is no overall explicit federal policy toward children out of their homes. The implicit policy reflected in federal funding priorities acts as a disincentive to the development of strong programs ensuring children their own or adoptive families. Federal protections for children at risk of removal or out of their homes are uneven; and weakest in child welfare legislation. There is an explicit policy supporting the deinstitutionalization of already institutionalized persons but there has been little systematic attention to its implications for children. Efforts to require state compliance with federal regulations and laws are virtually nonexistent. Administratively, responsibility for children out of their homes is diffuse and weak. The absence of useful national information about children out of their homes is a scandal, and prevents the monitoring of basic facts about the impact of federal dollars on the care of children.

Federal funding patterns provide incentives for long-term foster care.

- The AFDC Foster Care Program (Section 408 of the Social Security Act) pays for out-of-home care for children whose families are eligible for AFDC and who are placed, as a result of a judicial determination, in foster family homes or private nonprofit child care institutions. It pays only for room and board costs, not for services to prevent placement or reunite families, or for services to facilitate, as appropriate, termination of parental rights and adoption. Fiscal Year 1976 federal expenditures for the program were $176 million.

- One federal program funded under Title IV-B of the Social Security Act provides funds for a broad range of child welfare services, including services to prevent the removal of a child from his or her own home, but has been consistently funded far below the authorized ceiling of $266 million. For the past few years, the actual appropriation has barely exceeded $50 million. Further, states have used much of this money to pay for out-of-home care, not for services to prevent the removal of children from their homes or to reunite families.

- No federal funds are specifically targeted for adoption subsidies. Furthermore, the fact that a handicapped child in foster care who is often eligible for Medicaid would lose eligibility if adopted, serves as a disincentive to finding permanent adoptive homes for children with special needs.

Current federal policies fail to ensure adequate procedural and substantive protections to children at risk of placement or in care.

- None of the federal child welfare programs providing funds for children out of their homes requires:
  — Services to the family to prevent out-of-home placement
  — Placement priorities such as placement in the least restrictive setting appropriate to the child's needs and within reasonable proximity to the child's family
  — Periodic case reviews by those not providing services
  — A dispositional hearing to ensure children are returned home or freed for adoption when appropriate
  — Time limits on federally reimbursable foster care for children whose family ties are broken, with good faith efforts to provide a child with permanence

The federal commitment to deinstitutionalization has been haphazard.

- Despite national rhetoric favoring deinstitutionalization, federal funds are often not used to ensure care in the least restrictive setting. The availability of Medicaid funds often serves as an incentive to keep children with special needs in hospitals or nursing homes, when foster home placements might be more appropriate.

- Juvenile Justice and Delinquency Prevention Act requirements to deinstitutionalize status offenders and dependent and neglected children have been poorly monitored. And there has been little attention given to ensuring that appropriate services are available for children leaving institutions.

Only limited attention has been given at the federal level to the quality of care provided to children out of their homes.

- There are a number of federal programs that provide funds to meet the special needs of institutionalized children. But there has been no federal effort to follow the total federal dollars going into institutions to determine the extent to which they are meeting children's needs or whether in some instances the various programs may be working at cross-purposes. Frequently, inadequate attention is paid to the quality of the federally reimbursed care these children receive.

Federal enforcement of existing child welfare laws is virtually nonexistent.

- Despite recent GAO documentation of abuses in the AFDC Foster Care and Title IV-B programs,[11] HEW has taken no corrective action. Further, no one is systematically following up violations identified by the HEW Audit Agency in its extensive review of the AFDC Foster Care Program.[12]

Federal leadership in monitoring discrimination in programs affecting out-of-home children is minimal.

- Title VI of the Civil Rights Act of 1964 prohibits discrimination on the basis of race, color or national origin in federally assisted programs. To date, however, although states receive in excess of $2.5 billion in federal funds for social services, the Office for Civil Rights (OCR) in HEW has never published policy guidelines for the states to use in monitoring the administration of social services programs. OCR conducts periodic surveys of nursing homes and hospitals in order to assess their compliance with Title VI, but has never conducted comparable surveys of child-placing and child-caring agencies. Similarly, there has been no coordinated effort to monitor compliance with Section 504 of the Rehabilitation Act of 1973 which prohibits discrimination against handicapped persons in federally assisted programs.

The administration of relevant federal programs is fragmented and unwieldy.

- There are at least 34 federal programs administered by six different federal agencies that directly impact on the lives of children at risk of removal or in placement. Within HEW alone there are five different offices and numerous divisions with responsibility for these programs. But there is no formal mechanism for coordinating the agencies and offices with responsibility for these programs across federal departments. The division of responsibility between Washington and regional offices, with respect to individual programs, further fragments program authority.

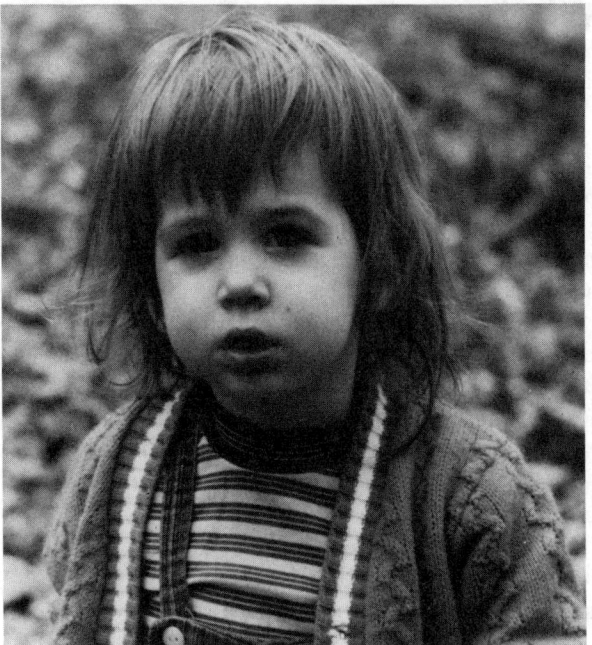

[11]See, for example, General Accounting Office, *More Can Be Learned and Done About the Well-Being of Children* (Washington, D.C.: GAO, April 1976), and *Children in Foster Care Institutions: Steps Government Can Take to Improve Their Care* (Washington, D.C.: GAO, February 1977).

[12]See, for example, reports by the HEW Audit Agency's Philadelphia Regional Office, *Review of AFDC Foster Care Program Administered by the Department of Public Welfare, Commonwealth of Pennsylvania* (Washington, D.C.: HEW Audit Agency, Audit Control No. 60253-03, May 1976), and *Report on the Aid to Families with Dependent Children Foster Care Program, Commonwealth of Virginia* (Washington, D.C.: HEW Audit Agency, Audit Control No. 60253-03, June 1976). A list of the 27 states where audits have been scheduled and the status of the audits as of June 1, 1978 is set forth in Appendix B.

Mechanisms for program and fiscal accountability for federal dollars are almost nonexistent.

- Few federal laws require administrative agencies responsible for children at risk of removal or in placement to report to Congress and the public on the status of these children and their families, or on the impact of federal programs affecting them. There is no current federal effort to develop a unified data system appropriate for problem identification, planning and trend analysis about children at risk of removal or in placement.

The federal data collection effort is haphazard and often meaningless.

- Very little useful comparable data are available on a national basis on children in out-of-home care, in spite of the fact that there are at least 20 data collection efforts conducted by or under contract with federal agencies which address this population. Reporting at the federal level concerning child welfare and adoption services has been voluntary and virtually useless.

- The Decennial Census conducted by the Census Bureau is the only effort to obtain periodic data on the race of children out of their homes across systems. No statistics, however, tell anything about the comparative types or lengths of placements for minority and non-minority children, nor the comparative numbers of such children being returned home or adopted.

What Can Be Done?

The realities facing many children now out of their own homes are grim. And so is the outlook for the next generation of children at risk of placement unless there is an intense, concentrated effort to restructure several key parts of the child care systems concurrently. Child care systems, despite the goodwill and concern of many of those who are a part of them, function to uproot and alienate children, not to foster their strengths. Piecemeal tinkering—a new training program here, some demonstration funds for preventive services there—will not work. Nor will money alone correct existing problems or prevent future ones. Legislative and administrative protections, quality services, and strong effective advocacy are required to reverse the destructive patterns now so common.

A concentrated effort on behalf of children out of their homes can pay off not only for the children, but for the taxpayers. Individual children and families can be reunited if special efforts are made; children lacking families can be ensured adoptive families; unsavory conditions in institutions can be challenged and changed; and data can be gathered and used in planning responsive programs. In short, the federal government and states *can* be held accountable for what happens to the Terris, the Timmys, the Alvins, and thousands of others like them.

The major directions which change at the local, state or federal levels must take are summarized briefly below. Specific recommendations for policy and procedural reforms are detailed in subsequent chapters.

State and Local Action

Each state should review efforts to ensure appropriate permanent settings for every child currently in out-of-home care. Priority should be given to children in placement for over 18 months. Plans for these children should be periodically monitored.

All out-of-state placements should be examined to determine if in-state placements, closer to the child's home, are appropriate.

Each state statutory framework must be examined and strengthened to: require affirmative documented efforts to prevent unnecessary out-of-home placements; ensure that each placement is in the least restrictive setting appropriate to the child's needs; ensure that for every child in out-of-home care there is a timely, decisive review of the child's progress and status independent of those providing services; mandate the collection of adequate aggregate information about children in out-of-home care; and require periodic reporting to the public and legislature.

Each state should take concrete steps to reverse anti-family practices and policies affecting children at risk of removal or removed from their own homes. These should include: revisions in regulations which discourage family contact; more effective monitoring of local practices; and substantive training for staff working directly with children and families.

Voluntary placement agreements should specify state and parental rights and obligations. Public officials should be required to encourage parent-child contacts and document the extent of such contacts. Specific funds for preventive and reunification services should be allocated.

Each state should examine the impact of its accountability mechanisms to ensure quality care to individual children. Licensing statutes should specify the rights of children in out-of-home care and sanctions if institutional abuse is uncovered. Purchase-of-service agreements should be monitored to ensure performance standards are met.

Each state should develop data collection systems that provide up-to-date information on what is happening to individual and groups of children at risk of or in out-of-home placement. Data should be comparable to the extent possible across all child-placing systems.

Each state should take steps to eliminate patterns of discriminatory treatment of children at risk of or in out-of-home care, by virtue of race, ethnic background or handicapping condition.

Each child-placing system should provide an ombudsman mechanism for parents, foster parents, children in out-of-home care, and their advocates, to ensure the children and families receive the services to which they are entitled.

Advocates at the state and local levels must assume a special responsibility to see that adequate funds to serve these children and their families are available; that priorities in the use of existing and future funds reflect a commitment to supporting families and ensuring permanence for children; that inequitable, discriminatory patterns of care within or across child care systems are ended; and that there is continuous monitoring of public agencies to hold them accountable for the lives of children and the taxpayers' dollars.

Federal Action

There must be immediate action at the federal level to respond to these most vulnerable children. Current federal moneys should be redirected and made available to strengthen each state's capacity to provide preventive and reunification services; conduct special reviews and planning for children who must be placed to ensure they are provided quality care and permanence; and develop adequate monitoring and enforcement mechanisms based on comprehensive data collection systems.

Federal funds for child welfare services should be increased and targeted for services to prevent unnecessary and inappropriate out-of-home placements, and to reunite children in care with their families. These funds must not be used for the maintenance of children in foster care, and must be kept apart from any general revenue sharing type funds.

The anti-family bias and fiscal disincentives to ensuring a child a permanent home should be eliminated from federal legislation. Limitations should be placed on the length of time federal reimbursement will be available for children in out-of-home care without good faith efforts to ensure the child permanence. Federal funds should be targeted for adoption services and subsidies. The Medicaid Program should be amended so that children with handicapping conditions will continue their Medicaid eligibility after adoption, regardless of the income of their adoptive parents.

Procedural and substantive safeguards for children at risk of removal or in out-of-home care should be required as a condition for receipt of federal funds. Such safeguards should include: requirements for preventive services; placement in the least restrictive setting within reasonable proximity to a child's family in accordance with any special needs he[13] may have; preference to placement with willing relatives; reunification services; semi-annual periodic reviews by a party not directly providing services to the family; a dispositional hearing within 18 months of placement by a court or independent body; and provision for a due process grievance mechanism.

Deinstitutionalization efforts across federal systems, agencies and programs should be coordinated and their impact on children analyzed. Specific attention should be given to tracing the federal dollars flowing into specific group care facilities to determine what differential impact they have on individual children.

Federal agencies should be required to move diligently to enforce the protections for which they are responsible. They should require states to

---
[13]CDF clearly recognizes that the children talked about throughout this report are both male and female. However, for readability, we often use only the pronoun "he."

comply with all procedural and substantive protections mandated by federal statute, regulations or the Constitution which affect children at risk of removal or in placement, and their families.

Reorganization of federal responsibility for children at risk of removal or out of their homes is essential to end the current fragmentation of effort and lack of leadership. A body should be designated within the Department of Health, Education and Welfare with clear centralized administrative responsibility for major programs affecting children at risk of or in placement. In addition, there should be clear statutory authority for an office with coordinating and monitoring authority for federal programs across agencies affecting these children.

Federal agencies providing funds to the states for services to children at risk of placement or in care should require the states to report periodically on the status of the children and families. States should be required to develop an integrated data collection system that provides meaningful, timely data to state and local officials on the status of children in their care, and provides useful data at the national level, comparable to the extent possible across systems, for ensuring compliance with existing federal policies and programs and planning future program directions.

How the Report is Organized

The report is organized in three major sections. *Part I, Defining the Problem,* describes the destructive forms of public neglect often resulting in the isolation of children from their families and from the purview of responsible public agencies. Chapter 1 focuses on implicit and explicit anti-family biases throughout the placement process. Chapter 2 describes the ways in which systems with official responsibility fail the children. Chapter 3 examines the extent of out-of-state placements of children and the special problems faced by children in out-of-state facilities.

Part II, State and Federal Responsibility, takes a comprehensive look at the state and federal role concerning children at risk of or in out-of-home placement. Chapter 4 covers state responsibilities and examines how well children in our seven study states are served. Chapter 5 describes the tangle of federal programs affecting the care of children at risk of or in placement, with special attention to statutory and administrative strategies that define—by default—a policy encouraging many harmful state and local practices.

Part III, Effecting Change, is concerned with how to change the ways child care systems now respond to children without homes and their families. Chapter 6 summarizes a range of successful programmatic, statutory, and administrative reforms. Chapter 7 provides guidelines for advocates who want to make change happen.

Each section of the report varies in its approach. *Part I* may be of particular interest to those just learning about the extent and complexity of problems facing children without homes. *Part II,* the most technical, should be useful to policymakers at all levels of government, as well as to professionals and others seeking a broader understanding of the variety of public programs and policies in this area. *Part III* is intended as a resource for program planners and child advocates. Extensive recommendations for change are included throughout the report.

....

The problems of children without homes will not go away. The time has come for political action at all levels of government. Parents, foster parents, concerned citizens, lawyers, legislators, professionals within the child care systems—all of us must speak out on behalf of these vulnerable children. Their needs must no longer be ignored. The cost is too great to the children and to society.

Part I.
Defining the Problem

Chapter 1
Families Don't Count

Chapter 2
Children Don't Count

Chapter 3
Children Placed Out of State

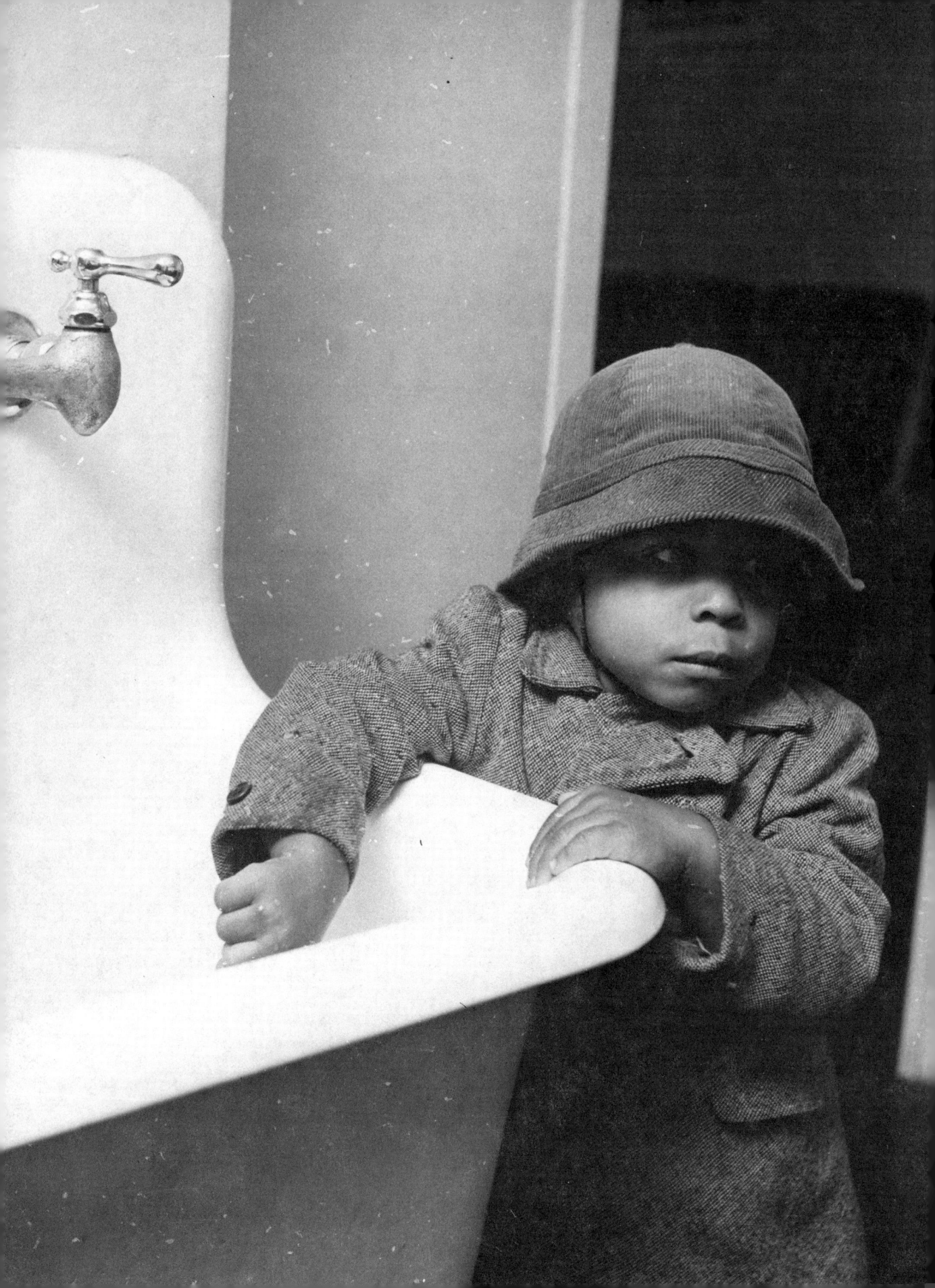

1 Families Don't Count

Severing Family Ties

Parents come in many different styles. Some are biological parents, some are adoptive parents, and some are adults who have established a continuing, nurturing psychological relationship with a child without benefit of a specific legal status. Parents are part of many different types of families and have many different beliefs about what is important for children and how children should be raised. They bring to the job of parenting a wide range of personal and financial resources. But regardless of these variations, one truth stands out. Parents are important both to children who live with them and to children who do not. Indeed the ties between children and parents are often strong and meaningful, even if the actual relationship is perceived by others as negative.[1]

Consequently, one would expect that if a child must be placed out of his own home, every effort would be made by responsible officials to maintain and strengthen parent-child ties, except where a relationship poses the risk of serious emotional or physical harm to the child. And when parent-child ties have irrevocably deteriorated or are nonexistent, one would expect that every effort would be made to help the child establish new ties. But this is not what happens.[2]

In every community we visited, we found policies and/or practices that overtly or covertly prevent or discourage parents from keeping children at home and from maintaining contact with children already out of their own homes. Similarly, we found policies and practices that make it difficult, if not impossible, for children without parental ties to establish new ones.

The severing of parental ties is the result of arbitrary decisions, inaction, and, sometimes, fiscal or administrative policies. But for children out of their homes, whatever the reason, the message is clear: no one cares.

Separating Children from Families

Mrs. G., a single parent,[3] *has five children, aged eight, five, two, and six-month-old twins. Her*

---

[1] See, for example, N. Littner, "The Importance of the Natural Parents to the Child in Placement," *Child Welfare* 54 (March 1975) and M. Meyer, "Family Ties and the Institutionalized Child," *Children* 16 (November-December 1969).

[2] Our analysis in this chapter focuses primarily on the child welfare system because we found that children placed by child welfare, as a group, appear to be most vulnerable to the severing of family ties.

[3] Female-headed families are potentially a high risk group. They are especially vulnerable to having their children placed out of home not because of parental inadequacies but because of the financial and other stresses associated with having sole responsibility for children. In this context, it is worth noting that between 1970 and 1973, there was an 18 percent increase in female-headed households, compared with a 24 percent increase during the entire preceding decade. K. Snapper, H. Barriga, F. Baumgarner and C. Wagner, *The Status of Children 1975* (Washington, D.C.: Social Research Group, George Washington University, 1975), p. 6.

two-year-old child is moderately retarded and requires a great deal of care. The twins are active, alert babies also requiring much attention. Mrs. G's older sister, with whom she was very close, was recently killed in a car accident and Mrs. G. has been too depressed and overwhelmed to meet her demanding family needs. She went to the local child welfare agency for help. As a result her children were placed in four foster homes scattered around the city in which she lives.

Mrs. R. is the mother of three pre-schoolers. She had been receiving federal welfare assistance for herself and her children until last winter. But last winter was a very cold one—and the furnace in her rented home broke. The welfare department said they had no way of giving her the $250 necessary for repairs. Instead, they charged Mrs. R. with neglect (one of the children had developed a severe respiratory infection), and placed her children in a foster home. Without her children, Mrs. R. was no longer eligible for federal welfare benefits and was transferred to a state relief program which was totally inadequate to enable her to find a place to live. She had to leave the state and return to her own parents in another state—a move which made visits to her children virtually impossible.

Placement by Default

What happened to Mrs. G. and Mrs. R. and their children are typical examples of placement by default.[4] In Mrs. G.'s case, her children were separated from her and each other because no alternatives to out-of-home care were considered, such as enrolling the two-year-old in a half-day day care program, offering Mrs. G. the assistance of a homemaker a few days a week to help care for the twins, or crisis counseling to help her grapple with her depression.

For Mrs. R., the alternative to removing her three children was obvious: $250 for repairing the furnace.

Theoretically, it is not difficult to imagine a range of services to prevent removal and enable families under stress to continue to function as family units. A poor family about to be evicted might need temporary shelter, money to prevent eviction, or a lawyer to challenge the eviction. A mother with a history of psychiatric illness, overwhelmed by the demands of a new baby, might need day care for her four-year-old or a homemaker to give her some afternoons of relief and prevent her rehospitalization. Day care, day treatment programs, adequate housing, legal services, homemakers, and family shelters are all part of what might be considered supportive family services. So too are parent education programs and respite facilities so parents of severely handicapped children may have some time off. Yet, in most communities few, if any, of these alternatives exist.[5] Consider, for example, what we found in the communities we visited.

- In early 1976, Los Angeles County, with a population of seven million, had 61 homemakers to assign to children and families. The program director was valiantly seeking funds to support more homemakers, but as he ruefully said, "It is, in L.A. as elsewhere, a low priority."[6]

- Only one county out of the 22 we visited had a family respite program providing temporary shelter to children, and sometimes to families experiencing significant stress.

- Most counties did have limited monies available to purchase day care for children who would otherwise

---

[4]Placement by default occurs when services to prevent placement do not exist or exist but are not used. Reported reasons for placement vary considerably by state and do not include a category for default. In studies of foster care in Arizona, California and Massachusetts, three of our study states, neglect or abuse was cited as the reason for placement in 51 percent, 46.3 percent and 13.6 percent, respectively, of the samples studied. Parents' mental illness or addiction was cited in 4.7 percent of the Arizona placements and 24.6 percent of the Massachusetts placements. (California did not report comparable figures.) S. Vasaly, *Foster Care in Five States: A Synthesis and Analysis of Studies from Arizona, California, Iowa, Massachusetts and Vermont* (Washington, D.C.: Office of Human Development, U.S. Department of Health, Education and Welfare, 1976), p. 23.

In an analysis of reasons for placement of approximately 27,000 New York City children, it was reported that 27.7 percent of the children were placed because parents were unable to cope, 7.3 percent because of inadequate housing and 4.5 percent because of inadequate finances. Even more startling were the data which related length of time in foster care to initial reasons for placements. For 10 percent of the children in care for 10-21 years, the reasons for initial placement included inadequate housing or inadequate finances. For children under two years of age, those reasons were identified for 19.9 percent of the children. Child Welfare Information Services, Inc., *System Level Reports*, May 31, 1975, cited as Appendix Tables 59 and 64 in T. Lash and H. Sigal, *State of the Child: New York City* (New York City: Foundation for Child Development, April 1976), pp. 176, 179.

[5]Vasaly reports that in the sample studied in Arizona, only 51 percent of the natural mothers and 30 percent of the fathers were offered services prior to the child's placement. In the Massachusetts sample, 59 percent of the natural parents were in contact with the agency for only two weeks or less prior to placing the child in foster care, and 66 percent of the parents said a specific crisis (which for 25 percent was financial) precipitated the placement. Vasaly, *Foster Care in Five States*, pp. 24-27.

[6]The program no longer exists. All homemaker services are now purchased from private agencies and no special training or emphasis is given to children and parents. San Francisco reported it had nine homemakers to be used for children and families, but only on an eight-to-five basis, and only if a parent was in the home.

have to be placed out of their homes, but in general, only children who had been or who were in danger of being abused were eligible.[7]

- Recent fiscal pressures have sharply cut into even the few services that are available to prevent out-of-home placement. An annual report from a county in our survey had this to say about a special program that had just been phased out: "When it was in operation, the unit had four caseworkers who specialized in providing intensive casework service for multi-problem families. The overall objective of the unit was to render protective services to children by preventing complete family breakdown.... During 1975, 215 families with 558 children received service.... We are of the firm belief that were it not for the services of this unit, many children from these homes would have been referred to the child welfare teams and probably some placed in foster care. The unit effectively responded to the needs of this client population ... less than 6 percent of the cases had to be transferred to the child welfare teams for wardships." (Wardship refers to out-of-home placement.)

No one knows exactly how many children who are now removed from their own homes could remain with their families if the necessary supportive services were available.[8] But the evidence is clear that where there are adequate resources for preventive services, they can and do make a difference.

- In 1976, the Lower East Side Family Union in New York City provided services to over 400 families, half of whom were identified as high risk families with problems comparable to families whose children had been entering foster care. Yet over the course of the year, foster placements only had to be obtained for children in 11 families. In six of these, the children returned home in less than two months. The project contracts with families and with local agencies to supply necessary services in an attempt to reduce pressures on the family that lead to family break-up. The Union's direct services include case management, homemaking, counseling, information and referral, escort and advocacy. In addition, it brokers with other agencies for additional services to its clients.[9]

- In 1973, The Boston Children's Service Association began the Treatment Alternatives Project (TAP) to demonstrate that with intensive service efforts the kind of children usually placed in residential treatment facilities can remain in their own homes. All the children involved in the TAP had been referred to the Massachusetts Department of Public Welfare for placement. A comparable control group was selected. At the point the report was written, 69 percent of the TAP children were able to remain in their own homes, compared to 24 percent of the control group.[10]

- In South Carolina, one of our study states, a study was conducted between October 1973 and March 1974 of 13 counties having special protective service units to enable children to remain in their families. It found a 25 percent decrease in the number of placements.[11]

- In New York State in 1974, the legislature funded a year-long demonstration project to determine the impact of intensive casework efforts on preventing initial placements and facilitating rehabilitation (the return home or adoption of children already placed). At the end of 18 months, 92 percent of the experimental group children initially at home remained at home, compared with 77 percent of the control group.[12]

The evidence suggests that maintaining children in their own families pays off not only for children, but

---

[7]Both in-home and out-of-home services to children at risk of abuse or neglect or already abused or neglected are generally called "protective" services. "Preventive" services to eliminate or reduce the need for out-of-home care theoretically should be available to all vulnerable children, not just those who are neglected and abused. In reality, fiscal constraints often limit eligibility for preventive services to children explicitly needing protection.

[8]A New York City case reading study of the appropriateness of the actual settings in which children were placed estimated that 7.5 percent of the children in out-of-home care should be in their own homes. B. Bernstein, D. Snider and W. Meezan, *Foster Care Needs and Alternatives to Placement: A Projection for 1975-1985* (Albany: New York State Board of Social Welfare, 1975), p. 25. Data based on interviews with parents whose children were placed suggest a substantially higher proportion of unnecessary removals. See, for example, A. Gruber, *Children in Foster Care: Destitute, Neglected...Betrayed* (New York: Human Services Press, 1978), pp. 140-141, in which almost one-third of the parents interviewed felt that had they had other options such as intensive family counseling or homemakers, placement could have been avoided; and S. Jenkins and E. Norman, *Filial Deprivation and Foster Care* (New York: Columbia University Press, 1972), p. 80, in which 22 percent of the 390 families interviewed felt placement was unnecessary.

[9]"Lower East Side Family Union Annual Report," New York: October 1977.

[10]"Treatment Alternatives Project Annual Report," Boston: Boston Children's Service Association, undated.

[11]Unfortunately, the control group data were gathered at a different time from the data on the service units, raising some methodological questions. The pattern of results, however, is consistent with other findings. South Carolina Department of Social Services, "Research Proposal and Results of Definitive Protective Service Units," South Carolina, undated. (Mimeographed.)

[12]M. A. Jones, R. Neuman and A. Shyne, *A Second Chance for Families: Evaluation of a Program to Reduce Foster Care* (New York: Research Center, Child Welfare League of America, January 1976), pp. 97-99, 122. See also M. A. Jones, "Reducing Foster Care Through Services to Families," *Children Today* 5 (November-December 1976): 6-10.

fiscally as well.[13] Yet it happens too rarely. The roots of the neglect of services to children in their own homes are complex, anchored in biases against the poor and the nearly poor,[14] conveyed in historical patterns of service delivery, and reinforced by current fiscal patterns. The result is that at the point out-of-home placement becomes a serious possibility, it is very likely to become a reality. This is not necessarily what either the parents, the children or the service providers want. It is certainly not what is conveyed in the theory and rhetoric of children's service systems which regard placement of a child out of his own home as "a last resort." But the fact is, it is often easier to place a child than to offer services to him and the family while the child remains at home, regardless of the consequences.

Placement by Coercion

Children are not only removed from their homes because there are no alternatives. Sometimes, they are removed coercively. There is no question that for those children who are at risk of substantial physical or emotional harm if they remain in the home, the state has and should have the power to protect and, where required, remove the children. But the coercive power of the state is not always used appropriately.

Mr. and Mrs. M. were told that in order to get services for Jimmy, who was having great difficulty in school, they had to sign a voluntary placement agreement transferring legal custody to the Department of Welfare. The parents signed the agreement without fully understanding it. For six months Jimmy did go to a special school, but then he was transferred to a foster home and enrolled in a regular school. The mother requested that Jimmy be returned to her but was refused.

The M.s lived in New York. In another state, we learned of parents who were told that for their child to remain enrolled in a special school they had to "voluntarily" place him in foster care. Four years later, the parents were still engaged in a court battle to regain custody of their child.[15] In other instances parents are forced to place their children "voluntarily" or be formally charged with neglect or abuse.

Children are also separated from their own families because someone in authority dislikes the lifestyle or child-rearing practices of a particular family.[16] Influenced by moral beliefs, political ideologies, or child-saving fantasies, those with decision-making responsibility sometimes fail to consider the psychological consequences to a child of removal from his family. In one rural county we learned of yet another struggle between a parent and a service system, this time the Department of Welfare.

The Department was seeking to remove five children ranging in age from 2 to 12 from their "mildly retarded" parents on the grounds that the home reflected general neglect. In this case, the father had sought the aid of a private lawyer, and so far had been successful in blocking the removal. In response to a question from CDF staff about why the home was so bad, the case supervisor said, "The stove does not have a grate and the father won't put one up. He wants the children to learn. The only thing there is in that family is love, and love is not enough." When asked how she could be sure the children would be loved in foster care, she paused and said, "I never thought of that."

We have no way of quantifying the extent to which coercive placements are made.[17] The high cost of foster care, the growing tolerance among the middle class for once suspect lifestyles and social sanctions against

---

[13]Studies support the cost-effectiveness argument. According to a study in New York City during the period 1966 to 1971, the cost of foster care appeared to be "about five times the expense a family on a low-cost budget would incur in rearing its own child." In the sample of 467 families studied, over $36 million was saved by the return of children to their own homes in about 60 percent of the families. D. Fanshel and E. B. Shinn, *Dollars and Sense in the Foster Care of Children: A Look at Cost Factors* (New York: Child Welfare League of America, 1972), pp. 17-25. In 1976, a study cited earlier calculated the dramatic cost savings from both preventing a child's entry into foster care and shortening a child's stay once in care. By providing intensive family services, a project in several New York counties, as well as in New York City, averted the need for out-of-home placements, resulting in a savings of $285,000 in foster care expenditures during the project period. Project staff further estimated that the children returned home by the project saved an additional two million dollars over a four-year period. Jones, Neuman and Shyne, *A Second Chance for Families*, pp. 97-101.

[14]For a thoughtful account of the class bias in the foster care system, see S. Jenkins, "Child Welfare As a Class System," and M. Rein, T. E. Nutt and H. Weiss, "Foster Family Care: Myth and Reality" in *Children and Decent People*, ed. A. Schorr (New York: Basic Books, 1974).

[15]See Opinion of the Supreme Court of Pennsylvania (E.D.) filed May 13, 1975, in *Lee v. Child Care Service Delaware County, et al.*, No. 350.

[16]A lawsuit in Alabama successfully challenged the procedure whereby a three-year-old child was taken from his mother, whose parental rights were subsequently terminated, solely because she was living with a black man to whom she was not married. *Roe v. Conn*, 417 F. Supp. 769 (M.D. Ala. 1976). In a case reported in a Florida newspaper, an Iowa woman who worked as a masseuse lost custody of her child because of her employment. Again there were no charges of neglect or abuse. "Nude Masseuse Told to Give Up Her Child," *Miami Herald*, 18 December 1975.

[17]For a further discussion of such placements, see R. Levine, "Caveat Parens: A Demystification of the Child Protection System," 35 *University of Pittsburgh Law Review* (1973): 1-52.

MAKING PREVENTIVE SERVICES WORK

Mounting a successful effort to prevent the removal of a child from home requires understanding of the family's strengths, the participation of the family and the capacity to mobilize community resources. Consider the following case history from the Lower East Side Family Union (LESFU).[1]

"This case involves a single parent 38 years old. She has had nine children; eight of them had been placed at the time we entered the case, and the ninth was on the verge of placement. The mother had a drinking problem.

"The case was referred to us by New York Foundling Hospital. The lone child remaining with the parent (a 5-year-old son) was being treated by the Hospital for a severe case of sickle cell anemia (the disease disabled the child who had trouble walking). The mother is extremely attached to this child and determined not to lose him as she had the others. Largely because of this, over the last year she has brought her drinking under control.

"The mother and son were living in a third floor apartment in a semi-abandoned building with no hot or cold water and no electricity. Moreover, through a bureaucratic foul-up, the family had been illegally cut off welfare and had been begging food from neighbors and friends. When the hospital discovered these conditions, it refused to release the child. After weeks of trying to find housing and get the welfare situation resolved, the hospital social worker in 'utter frustration' contacted LESFU to see what we could do.

"We developed a written, signed contract with Brooklyn Home for Children that the child would be placed temporarily until we were able to secure suitable housing for the family. Then the child would be returned to the mother. We also secured agreement with Legal Services to help get the mother back on income maintenance and with NY Infirmary and NENA for after-care of the disabled child.

"The child remained in placement for a short period during which time we helped the mother find suitable housing and assigned a homemaker to work with the mother on child nurturing. Two days after we secured adequate housing, Brooklyn Home, as per the contract, returned the child to the mother. By this time, Legal Services had straightened out her problem with Income Maintenance. NY Infirmary and NENA provided after-care as previously arranged.

"The mother has been gaining strength and may well be able to assume parental responsibility for some of the children now in foster care. Through our efforts several of the children have already come home for overnight visits. These have been extremely satisfactory and bode well for future efforts to reunite the children with their mother."

---

[1] Reprinted with permission from "Lower East Side Family Union Annual Report," New York: October 1977, pp. 47-49.

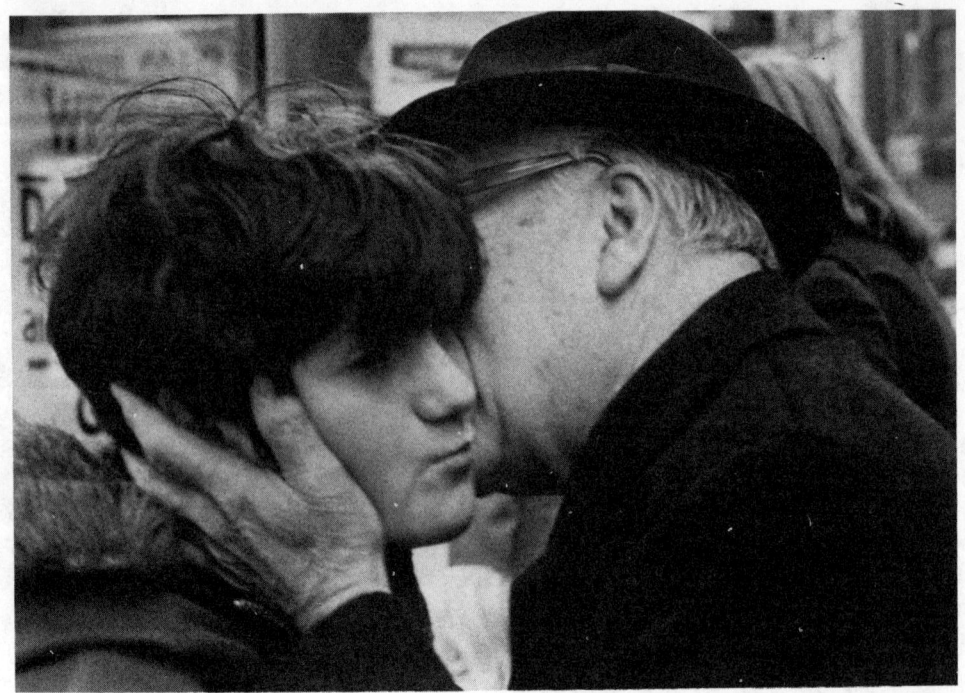

overt racism, may be reducing the problem of inappropriate coercive placements among the most vulnerable groups.[18] But as litigation and our interviews indicate, coercive placements still occur. These must be eliminated by clearer placement criteria and due process procedures.[19]

Ignoring the Homes of Relatives

Dear Grandma:

Hi, sorry I haven't written sooner. I must ask you something. Can you take me with you when you come down, I really need you right now. My home is coming down. I may be placed in a receiving home, foster home, please come get me. I only have five minutes before the mailman comes, so, when you come down, or write me back, I'll "explain." O.K., PLEASE HURRY! You're my "LAST" hope.

Love,

This teenage girl had been in two foster homes and had just been told by a third she had to leave. Her grandmother had wanted to care for her all along, but could not afford to without increased financial aid. In her state the welfare department was not allowed to pay the grandmother the same rates it could pay strangers for taking care of a grandchild she loved and who loved her.

It is popular to talk of the degeneration of the family, and the disappearance of the extended family. But we have seen something else. We have seen relatives making valiant efforts to care for children who could not remain with their natural parents. And we have seen these efforts defeated by administrative regulations, by state laws, and sometimes by the

---

[18]The issue of coercive placements also arises in relation to children committed to mental hospitals. Abuses have been documented and two cases challenging the voluntary commitment of children to mental hospitals by their parents are before the U. S. Supreme Court. See, *Bartley* v. *Kremens*, 402 F. Supp. 1039 (E.D. Pa. 1975), *vacated on other grounds*, 43l U. S. 119 (1977), *on remand*, Civ. No. 72-2272 (May 25, 1978), *prob. juris. noted, sub nom. Secretary of Public Welfare* v. *Kevin S.*, 46 L. W. 3776; (June 19, 1978) (No. 77-1715); *J. L. and J. R.* v. *Parham*, 412 F. Supp. 112 (M.D. Ga. 1976), *prob. juris. noted*, 97 S.Ct. 2647 (1977) (No. 75-1690); reargument scheduled 98 S.Ct. 761 (1978).

[19]There have been attempts to define appropriate criteria for the initial removal of a child from the home. For a discussion from a legal perspective, see M. S. Wald, "State Intervention on Behalf of 'Neglected' Children: Standards for Removal of Children from Their Homes, Monitoring the Status of Children in Foster Care, and Termination of Parental Rights," *Stanford Law Review* 28 (April 1976): 623-706. See also Institute of Judicial Administration and American Bar Association Joint Commission on Juvenile Justice Standards, *Standards Relating to Abuse and Neglect* (Tentative Draft) (Cambridge: Ballinger Publishing Company, 1977), and for a thoughtful critique of the standards, R. Bourne and E. H. Newberger, "'Family Autonomy' or 'Coercive Intervention'? Ambiguity and Conflict in the Proposed Standards for Child Abuse and Neglect," *Boston University Law Review* 57 (July 1977): 670-706.

arbitrary decisions of individuals.

Samantha and Josh, ages eight and twelve, were living with their older brother and his family. The children's parents had been killed. The brother wanted very much to keep the family together, but after six months he lost his job, and could not afford to. There was no alternative but to place the children. In the metropolitan county in which these children lived, a district director of child welfare estimated that five percent of the children entering care entered because relatives could no longer afford to care for them without more adequate financial assistance.

Coretta and Dalton, ages eight and ten, had already had a difficult time with a mother who had severe nervous breakdowns and was a chronic alcoholic. At various times the children stayed with relatives in unfamiliar cities, but mostly they stayed in their own neighborhood with an aunt who loved them and whom they loved. The aunt applied to become a foster parent (which was possible in her state). But the caseworker told the aunt, who was attending college, she would not approve her request to be a foster parent and would have the children placed either in foster care or in an institution within two weeks. Her reason: the aunt could not go to college and care for the children at the same time (although she made perfectly adequate provisions for her own children and planned to do the same for her niece and nephew). Only because the aunt was resourceful and her city had concerned advocacy groups were these children prevented from a cruel and unnecessary severing of family bonds.

The failure of child-placing systems and particularly the child welfare system to turn to interested and willing relatives at the point of placement, or to enable relatives who have been informally caring for children to continue to do so,[20] violates every principle of good child development. Children need to feel a part of some kind of unit, and they need to feel loved. Kinship can be a powerful means of giving a child a sense of stability and caring. Yet many policies and practices disregard the force of kinship, even when this has been demonstrated by the efforts of relatives to reach out to children who cannot remain with their parents.[21]

This happens for a number of reasons. Sometimes agency workers just do not think about relatives as a resource.[22] Few places require evidence that relatives have been considered before placement with a stranger is approved. Sometimes, as in the case of Coretta and Dalton, the workers make arbitrary and capricious decisions about relatives' lifestyles, even as they do about parental lifestyles, although going to college is not usually seen as suspect.

The reluctance to turn to relatives also grows in large part out of an unrealistic assumption that relatives ought to care for children out of love and not for money. That may be a sound argument when there is money to support an extra child. Often, however, the money is not there. As a consequence, the child is deprived of the opportunity to remain with familiar adults and is forced to adapt to strangers, often believing that those who might have cared for him did not want him.[23]

---

[20] In a study of 467 families with children entering care for the first time in 1966, only 51 percent of the children placed were actually living with their mothers at the time of placement. However, 30 percent of the children were living with various relatives. Jenkins and Norman, *Filial Deprivation*, pp. 88-90.

A study of informal placements among black families reported 800,000 black children are being raised by relatives; two-thirds by grandparents, the rest by aunts and uncles. Hill further estimated that 64 percent of these children are six or older. See R. B. Hill, *Informal Adoption Among Black Families* (Washington, D.C.: National Urban League, 1977), pp. 35, 42.

[21] There is also evidence that parents prefer to have children placed with relatives. See H. J. Leichter and W. E. Mitchell, *Kinship and Casework* (New York: Russell Sage Foundation, 1967) and C. R. Stack, *All Our Kin: Strategies for Survival in a Black Community* (New York: Harper & Row, 1974).

[22] In a special examination of agencies serving 624 New York City children whose careers in foster care were traced in a major longitudinal study, the author noted, "Workers appeared to regard relatives as dubious resources and had little motivation to work with them." D. Shapiro, *Agencies and Foster Children* (New York: Columbia University Press, 1976), p. 30. Leichter found, in comparing client and worker definitions of family, that workers thought of the nuclear family, clients of the extended family. Leichter and Mitchell, *Kinship and Casework*.

[23] In some states related foster parents are paid at a lower rate than foster parents unrelated to the children in their care. The Department of Health, Education and Welfare has issued a program instruction concluding that foster care provided by relatives is included within the scope of the federal foster care program. U. S. Department of Health, Education and Welfare, Social and Rehabilitation Service, Program Instruction APA-PI-75-9, October 25, 1974. The majority of states provide assistance under that program to otherwise eligible children who are placed in relatives' foster homes. However, some states refuse payment of federal foster care benefits to such children and instead only provide financial assistance at the generally lower public assistance rate.

There have been a number of court decisions requiring states to pay foster care rates to non-legally liable relatives. In a recent case in Oregon currently on appeal, the court ruled that the state law precluding payment of foster care rates to relatives was invalid, and ordered full foster care payments on behalf of children placed in the homes of relatives. *Jones v. Davis*, D. Ore., Civ. No. 76-805, decided January 31, 1977, appeal docketed C.A. 9, No. 77-254. See also, *Clampett v. Madigan*, S.D. _____ S.D., decided May 24, 1973, and *Jackson v. Ohio Department of Public Welfare*, N.D. Ohio, Civ. No. C72-182, decided April 17, 1972. The question of whether a state may deny foster care benefits under the federal foster care program to otherwise eligible children placed in the foster care of relatives is currently before the Supreme Court, *Miller v. Youakim*, 431 F. Supp. 40 (N.D. Ill. 1976), 562 F. 2d 483 (7th Cir. 1977) *prob. juris. noted*, 46 L.W. 3513, (No. 77-742). In spite of the advantages of placements with relatives for many children, the uncertainty of federal reimbursement and generally lower payments available clearly serves as a deterrent in some states.

Reducing Family Ties After Placement

Once a child is in placement, the systems responsible for the children fail almost universally to enable them to remain in contact with either their immediate families or other relatives, thus compounding the initial harm. The policies and practices that culminate in reduced or terminated family contact take many forms.

Visiting: No Parents Allowed

Children need parents to know that they are loved. They need parents in order to develop a sense of self, to try new tasks, and to be sure that someone cares about them. Even parents who may not always appear to others to love their children are important to them. Visiting between parents and their children in placement is perhaps the most significant way to ensure that a relationship is maintained. In a five-year study of 624 children who entered foster care for the first time in 1971, Dr. David Fanshel found that patterns of parental visiting proved to be the best predictor of whether the child returned home.[24] Sixty-one percent of the children whose parents failed to visit during the first year were still in care at the end of five years. In contrast, only 27 percent of the children whose parents visited regularly were still in care.[25]

In the face of the apparently strong relationship between parental visiting and outcomes to children out of their own homes, it is discouraging that we found over and over again policies and practices that make it difficult, if not impossible, for parents to visit their children.

First, there was a massive failure of agencies to articulate specific policies about parent-child visiting. Of the reporting counties in our survey of child welfare offices, 50 percent had *no* written policies about visits between children and parents.[26] Thus, there was no expectation that workers would explain to parents why visiting was important, and what a failure to visit would mean to a child. Parents were not expected to plan for regular visiting. In fact, parents' visits were all too often viewed by foster parents, the agency worker, or (in residential facilities) the responsible child care staff as a nuisance—something to be avoided if at all possible.

Second, when specific policies did exist, they were often restrictive, implying that the majority of parents could not be trusted with their children. In one survey county, children were allowed visits from their parents "on birthdays and other special occasions." In another, visits were held in the courtroom—hardly a setting to elicit spontaneous interactions between parents and their children.[27] A parent whose child entered foster care when her marriage was dissolving was told she could visit once a month, but a soft-hearted foster mother allowed her to visit once a week. Elsewhere, parents were not permitted evening visits. Some places required that caseworkers be present. Not only was this likely to inhibit both parents and children, but it was unrealistic given typical caseloads.

Third, even where state policies specified visiting requirements, they were generally disregarded in practice. For example, Massachusetts state regulations[28] required that the social work staff develop a visiting plan for a child in care. But none of the local offices CDF staff visited reported such a policy. Officials said they generally tried to have parents arrange for the visits directly with foster parents, because they did not have time.[29]

Fourth, perhaps the most widespread disincentive to parental visiting was the failure of agencies to make provision for or reimburse parents for transportation. Most parents whose children are out of their homes

---

[24] D. Fanshel, "Parental Visiting of Children in Foster Care: Key to Discharge?" *Social Service Review* 40 (December 1975): 493-514. For a further discussion, see D. Fanshel and E. B. Shinn, *Children in Foster Care: A Longitudinal Investigation* (New York: Columbia University Press, 1978).

[25] A study of over 5,000 children in Iowa reported similar results. Continuing parental contact seemed related to shorter stays in foster care for the child. For example, of the children with significant contact, 66.5 percent were in care under ten months; 3.8 percent for 40 months or more. Vasaly, *Foster Care in Five States*, pp. 63-64.

[26] For a full summary of the CDF survey findings see Appendix C.

[27] We learned of another county, that was not part of our survey, which had a policy of *forbidding* visits in the home of natural parents.

[28] Massachusetts Office for Children, Regulations, Chapter 4, Section 400.01.

[29] In New York City, where a special parents' rights unit had been set up within the child welfare agency, a large percentage of the requests for help during a typical month concerned parents' requests for more visiting and complaints about agencies' failures to allow visits. This unit is described in Chapter 6. Further, the child welfare agency in New York City, the Office of Special Services for Children, has developed an explicit, comprehensive written policy on parent-child visiting. It is included in Appendix D.

have marginal or poverty level incomes. Many are welfare recipients whose aid is reduced, sometimes sharply, when a child enters placement through the child welfare system. They may wish to visit, but simply lack financial resources to do so. Rarely can these parents request and receive aid from any of the service systems for visiting their children. Lacking the funds or transportation, the parent is dependent upon the caseworker, probation officer, or sometimes a legal aid lawyer. If the person responsible for the child has a small caseload and the child is close by, this approach may work, although the parent may have to lose an afternoon or even a day's work. But it usually does not work. Typically, the pressures of too many children in a caseload scattered over large areas, coupled with the daily crises that beset the staff of child welfare and probation offices or legal aid lawyers, make arranging even sporadic parent-child visiting difficult.[30]

In a few places we surveyed, agencies had managed to find special funds for transportation. One county reported that 12 drivers were employed to provide transportation for parents and children. A probation office in an Arizona county had established a "special slush fund" for transportation costs. In another Arizona county, probation officers encouraged parents to visit their children day or night, providing transportation as necessary. But these were exceptions. For the most part, transportation arrangements were haphazard and informal, and they did not work.

Discouraging Other Contacts

There are other ways families don't count. Parents are denied information about their child in placement. They do not routinely receive progress reports. They may not be told when their children are transferred from one placement to another. Sometimes they are not even told of transfers across state lines. They are not expected to participate in decisions about their children's medical care. They are not expected to raise questions about what is happening to their children. Nor are they told of their responsibilities. Indeed, parents who want to exercise parental responsibility[31] must often fight the agencies that ignore their strengths and concerns.[32]

Trial visits by children to their own homes are difficult to arrange. Unless the family has resources to assume additional costs for food and other incidentals, such visits are unlikely to happen. The welfare department is not able to transfer funds from the foster parents to the natural parents for a weekend. A group facility risks loss of a per diem reimbursement if the child is not there overnight. And yet such a visit can be significant in testing the feasibility of the child's return home, and in easing the transition back home for a child who has been in a lengthy placement.

Barriers to parent-child contact are pervasive not only in public systems, but also in the private facilities from which public systems often purchase care. In 1973, the National Society for Autistic Children surveyed 450 facilities serving children with severe mental illness. They found that 15 percent of the facilities that accepted such children imposed rigid restrictions on parental visiting (including forbidding visits to a child's eating and sleeping quarters), and on parental access to information about children (including prohibiting parents from talking with the child's teacher or therapist). At the same time, 28 percent of the facilities *required* parents to undergo therapy while the child was in the program.[33]

A citizens' committee in New Jersey studied private residential treatment facilities accepting less severely handicapped children. They found the facilities paid little attention to parents, failing to involve them in the child's treatment, share progress reports with them, or

---

[30]The problem is further compounded for those children who are placed far distances from their homes. In the CDF survey, nine percent of the children in out-of-home care were placed outside their own counties. In San Francisco, a review of probation, child welfare and mental health placements revealed a staggering proportion of out-of-county placements: 40 percent of child welfare foster home placements, 75 percent of child welfare residential placements, and 63 percent of mental health, mental retardation placements. Interview with staff of the San Francisco County Welfare Department, February 1976. The barriers to visiting imposed by distant placements, as we shall show in Chapter 3, are virtually insurmountable.

[31]While natural parents of children in foster care have no federally protected right to participate in decisions affecting their children, parents of children with special educational needs are now, as a matter of public policy and law, empowered to act as their children's advocates. For a discussion of the rights afforded to children and their parents under Public Law 94-142, see Children's Defense Fund, *94-142 and 504: Numbers That Add Up to Educational Rights for Handicapped Children—A Guide for Parents and Advocates* (Washington, D.C.: Children's Defense Fund, 1978).

[32]A study of over 400 families with children in placement found that parents worried about whether they had lost their children forever and were concerned because agencies did not keep them informed regarding their children's progress. Jenkins and Norman, *Filial Deprivation*, pp. 227-233.

[33]For further results of this survey, which covered residential and day treatment, school and camp programs, see R. C. Sullivan, "Report of Data Analysis Project," West Virginia: Information and Referral Service, National Society for Autistic Children, December 1975. (Mimeographed.)

encourage visiting.[34]

The severing of parental ties is not always the result of faulty policies or practices. Sometimes parents abandon children; sometimes they move, telling neither the child nor the agency where they are going. Most parents, however, do care.[35] Yet, because of the ways in which current policies and practices ignore them, these parents, in the eyes of both their children and the child care systems, often are indistinguishable from parents who do not care.

We also found repeated instances in which grandparents, aunts, uncles and even siblings have been arbitrarily and capriciously denied contact with a child in placement.

In a southern state, a grandmother of a 12-year-old boy in foster care sent her grandson a birthday card, but he never received it. When the card reached the child welfare office, it was intercepted by the supervisor who saw no need for the child to have it. She simply stamped it "date received" and put it in the child's case folder.

Two brothers from an eastern state, ages 8 and 11, were placed in separate children's institutions located in the same two-block area. The brothers, however, were not permitted to visit because the staff said they would be a "bad influence on each other," and that the visits required too much supervision. In other words, the staff found it inconvenient.

In Ohio, we found perhaps the most bizarre example of abuse to children and their relatives. Two boys who had been declared dependent and neglected had spent a happy year with a loving aunt and uncle who wanted to adopt them. Without explanation or notice, the aunt and uncle were suddenly told by the caseworker the boys were to be moved. Seven days later, the two were sent to a residential school many miles away. At the school the boys were harshly treated, and the aunt and uncle were not permitted to phone or write. The boys were there for five years, requesting repeatedly to return home, but to no avail.

It was only after the Children's Defense Fund brought a lawsuit that they were returned to their aunt and uncle.[36]

These dramatic illustrations are not atypical. Too many children out of their homes are cut off from whatever existing family and community supports they have.

No Help for Parents

The majority of children who enter out-of-home placement, at least through the child welfare system, are placed because of parental problems or actions.[37] Yet parental problems, which are frequently related to poverty, are widely ignored while the child is in care. Regulations often do not mandate any caseworker-parent contact, and so, except for an occasional visit by a caseworker, families are typically left to fend for themselves.[38]

If an effort is made to work with the family, often the case is "split" between two caseworkers—one assigned to the child, the other the parent, with little or no communication between the two. Such a practice often hinders eventual reunification. Or, if a parent is referred to another agency (the local community mental health center, for example) little effort is made to see that services are provided or that the person helping the parent knows about the child. The service response to the family while the child is in care is

---

[34]Citizens Committee for Children of New Jersey, *Long-term Residential Care of Children in New Jersey* (Montclair, New Jersey: Citizens Committee for Children of New Jersey, December 1975). An updating of that report is currently in progress.

[35]For example, in a Massachusetts study, about 60 percent of 160 natural parents who reported some contact with their children felt they did not see enough of them. The reasons varied. Of the 93 parents, 19 percent said foster parents discouraged visits and 38 percent said caseworkers prohibited visits. Gruber, *Children In Foster Care*, pp. 144-145.

[36]*Sinnet, et al.*, v. *Mountain Mission School, et al.*, C.A. No. 75-0306(a) (W.D. Va., final order entered June 23, 1975).

[37]Vasaly reported, for example, that only 2.1 percent of the children in Arizona, 9.6 percent in Massachusetts and 19.2 percent in California were placed in foster care because of the child's behavior or disability. Vasaly, *Foster Care in Five States*, p. 23. Lash cites figures showing that 39 percent of New York City children were placed for "child reasons" (e.g., school, home or community behavior). Lash and Sigal, *State of the Child*, p. 176.

[38]Vasaly reported that of 462 cases reviewed in Arizona, 56 percent of the mothers were not offered services while a child was in placement. In a study in Iowa of 5,481 children, 65 percent of the mothers had had no contact with the placement agency for six months or more. There was a similar pattern in Massachusetts. Vasaly, *Foster Care in Five States*, pp. 32-36.

In a study of the federal foster care program, the General Accounting Office reported that 40 percent of the natural families of the children it studied had not been visited by caseworkers during the six-month study period. General Accounting Office, *Children in Foster Care Institutions: Steps Government Can Take to Improve Their Care* (Washington, D.C.: General Accounting Office, February 1977), pp. 10-11.

In a more complex analysis of caseworker, parent and child interactions, Shapiro found the longer the child is in care, the less likely a worker is to maintain contact with the child's parents. But, significantly, the study also found that the proportion of children returning home increased with the frequency of contact between the parents and workers. The author added, "It is worth noting that the families with maximum contact showed a much higher proportion of improvement than the next closest ('above average') category." Maximum contact was defined as two times a month. Shapiro, *Agencies and Foster Children*, pp. 73-75, 81-82, 85-88.

When Out-of-Home Care Ends: Is There Any Family?

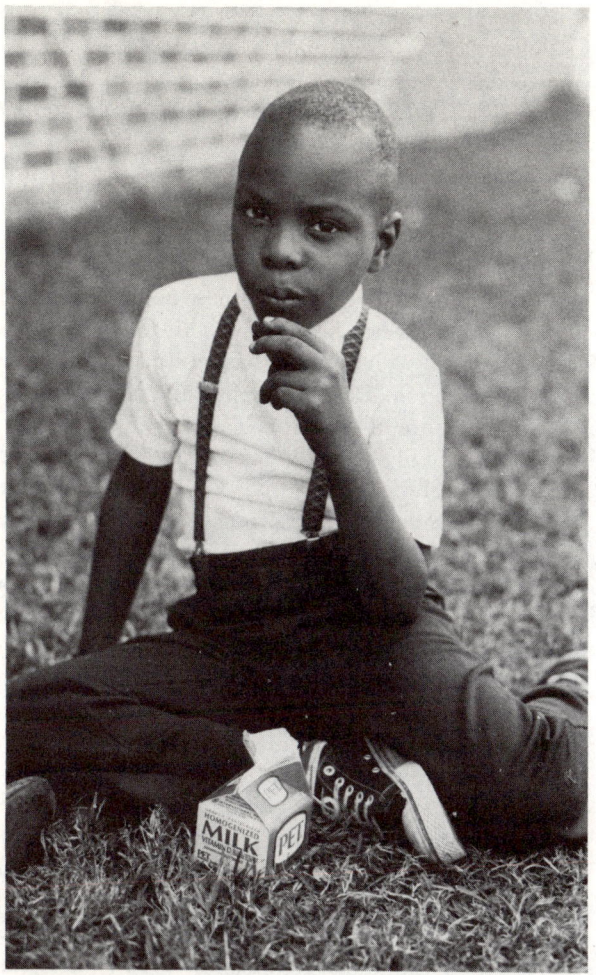

A child's placement in out-of-home care may be ended in one of three ways: return to the child's own family, adoption by a new family, or discharge from care when the child has simply grown too old and is no longer a minor.[40] The sad fact is that for many children out of their homes, there is no end; they simply grow up in the foster care system—never certain of their status. A number of studies have reported the average length of time in foster care to be about five years.[41] Our own survey found 20 percent of the children in the reporting counties had been in foster care for over six years. Efforts to facilitate reunification with the child's own family or to ensure simply not structured to support the strengths of the family or to ensure a speedy reunification of the family unit whenever possible. Yet there is no question that when concerted efforts are made to facilitate reunification, the results are frequently positive.[39]

---

[39] A program to reduce foster care in two counties in New York State and in New York City discussed earlier demonstrates the effectiveness of intensive family services in shortening the length of placement for children. Thirty-six percent of the 549 cases included in the project were cases where the children were already in placement. By the end of the project, 47 percent of this experimental group (and 38 percent of the control group) had returned home. Within another six months, a total of 62 percent of the experimental group and 43 percent of the control group were at home. The experimental group received significantly more services than the control group. Essential elements of those services included small caseloads to allow close contacts with nuclear and extended families and work with other agencies, supplementary support services such as day care and homemakers, as well as case management and advocacy skills. For a detailed description of the program and conclusions drawn from it, see Jones, Neuman and Shyne, *A Second Chance for Families*. For another family support effort, see D. A. Murphy, "A Program for Parents of Children in Foster Family Care," *Children Today* 5 (November-December 1976): 37-40.

[40] Some states have created a category of "permanent long-term foster care" in which a child is placed on a planned basis in a foster home that receives minimal agency supervision. The use of permanent foster care homes is particularly appropriate for adolescents who cannot, or do not, wish to be adopted. However, there has been no broad-based evaluation of the use of the strategy to determine if, in fact, it is being used properly.

[41] In New York City in 1975, for example, the average length of time a child had been in foster care was 5.4 years. Twenty percent of the children had been in care 10 years or more. D. Fanshel and J. Grundy, *Computerized Data for Children in Foster Care: First Analyses from a Management Information System in New York City* (New York: Child Welfare Information Services, Inc., November 1975), p. 7. Massachusetts and New Jersey also reported five years to be the average time in placement. See Vasaly, *Foster Care in Five States*, p. 21, and New Jersey Division of Youth and Family Services, Case Review Unit, "Report of New Jersey Administrative Case Reviews," undated. (Mimeographed.) In a survey of 50 states and the District of Columbia, the average length of time in foster care ranged from four months to ten years. J. D. Culley, B. Settles and J. B. Van Name, *Understanding and Measuring the Cost of Foster Care* (Delaware: University of Delaware, 1975), pp. (7)14-(7)54.

For some children, the limbo is planned. Wiltse and Gambrill, analyzing case plans of 772 children, found that 19 percent of the children were to be returned to their own homes or the homes or relatives; six percent were to have parental rights terminated; 13 percent of the children had no definite plan; and 62 percent were slated for "long-term care." K. Wiltse and E. Gambrill, "Foster Care, 1973: A Reappraisal," *Public Welfare* 32 (Winter 1974):8. In New York City, discharge plans were either unknown or unreported for a startling 31.2 percent of the children in care. For the other children, 19.7 percent were to be discharged to parents, 2.8 percent to relatives, 20.2 percent were to be adopted, and 26.2 percent were to be discharged to their own responsibility, that is, released when they reached the age of majority. Child Welfare Information Services, *System Level Reports*, May 31, 1975, as cited in Lash and Sigal, *State of the Child*, p. 69.

Evidence regarding whether children placed by court order remain in care longer than children placed voluntarily is inconsistent. A study in Santa Clara, California, found that the mean length of placement for 103 children placed voluntarily was 6.5 months, compared with 13.6 months for 87 children placed by court order. Santa Clara County, Department of Social Services, "Dependent and Voluntary Foster Home Placement," California: Social Service Analysis Report No. 74-A, June 13, 1974. (Mimeographed.) In contrast, a study of 317 case records in six California counties found that, on the average, children placed voluntarily remained in care as long as children placed by court action. Office of the Auditor General, "Report on the State's Role in Foster Care in California," Sacramento, California, January 1974, pp. 11-12.

the child permanence[42] at a time when it can still be meaningful to him or her are often limited.

Obstacles to Reunification

There are no national data available on the number of children who are placed out of their own homes and eventually returned home. Sometimes children, particularly adolescents, are returned home simply because no one else will take them. Sometimes—ignoring the length of time the child has been out of the home, the nature of the intervening contact with the natural family, the child's relationship with psychological parents, or the child's wishes—the court orders the child's return as a way of compensating parents for past wrongful actions by the responsible agency. Rarely, however, is anyone fully prepared for the child's return, whatever the reason. Some families, because they are strong and resilient, can readjust even if they have had minimal or no contact. Others do not fare so well.

Just as funds for preventive services are lacking, so typically are funds for special "restorative" services. These are services designed to encourage family reunification and transitional services to help the family and child readjust to one another. Such services need not be elaborate: helping the family find a new apartment, calling a mother once a week to see how things are going, or helping a mother get public assistance benefits reinstated.[43]

Dilemmas of Terminating Parental Rights

Child: *I came here because they couldn't find my mom. When they find my mom, I'll go back....They need to find my mom.*
Interviewer: *If you had one wish, one thing that you could get, just one wish, what would you wish for?*
Child: *It's never came [sic] true, but I've wished to go home a lot of times.*
Interviewer: *Have you ever thought how it would be if...[your foster parents] adopted you?*
Child: *Then I wouldn't be saying I wish I was at my real mom because I would be at my real mom.*[44]

Red, whose words are quoted above, has been in foster care for five years. He is now nine. His mother abandoned him when he was four. Since then she has had no contact with him, but has refused to relinquish him for adoption. Despite the passage of five years, which in the life of a child is a very, very long time, the state has only recently begun action to make his wish for a real mom come true. Yet the state's statute permits the initiation of desertion proceedings if there has been no parental contact for three months.

For children like Red who cannot or should not return to their own homes, ensuring an alternative permanent home should be a three-step process: (1) timely identification of the children by workers or as a result of independent periodic review procedures; (2) timely initiation of proceedings to determine if legal severing of the rights of the natural parent is appropriate, either by voluntary relinquishment of the child or by court-ordered termination; and (3) timely adoption of the child by a new parent or parents. In almost every county we visited, however, we were told that termination of parental rights was infrequent.[45] While there is no question that termination of parental rights is a serious, difficult step, it is equally true that indefinitely avoiding the issue results in a grave injustice to both the child and the family. We found that often the child's right to permanence was denied because of complex psychological assumptions about parents and children, and because of administrative, fiscal and statutory constraints. These factors are examined next.

---

[42]In this discussion, we are using the term "permanence" to refer to a child's continuing contact with his own family or the establishment of ties with a new psychological family. We also believe that while in the foster care system, children should be entitled to stability and permanence in an out-of-home setting. By and large, this does not happen, and children, as we show in the next chapter, are subject to yet another disruptive form of impermanence: movement from one out-of-home setting to another.

[43]For instance, federal public assistance payments to a parent under the Aid to Families with Dependent Children Program cease if there are no children in the home. States usually substitute some form of home relief which provides lower benefits. When the child or children return to the mother, a new application for AFDC must be made.

[44]Reprinted with permission from CBS, "60 Minutes," 30 May 1976, "Unwanted."

[45]For instance, despite the length of time children in the CDF survey had been in care, only 18 percent of the children were in the permanent custody of the state: eight percent of the children had been voluntarily relinquished by their parents, ten percent had had parental rights terminated. In another study, there were plans for severing of parental ties for six percent of the sample, two percent by voluntary relinquishment, four percent by court proceedings. These figures did not include 75 percent of the sample: that is, children for whom there were no plans or for whom long-term care was "planned." Wiltse and Gambrill, "Foster Care, 1973," pp. 8, 10-12.

Protecting the Parent at the Child's Expense

There is a "catch-22" quality about the reluctance to consider termination. While the child is in placement and even prior to placement, the child's natural family is rarely seen as a resource to help the child. But when the termination of parental rights is at issue, this stance is reversed. Regardless of the reality of the current situation for the family or the child, there is a widespread unwillingness to initiate proceedings or to actually terminate the rights of biological parents. It is a tragic irony that only at this point is a bias toward the child's natural family visible.

Behind this systemwide avoidance of termination proceedings lies some complicated reasoning. Many judges with whom we spoke took the position that while the biological parents were often inadequate, termination is an extreme act, and something might happen in the future to make the parents more adequate. Usually the hope centered on changes in parental behavior: sustained remission of alcohol-related violence, improved parenting, abatement of chronic mental illness. One judge, who had repeatedly refused either to terminate the parental rights of a retarded mother or to return her child to her, said to a CDF staff member: "Who knows, perhaps some day they will develop a miracle drug for retardation."

The overemphasis on biological ties, without consideration of the psychological cost to the child, can place children in serious psychological jeopardy.[46] Consider, for instance, the roller coaster childhoods of three children living in one of our study states.

Jimmy, Michael and Sara are five, six and ten. During the past five years their mother has been hospitalized for alcoholism three times: first for an eight-month period, then for a ten-month period, and then for a three-month period. During the five years, the children were in foster care for a total of 45 months, once for a two-year period when they were removed from their mother's care because she became violent and abused them, and the other times while she was hospitalized. During this period, on four separate occasions four different caseworkers sought permanent custody of the children (in that state a precursor to the termination proceeding). Each time the judge returned the children to the mother. The children are now back in foster care again.

Buffeted back and forth between their mother and foster homes, Sara, the oldest child, shows signs of depression and deteriorating school work. She has had the burden of protecting the younger children from their mother's violence when all three have been in their own home. At times, she has gone to the police station; at times she has sought aid from neighbors; and often she has slept in the boys' bedroom to ensure their mother did not harm them. After Sara's first stay in foster care she was eager to return home; since that return failed, her feelings have changed. In her words, "I'm a foster child—nobody wants me." The other children respond now to their sporadic encounters with their mother with bedwetting, anxiety and speech difficulties. The youngest child speaks of his mother as "that lady who drinks" and shows no signs of affection for her. Jimmy and Michael's foster parents would like to adopt both of them, but there can be no adoption proceedings without termination.

In a variant of an over-zealous commitment to biological parents, some judges require extensive, time-consuming searches for putative fathers who have shown no interest in their children. We learned, for instance, of a child who had been in foster care for ten years and whose foster parents wanted to adopt him. His own mother had had no contact with the child for six years, and his father for eight years. Yet, the judge insisted that the father be found before he would proceed.[47] Little consideration was given to the impact of the passage of time on the child and his need for a permanent psychological parent in the absence of a caring biological one.

Judges are not alone in perpetuating this reluctance to

---

[46] At the same time, there are also instances in which termination proceedings are brought inappropriately—in the face of parental interest. Sometimes this occurs when services have been provided to the parent, sometimes even when they have not. The legal and ethical issues in these cases become particularly complex if the child has formed new psychological ties, and/or the initial removal of the child from the home was inappropriate.

[47] In part, this suggests an over-reading of the U.S. Supreme Court decision in *Stanley* v. *Illinois*, 405 U.S. 645 (1972), which involved the rights of a putative father in a dependency proceeding. In *Stanley*, when a mother died and the Department of Welfare sought permanent custody of her children, the putative father argued that he had a right to notice and to be heard on the issue of his fitness as a parent. Although the state court disagreed, the Supreme Court upheld the father's position, noting that he had lived with and supported the children and their mother for many years. However, the decision in *Stanley* has been interpreted by some states as requiring extensive efforts to track down putative fathers prior to terminating parental rights, even when they have not acknowledged paternity or shown any interest in a child. For a discussion of post-*Stanley* statutes in Illinois, Michigan, New York and Wisconsin, see N. L. Freeman, "Remodeling Adoption Statutes After *Stanley* v. *Illinois*," *Journal of Family Law* 15 (1976-77): 385-422.

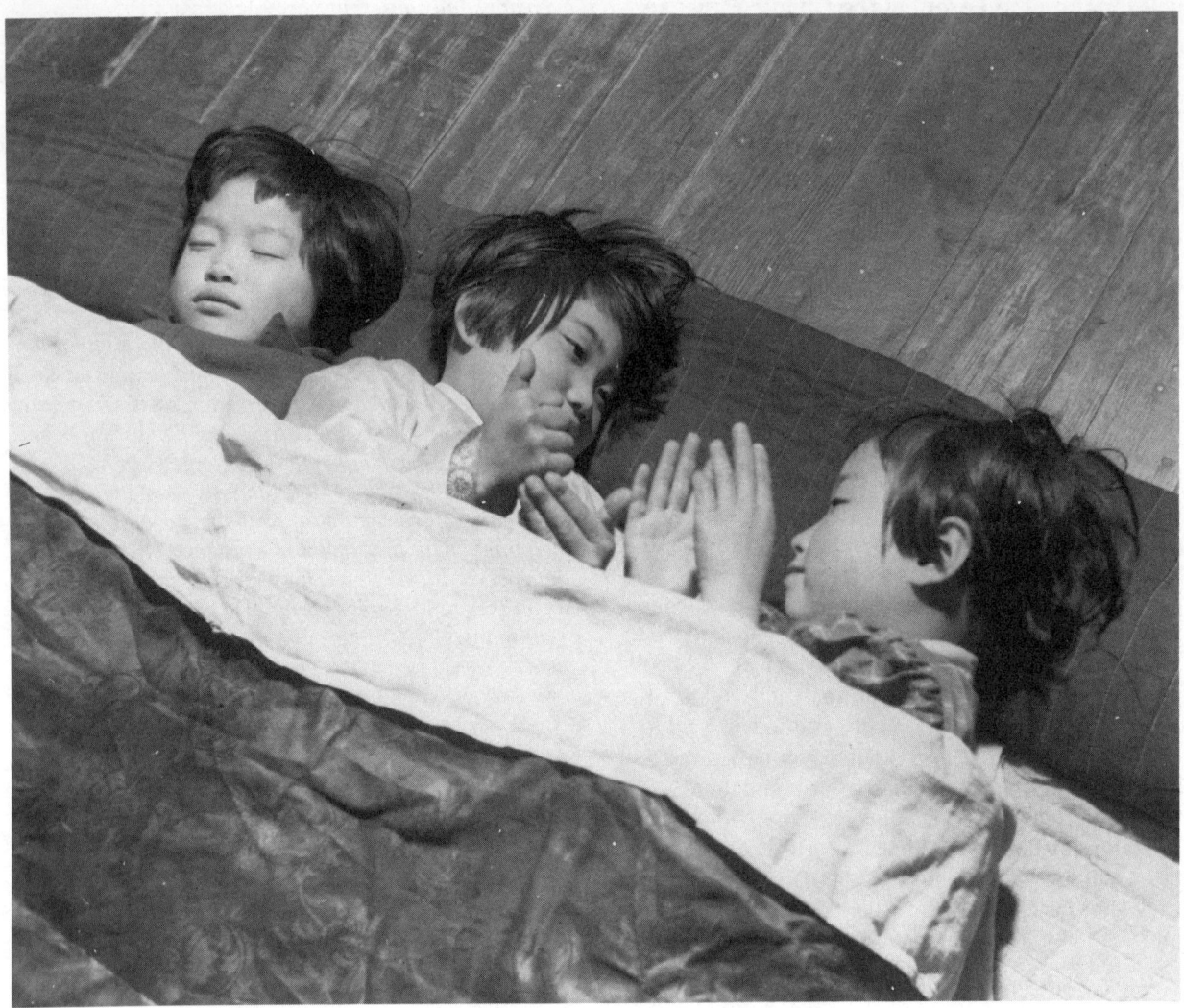

terminate parental rights. Partially in expectation of judicial reluctance, and partially as a result of their own failures, caseworkers often do not bring potential termination cases to court. Case documentation that efforts to work with the parents have been tried and have failed is crucial to the success of a termination effort. Often, as we showed earlier, such efforts do not take place, or if they do, they are poorly documented. Caseworkers feel that if they bring a petition, natural parents or their lawyers can correctly argue that they were not given a chance. As a compensation for past agency failures, the parent is protected at the expense of the child and his current situation. This is the tragedy behind the still unresolved case of Lee.

Lee is a completely deaf six-year-old Chinese child who, at two-and-a-half, was hospitalized as a battered child. She remained in the hospital for ten months while the hospital sought an agency willing to try to find a foster home for her. During that time, Mrs. T., a teacher of deaf children, began to visit Lee, learning of her through a friend working at the hospital. After ten months, a private agency finally agreed to find a home for Lee. Having grown to love the child, Mrs. T. applied and became Lee's foster parent. For the next five years Lee made tremendous progress, growing into a charming, friendly, happy child, deeply attached to Mrs. T. On several occasions agency workers asked Mrs. T. if she would like to adopt Lee. She said yes, and workers agreed to try to encourage Lee's parents to relinquish the child for adoption.

In the meantime, Mrs. T. sought permission from the agency to take Lee out of the state to enroll her in a school with a unique program for deaf children. With no explanation, the agency denied permission. Two weeks later, Mrs. T. was to appear in court. She found both natural parents with lawyers. The father was agreeable to relinquishing Lee, if he could still see her. The mother, who during the last five years had seen her daughter only five times (each of which was extremely upsetting to Lee), was unwilling. At the hearing, the agency did not support Mrs. T.'s request to adopt the child. The judge equivocated, saying only that Lee should remain in care. Later, an agency worker commented, "It would be unfair to the mother to honor the adoption request because they had not tried hard enough to work with her in the past."

While the legal process drags on, Lee cannot be enrolled in the special program and Mrs. T. is continually anxious and fearful that ultimately this permanently handicapped and once-abused child, whom she has nurtured and cared for for five years, will be taken from her.

Again, this is not an isolated case. It is a tragedy made more poignant by Lee's deafness. But even with non-handicapped children, agencies too often ignore positive changes and dismiss the strengths of new psychological relationships in order to compensate for their failures to work with the parents. In lawsuits in which one party has injured the other, the injuring party is typically ordered to pay damages. In cases like Lee's, the damage award to the injured parents may not be money, but the child, at the expense of her rights and psychological needs.

The failure to respond to the child's needs takes other forms as well. For instance, in a study of barriers to permanence for children in foster care in Oregon, researchers found it was possible to predict what permanent plans would be made for a child simply by knowing in which county he was placed. In other words, the child's own characteristics exerted very little influence over the caseworker's decision whether to terminate.[48]

To illustrate the reluctance to make hard decisions about natural parents and consequences for children, we have discussed the roles of judges and caseworkers. But other professionals have similar biases. For example, in a case in which a mother had been in and out of psychiatric hospitals 15 times prior to and since the birth of her child, a psychiatrist refused to say the mother would "never" make a good parent. Therefore, the judge refused to free the child for adoption, although the child, now five, had *never* lived with the mother.[49]

We have also seen a variant on the theme expressed by lawyers. Sometimes, in their attempt to redress earlier and real wrongs against the parents of children in foster care, including the initial failure to provide services to parents or properly inform them of conditions leading to potential loss of their child, they too may ignore the consequences of moving a child from foster parents who have become the child's psychological parents. On the other hand, we were also told that state or county attorneys often would not bring a termination petition unless the parents were egregiously inadequate, regardless of the current circumstances of the child.

The termination of parental rights is a serious action. It represents a relatively unique situation in which, in fundamental ways, the needs and rights of parents and children may be in irreconcilable conflict. There is no question, as we have shown, that children are removed from their homes unnecessarily, and sometimes arbitrarily. Nor is there any question that natural parents are individually, and as a group, often ignored or abused by those with responsibility for their children. But to correct this by creating new hardships for children is not the answer.

Lack of Criteria and Funds

Part of the problem is that adequate criteria for termination decisions are lacking.[50] Guides by which to judge when an individual child's needs and rights should take precedence over the residual rights of

---

[48]The Oregon study is described more fully in Chapter 6.

[49]We do not believe that mental illness, mental retardation or incarceration in and of themselves should ever be automatic grounds for termination. However, they are factors to be weighed in making a decision.

[50]See Wald, "State Intervention on Behalf of 'Neglected' Children," and Institute of Judicial Administration and American Bar Association Joint Commission on Juvenile Justice Standards, *Abuse and Neglect*.

natural parents must be articulated explicitly. They must take account of the child's developmental stage, and his or her past and present relationships with natural and psychological parents. All of the following factors should be considered in making an individual determination.

— The length of time the child has been out of the home
— The strength of the child's past relationship with the natural parent
— The child's response to current visits and trial stays at home
— The strength of the child's psychological relationship with foster parent(s) if such a relationship has been formed
— The child's wishes, depending on his age

At present, grounds for termination are often only loosely defined in state statutes and procedural protections are inadequate for the child and the parents.[51] A few states require *separate* counsel for the child and parents in termination proceedings. In a greater number of states, separate counsel for the child may be appointed only when there is conflict between the child and his parents or it is felt to be necessary to protect the child's interest.[52] Administrative guidelines and training for staff regarding termination are either inadequate or nonexistent. In addition, there are fiscal disincentives to terminating parental rights. Legal proceedings are likely to be costly. In many places, private or public agencies initiating termination proceedings must either assume the costs or rely on already overburdened district attorneys' offices for counsel.

Finally, even if termination proceedings are brought they may be drawn-out and complex, often involving appeals taking several years.[53] No system of priorities assures speedy completion of the court proceedings. Meanwhile, the child either remains in psychological limbo, or strengthens his or her psychological ties to natural, foster or potentially adoptive parents—ties that may eventually, depending upon the court decision, be disrupted.

The picture is not uniformly bleak. At least two of the states we visited, along with several others we identified, are implementing institutional mechanisms to reduce the denial of permanence to children. Chapters 4 and 6 detail these efforts. But no mechanisms will smooth out all the dilemmas around the severing of parental rights. The fact is there are few easy cases when termination is at stake. In the case of Lee, the judge's reluctance to terminate was also influenced by an ideological position that children should have parents of the same ethnic background. For him, this weighed as heavily as the evidence that this particular child's mother showed no sustained interest in her, and that under the care of a foster mother with a different ethnic background, the child flourished. Tensions may arise between natural and foster parents—particularly when, after little initial contact, the natural parent has been able to rehabilitate herself or himself and genuinely wants to care for the child. In other instances the dilemma revolves around how to assess the extent of parental interest in the child. But each of these issues must be addressed directly in policy and practice if individual children out of their homes are to be assured of a right to permanence.

Barriers to Adoption

Terminating parental rights is often a means to an end—the eventual adoption of a child. But even if termination proceeds appropriately and smoothly, obstacles remain. Adoption efforts are limited by several persistent, widespread problems: the failure to identify children for adoption; the failure to complete adoption proceedings; and the failure to subsidize adoptions to ensure that money is not a barrier to a child's having a caring home.

---

[51]The Children's Bureau in the Administration for Children, Youth and Families in HEW is in the process of finalizing a model termination of parental rights statute. The proposed draft mandates counsel for the parent and separate counsel for the child in all involuntary termination proceedings. For a discussion of termination statutes in the CDF study states, see Chapter 4.

[52]In neglect proceedings, most parents have a right to be represented by counsel and in some states to appointed counsel if they are indigent. A handful of states provide for mandatory separate counsel for the child without any qualifications in neglect proceedings, although a number provide for the appointment of either mandatory or discretionary counsel under specified circumstances: for instance if there is a conflict of interest between the parent and child. For a state-by-state description of statutory provisions for counsel in termination and dependency and neglect proceedings, see Appendix E.

[53]For example, a study in New York State revealed that 20 percent of the court proceedings for termination petitions initiated in 1973 had not been completed by May 1975. Temporary State Commission on Child Welfare, *Barriers*, Appendix II, Tables 1 and 10.

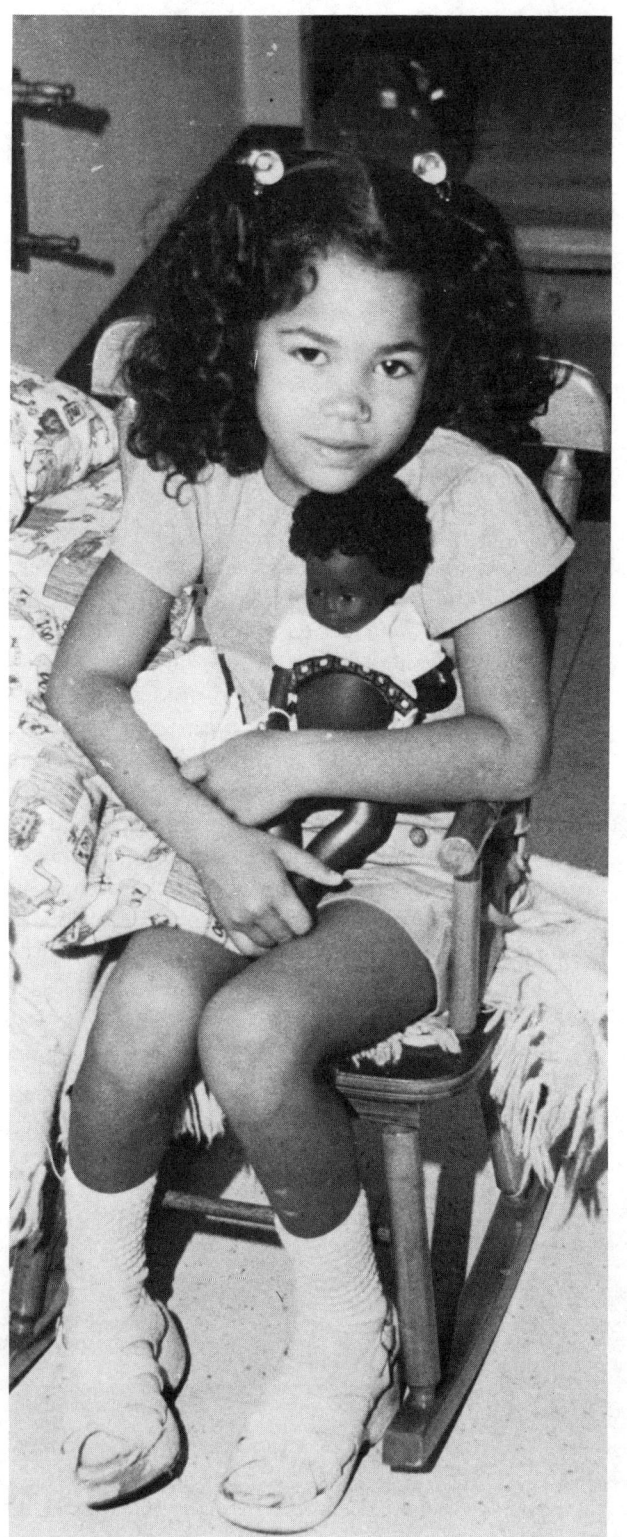

Failure to Identify Adoptable Children Appropriately

Mark was placed in foster care in 1971, at age six, along with four of his seven siblings. His mother, who had a history of serious drug addiction, failed to respond to any efforts by the welfare department to contact her. Eighteen months after the initial placement in a foster home, the child welfare agency's foster care unit referred Mark to the adoption unit. He was then eight. The adoption unit noted: "Child is not at an age where he is an easy candidate for adoption. Special education problems and adjustment problems due to his neglectful past might constitute problems to any adoption plan."

But in the very same case folder Mark is described as follows: "Child seems to have developed very positive relationships with his peers in the community. He has friends and gets along with the other children in the group home. Child is an attractive, friendly boy who has made friends in the community. He has made a fine adjustment to this community and family oriented group placement. We feel the child's placement is appropriate in terms of a permanent home environment."

Notwithstanding the above comments, this eight-year-old boy was then transferred from one group home to another. In the six-month progress report, the following comment appears: "Child is doing well in his present placement (group home). He has all the love and attention he requires from Mr. and Mrs. G. If the group parents were to adopt, they would lose salary." Three years later, Mark was still in the group home, having had four sets of "house parents" and no contact with any member of his natural family for over five years.

The question is: how many "unadoptable children" like Mark exist? One aspect of the problem of identification has to do with the tacit writing-off of particular groups of children as inappropriate for adoption either by adoption or foster care workers. The general wisdom and attitude, which sometimes hardens into guidelines and policies, is that certain handicapped children, sibling groups, black or other minority children, and children older than four, five or six are "unadoptable." Yet when special efforts are made on behalf of these children, permanent homes can be found.

The responsibility to identify children for adoption rests in large measure with the public agencies providing care. It is a responsibility that is often inadequately met. However, there is another aspect to the problem.

Private facilities, which are funded by public agencies, also fail to identify children who should be adopted, and even actively block adoption efforts.

Kerry, now nine, has lived in a children's home (a euphemism for an institution for dependent and neglected children) since she was six. She entertained herself by making frequent visits to a nearby firehouse. One of the firemen became particularly fond of her and introduced her to his wife. When they gave the child presents she asked if she could keep them at the firehouse because, "If I took them back home, they would not let me come back" —a telling comment about the atmosphere in this "children's home." Over a year ago, the couple went to the home to make a formal request to adopt the girl. Since then, they have been sent from the home to county agencies and back again. Kerry remains in the institution. No adoption proceedings have been initiated.

Eight-year-old Robert is a black child in the care of a private nonprofit agency providing adoption services as well as residential care. Several black parents sought to adopt Robert who is healthy and normal in all respects but, without explanation, the agency told the parents they were not appropriate.[54] *As a result, Robert remains in the institution.*

In both these cases, the local public agencies made no effort to challenge the private facilities' failure to encourage adoption, although they were paying the agencies for the care of these children. The reasons for such inaction vary. In some instances, there may be tacit collusion between public and private agencies, perhaps in order to maximize a per diem reimbursement.[55] Overt prejudice may also account for the resistance to adoption. In other instances, because of red tape or changing staff, there may simply be no one either in the public agency or the private facility to act on behalf of the child.

Failure to Complete Adoption Proceedings

Sam, age four, was removed by the state from the foster home in which he had been living after he was freed for adoption. His foster parents were not interested in adopting him, although they provided him with care and affection. He was placed in a facility for dependent and neglected children "temporarily" by the state adoption unit, and remains there three years later. He has not been adopted, and his ties with his foster parents have been broken.

Susan is a 12-year-old who was freed for adoption three years ago. She has been living with foster parents who have been anxious to adopt her since she was seven. The foster care worker, who feels these parents would make excellent adoptive parents, referred the case to the state's adoption unit for formal study three years ago. No one from the adoption unit has ever visited the foster parents, despite persistent reminders from the foster care worker. The foster father recently lost his job, so the foster parents are very worried that they will not be approved if the adoption study should start now.

Sam, in a flurry of activity, was removed from a familiar home and institutionalized as a "precursor" to adoption. There he has been stranded, with no one monitoring his progress or the caseworker's efforts. Susan was a victim of an understaffed, underactive adoption unit that failed to follow through even on the easy cases. Still other children may be identified as adoptable in case plans, but no steps are taken to ensure they are adopted.[56]

Inadequate Adoption Subsidies

Another significant obstacle to adoption is the lack of adequate funds to help in the adoption of children with special needs. These funds are particularly crucial to enable potential adoptive parents to care for handicapped children, siblings and children who

---

[54] A New York City audit of foster care agencies' efforts to find permanent homes for children reported that although many potential adoptive parents seek older children, minority children and children with various "handicaps," they are frequently rejected by agencies or discouraged from efforts to adopt, often for questionable reasons. New York City Comptroller's Office, *The Children are Waiting* (New York: Institute of Public Affairs, 1977), pp. 26-29.

[55] On the other hand, we also heard of efforts in which public and private agencies are working together to ensure children are provided permanent adoptive homes. New York Spaulding for Children, a private adoption agency specializing in the adoptive placement of children with special needs, is working with the Office of Special Services for Children in New York City to find permanent adoptive homes for 100 children with special needs who have been legally free for adoption for at least one year, and is also providing training for workers responsible for the children.

[56] In New Jersey, an administrative review of children in foster care resulted in the identification of large numbers of children for whom the goal of adoption was in the case plan, but who had never been referred to the state adoption agency. Interview with Director of New Jersey Bureau of Resource Development, May 1976.

In Arizona, a 1974 study reported that for 52 percent of the children for whom adoption was identified as a goal, and whose parents' whereabouts were unknown, no termination petitions had been filed. The Governor's Community Coordinated Child Care Committee, *The Neglected Family* (Arizona: State 4-C Committee, 1976).

In New York City, CWIS reports indicated that almost 50 percent of the 5,600 children for whom adoption was the goal had not been freed for adoption. Fanshel and Grundy, *Computerized Data*, p. 27.

would not otherwise be adopted. They are also important for foster parents who want to adopt children for whom they have cared for long periods. Consider the case of Jenny.

Jenny, a handicapped child in Ohio, had been in the same foster family for a long time. When the family sought to adopt her, the director of the children's agency found herself in the uncomfortable position of discouraging them, because Jenny would no longer be eligible for services she needed and now received, and the family could not afford to provide them privately.[57] *In her county there were no funds for subsidized adoptions.*

The commitment to subsidize adoptions is, at present, solely up to the state. There is no specific federal legislation targeting funds for subsidized adoption and consequently no federal incentive for states to provide subsidies.[58] State statutory provisions for subsidy vary considerably.[59] Only four states, including two of our study states, Arizona and South Carolina, define eligibility to include the existence of significant emotional ties between child and foster parents seeking to adopt.[60] States also vary according to whether a child who is placed in an adoptive home outside the state or whose adoptive parents move can continue to receive a subsidy from the original state.

Moreover, although many states have passed subsidized adoption statutes, fewer have provided adequate funds for subsidy or administration.[61] In Ohio, for instance, all subsidy funds must come from the county. In fact, the state has exerted so little leadership that it could not readily furnish us with a list of counties which had appropriated monies. One state official expressed concern that only children who were ineligible for federally and state-reimbursed foster care payments were likely to be considered, particularly in rural counties.

There has been no systematic or extensive evaluation of the impact of subsidized adoptions on ensuring children permanence. But available evidence does suggest that subsidies can increase the number of children, especially older children, assured permanence,[62] and that they are cost-effective.[63]

During the past few years, there have been a number of significant changes in adoption patterns for children. Pro-adoption child advocacy groups have been and continue to be very active, and significant gains have been made. Special attention has been focused on hard-to-place children; foster parents have been given standing and sometimes priority to adopt a child they have cared for; most states have some form of subsidized adoption law; and a number of local, state and regional adoption exchange systems have been established.[64] At the same time, in this area more than any other, we saw marked variations in efforts to find adoptive homes for children and in the leadership efforts of those charged with responsibility to do so. The uneven patterns of success speak to the uneven structural incentives for success. These must be changed.

---

[57]There are two aspects to the problem. In the first place, adoptive parents often cannot get medical insurance coverage for the child because the child's pre-existing medical condition makes him ineligible. In the second place, if the adoptive family is not eligible for Medicaid, the Medicaid benefits often available to the child in foster care cease.

[58]Because federal reimbursement is available for foster care maintenance payments but not for adoption subsidy payments, it may be to a state's benefit to continue the child in the federally-reimbursed program rather than referring him to a 100 percent state or locally financed program.

[59]The Children's Bureau within HEW has developed a Model State Subsidized Adoption Act and Regulations. The Act and Regulations, as well as a comparison of the Model Act with state subsidy laws in effect in 42 states in August 1976, are published in *Subsidized Adoption in America* (Washington, D.C.: HEW, August 1976). For a list of citations to current state adoption subsidy statutes, see Appendix F.

[60]There is, of course, a danger of pressuring foster parents to adopt a child when they do not want to, but when they genuinely do, there must be statutory and administrative support.

[61]Those states that have, have used money from a number of sources such as special appropriations or reallocation of foster care funds.

[62]For example, in New York City in 1969, prior to the enactment of a subsidy law, 5.7 percent of the children adopted were between 5 and 11. In 1973, 31.3 percent of the children adopted were between 5 and 11. They were 18 percent of those not subsidized, and 54.5 percent of those subsidized. New York State Department of Social Services, Bureau of Research, "Adoptive Discharges from Foster Care," cited as Appendix Table 67 in Lash and Sigal, *State of the Child*, p. 180.

[63]For example, during the period 1975 through 1976, 267 children in Los Angeles, California, who had been in long-term foster care were placed in adoptive homes with subsidies. The county estimated that to continue those children in foster care until age 18 would have cost the county $16.7 million in maintenance costs alone, excluding costs of service and administration. Senate Report No. 95-167, 95th Congress, First Session (1977), p. 21. It is clearly most cost-effective to have a child adopted with no subsidy. However, the administrative costs associated with a subsidy program are far less than the administrative and supervisory costs incurred when a child is in foster care.

[64]These systems serve as a clearinghouse through which attempts can be made by agencies to link prospective adoptive families with hard-to-place children. In addition, the North American Center on Adoption, a special project of the Child Welfare League of America, has operated a national exchange, the Adoption Resource Exchange of North America (ARENA), since 1967. Agencies from around the country may register with ARENA those children for whom they are unable to find adoptive homes locally or in their own states as well as families who are waiting for children. ARENA also engages in its own outreach efforts to identify children in need of adoptive homes. See Appendix G. for a list prepared by ARENA of existing exchanges.

For a description of numerous adoption resources, see D. S. Levine, *Adoption Resource Handbook* (Washington, D.C.: Children's Bureau, U.S. Department of Health, Education and Welfare), scheduled to be published by the close of 1978.

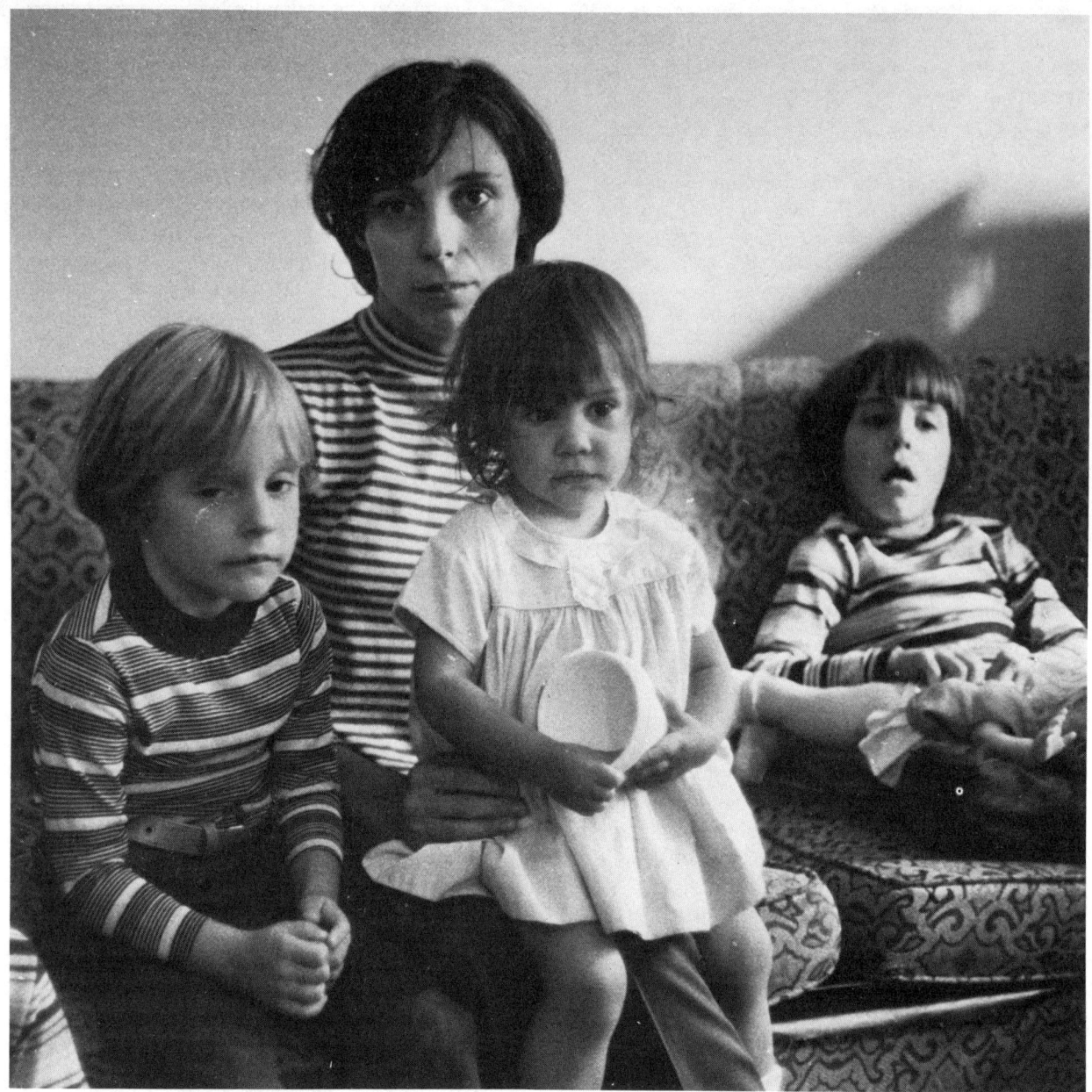

What Can Be Done?

To correct the abuses resulting from an anti-family bias throughout the placement process, a series of changes are necessary. Some must be directed toward children now in care, others toward protecting children who are likely to be at risk of separation from their own families or placed out of their homes. Changes are needed at all points. Reforming adoption procedures without ensuring that children are not needlessly removed from their homes will not be sufficient—nor will enhancing efforts to maintain a child's contact with his family be useful without also providing for restorative services. Our specific recommendations follow:

1. No child should be removed from his home unless services designed to prevent unnecessary out-of-home care have been provided to the family, or offered and refused. The only exception should be in emergency situations, when the child is in danger of substantial physical or emotional harm.[65]

2. If the child is placed "voluntarily," i.e., without court involvement, there should be a written agreement spelling out the obligations and rights of both the parents and the agency. The parents should be informed both verbally and in writing of their right, upon request, to the return of a voluntarily placed child within a reasonable period unless the state files a dependency, neglect or abuse petition.

3. If the placement is involuntary, i.e., as a result of a court proceeding, the parents and child should have the right to counsel.

4. If a child must be placed, priority should be given to the formal placement of the child with willing relatives with reimbursement at the foster care rate. If such placement is not possible, the child should be placed in the least restrictive setting appropriate to his needs, within reasonable proximity to family and home community.

5. While the child is in placement, the public agency with responsibility for the child should have a statutory obligation to maintain and encourage, whenever possible, parent-child ties; document the extent of parent-child contact; and provide specific restorative services designed to reunify the family. Parents should have a statutory right to receive progress reports.

6. There must be independent (of the agency or person providing services) reviews of children out of their homes at least every six months to determine progress toward reunification.

7. No later than 18 months after entry into care, there should be a dispositional review conducted by a court or specially designated board, independent of service providers and appealable to the courts. The purpose of this review should be to determine whether the child should be returned home; continued for a specified period in foster care until reunification; freed for adoption; or in special circumstances, placed in permanent foster care. All interested parties should be notified of this review and have the right to participate. A mechanism should be mandated to ensure recommended dispositions are carried out.

8. Statutory provisions regarding termination of parental rights and adoption subsidy should be reviewed and strengthened as necessary. All children should have separately appointed counsel in termination proceedings.

9. Parents, foster parents and children should have access to grievance mechanisms to register complaints about the care or treatment they are receiving.

10. Community advocacy groups should closely monitor, evaluate and seek to correct inadequate policies and practices toward children at risk of or in placement and their families. Budgets should be reviewed to ensure adequate funds for preventive, restorative and adoptive scrvices, as well as for review procedures.

---

[65] If an emergency removal is necessary, a court hearing should be held no later than 72 hours after the removal.

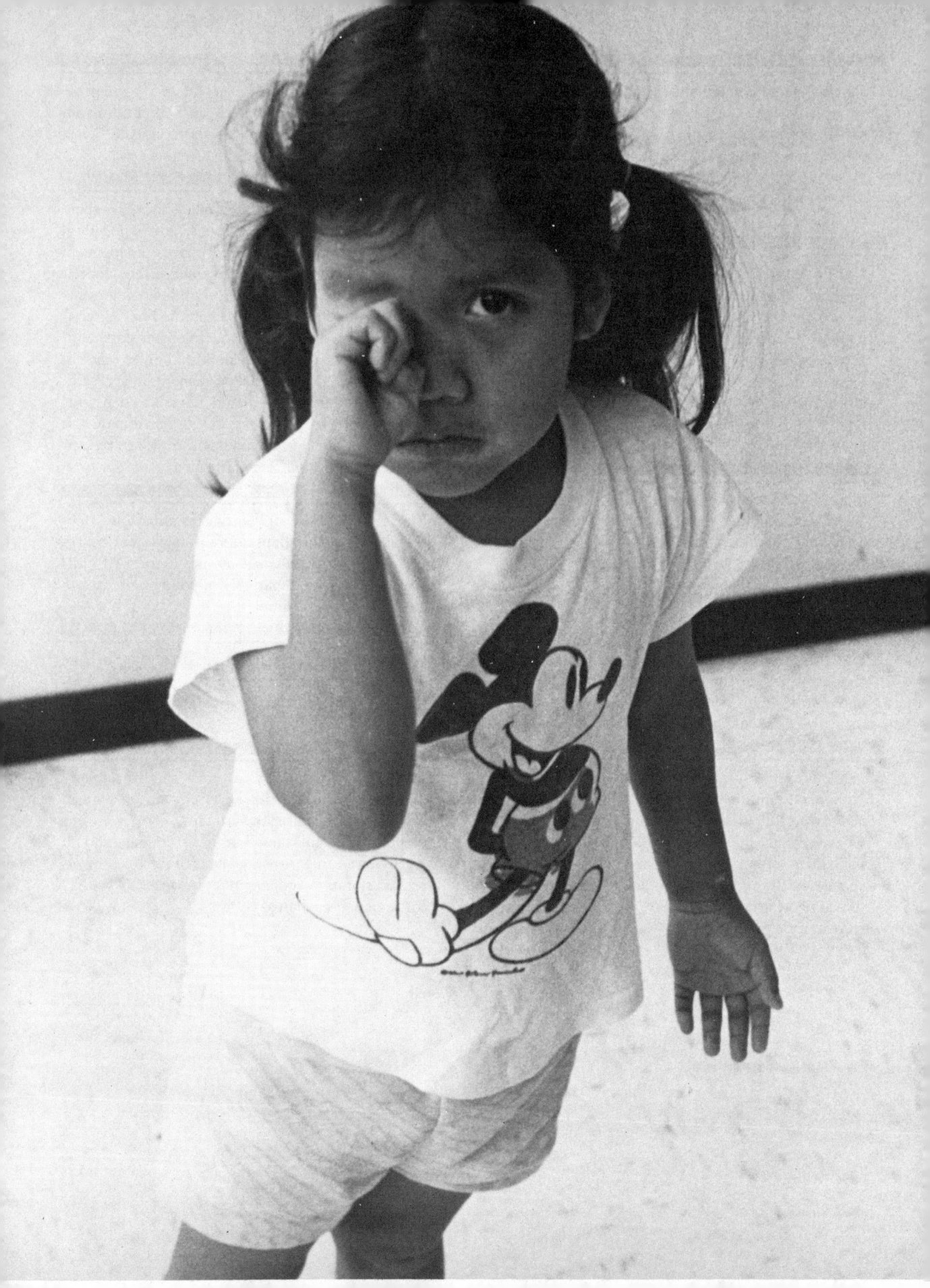

2 Children Don't Count

Patterns of Public Neglect

I have an allocations worker, I have a caseworker, and I have my caseworker's supervisor. None of them ever met me. They don't know what I look like. All they know is what my psychological test said. . . .The allocations worker is supposed to find a group home that is right for me, but she's never met me, she doesn't know what kind of a person I am. How can she find a group home. . . .And this is the same for all the people there. . .I'm not just one special case.

Interview with Thelma, age 15, by the Children's Express, *published in the* New York Times

What Public Neglect Looks Like

Not only are children who enter into out-of-home care isolated from their own or adoptive families, they are often also denied a chance to experience security and caring from any adult. Because the child-placing network is complex and options for placement are limited, placement decisions rarely take into account the special strengths and needs of a particular child. Thus, public neglect of family-child ties is often compounded by public neglect of the quality of life while the child is in out-of-home care.

Inappropriate Placements

There is a widespread belief, strengthened in recent years by legal decisions, that the most appropriate placement is in the least restrictive, most family-like setting appropriate to the child's needs. In addition, evidence suggests the least restrictive alternative is also the least costly.[1] Such a placement requires knowledge of the child; knowledge of what different settings actually provide; and a determination of the appropriate mesh between the two.

Some have interpreted the concept of the least restrictive alternative to mean that no child should be placed in an institution, regardless of the special needs of the child. This is overly simplistic. Some children

---

[1] A study of foster care needs and alternatives to placement in New York City which set forth the range of per-child, per-diem costs for various types of foster care placements reported that long-term institutional care was considerably more costly than foster home care. Generally, the various services which could provide alternatives to out-of-home care, such as casework, homemakers and center day care, were also less costly than any out-of-home placements. B. Bernstein, D. Snider, and W. Meezan, *Foster Care Needs and Alternatives to Placement: A Projection for 1975-1985* (Albany: New York State Board of Social Welfare, 1975), pp. 44-45. The data we obtained from three of our seven study states revealed similar cost patterns. Further, demonstration projects which have made alternative services available to families and eliminated the need for more costly out-of-home care have resulted in cost savings. See footnote 13, Chapter 1.

simply cannot cope with the demands of too intimate a setting, and some children need care from trained child care workers in special residential treatment facilities. On the other hand, evidence suggests that too often placements are, in fact, inappropriate and unnecessarily restrictive.[2]

Nationally, for instance, children in startling numbers live in jails.[3] Over 3,000 children live in nursing homes; some in pediatric nursing homes; and some in nursing homes for the elderly.[4] Other children spend their youth in public hospitals.[5] Adolescents are especially vulnerable to inappropriate placement in residential facilities and psychiatric hospitals. For them, it is often assumed they are too troubled to be cared for in foster family homes or small group homes, or these options just don't exist. A 1975 New York City study which reviewed case records of 1,250 children in out-of-home care concluded that a staggering 55.3

WHERE A CHILD IS PLACED: SOME DEFINITIONS

Foster Homes. Foster homes generally serve up to six children. Foster parents, who care for the children, usually receive payment for their room and board. Payments often vary with the age of the child. There are also specialized foster homes in which foster parents receive specialized training and/or support in caring for children with particular needs, including physical or mental handicaps.

Group Homes. Group homes, which often have salaried house parents, range from those providing treatment services to those providing only room and board. The goal underlying the emergence of group homes is to enable a child to receive care in his own community, drawing on as many of the available community resources as possible. Halfway houses usually refer to group homes for children who have been released from institutions or other closed settings. Group homes generally accept between 7 and 16, and sometimes up to 25 children. The larger group homes serving 13-25 children are often called group residences.

Institutions and Residential Treatment Centers. The term "institution" is usually used to refer to large congregate custodial care facilities for children, although sometimes it is used interchangeably with the term "residential treatment center." Child care institutions typically provide only custodial care and education, sometimes only the former. They are usually isolated physically and psychologically from community life and resources. Training schools, state psychiatric hospitals, and state schools for the retarded, some of which are now called developmental centers, are examples of institutions.

Theoretically, residential treatment centers offer an array of individualized treatment services to a child. In reality, however, the term "residential treatment center" is now used by programs varying tremendously in quality, cost, orientation to the child's family, reliance on drug treatment, therapeutic style and fiscal procedures. Some are run by state or county agencies; some are run by private nonprofit agencies (also called voluntary agencies); others are run by private agencies for profit.

---

[2] The proportion of children placed in foster homes and institutional settings varies by system and community. In the CDF survey, child welfare agencies reported 50 percent of the children were in foster homes; 24 percent in group homes; and 12 percent in institutions. Of the remaining 14 percent: seven percent were with relatives, three percent in adoptive homes and four percent in other settings. Precise figures from the probation agencies were not available because over 73 percent of the children were referred to other agencies for care and probation records did not contain data on the types of placements. Probation agencies did report that 16 percent of the children for whom they had responsibility were in training schools; 1 percent in mental hospitals. In New York City in 1974, 69.7 percent of the status offenders and 73.9 percent of the juvenile delinquents referred by probation to the child welfare agency for placement were in institutional care; 14.3 and 9.1 percent of the respective groups were in group or boarding home care; and 16 and 17 percent in other settings. T. Lash and H. Sigal, *State of the Child: New York City* (New York: Foundation for Child Development, April 1976), Appendix Table 81, p. 188.

Other data sources suggest different patterns. For example, in California in 1974, 80.6 percent of the children in the child welfare system were in family settings; 3.3 percent in group settings of 7-12 children; and 15.5 percent in larger group care or other institutional settings. Comparable figures for non-child welfare out-of-home placements were: 59.8 percent for family-like settings, 4.5 percent for group settings for 12 or fewer children, and 22.7 percent in larger group or institutional settings. California Department of Health, Center for Health Statistics, "Children in Foster Care," Sacramento: Data Matters Topical Reports, September 1974, p. 5

[3] A CDF report, *Children in Adult Jails*, found that only 11.7 percent of the children held in the 440 jails visited were charged with serious offenses against persons. The other 88.3 percent were charged with property or minor offenses, or else had no place else to go. See *Children in Adult Jails* (Washington, D.C.: Children's Defense Fund of the Washington Research Project, Inc., December 1976).

[4] U.S. Bureau of the Census, Census of Population: 1970, *Persons in Institutions and Other Group Quarters*, Final Report PC(2)-4E (Washington, D.C.: U.S. Government Printing Office, 1973), Table 6.

[5] Susan Jacoby in "The $73,000 Abandoned Babies," *New York Times Magazine*, 6 March 1977, reported on the nearly 300 children growing up in New York City hospitals. There has been no attempt nationally to identify other children living in urban hospitals. CDF is currently involved in a class action lawsuit challenging the boarding of handicapped children who have been adjudicated neglected and are in the custody of the District of Columbia Department of Human Resources in hospitals or other institutional settings when their needs could be met in less restrictive settings. *Bobby D., et al.* v. *Washington, et al.*, No. 16-77 (D.C. Super. Ct., Family Div., filed November 21, 1977).

percent of the children were inappropriately placed at the time of their *initial* placement, and that 42.8 percent of the *current* placements were inappropriate.[6] The study also found that the older the child, the more likely an inappropriate placement.[7]

Although the majority of the children in our study states were in foster family homes, officials repeatedly cited evidence to us of inappropriately institutionalized children[8] (See Figure 1).

- There were over 700 children in California psychiatric facilities, but 50 percent of them reportedly were not mentally ill, but had academic and behavioral difficulties. Moreover, even for those children who were mentally ill, there was no evidence that, within the hospitals, the children were in appropriate programs.

- Arizona officials reported that the majority of hospitalized children were neither autistic nor psychotic, but adolescents with behavioral problems such as running away, drug or alcohol abuse, or difficulties with authority.

- In New Jersey, based on case record information, 16 percent of the children referred to psychiatric hospitals during one month in 1973 by the child welfare agency were severely emotionally disturbed or psychotic. Eighty-four percent were not.[9]

- In Ohio, the director of a state school for the retarded reported finding over 50 children with IQs between 80 and 100 in his institution. But he also found, after meetings with the parents, that many of them refused to take home these children who never should have been institutionalized in the first place. Arizona also reported finding 13 children in state schools for the retarded who were of normal intelligence.

- In California, officials in the Department of Health estimated there were up to 800 children in nursing homes. Supposedly, the children were all non-ambulatory and chronically physically disabled. But when we asked state officials, no one could confirm that the children were, in fact, severely handicapped. In Ohio, we learned of a handicapped child whose psychotic mother voluntarily placed her in a nursing

	Foster Home	Institution
Arizona	74%	26%
California	75	25
Massachusetts	NA	NA
New Jersey	79	21
Ohio	69	30
South Carolina	79	21
South Dakota	NA	NA

Figure 1. Percentage of Children in Foster Home and Institutional Care under Child Welfare Auspices in Seven Study States[1]

[1]Arizona data are from Arizona Department of Economic Security, *Annual Report, July 1, 1974-June 30, 1975*, and figures from DES report of June 1975 on institutional placements cited to CDF staff by DES officials. The California data are from California Department of Social Welfare, "Caseload Movement and Expenditures Reports, 1975"; Ohio data are from Ohio Department of Public Welfare, "Ohio Public Welfare Statistics," January-March 1975; New Jersey data are from the New Jersey Department of Institutions and Agencies, Division of Youth and Family Services, Case Review Unit, "Summary of Case Review Reports," April 7, 1976. The South Carolina data, effective as of December 31, 1975, were reported to CDF by South Carolina officials.

[9]An analysis of 674 children placed, or in need of placement, during October 1973, in New Jersey indicated that 42 children were referred by child welfare district offices to psychiatric hospitals. Of these, only seven were psychotic or severely emotionally disturbed; the others exhibited various behavioral disorders. New Jersey Department of Institutions and Agencies, Division of Youth and Family Services, Bureau of Research Planning and Program Development, "A Needs Resource Analysis of New Jersey's System for Providing Residential Treatment to Delinquent and Disturbed Children," New Jersey, June 1974, p. 30. (Mimeographed.)

---

[6]Bernstein, Snider, and Meezan, *Foster Care Needs and Alternatives to Placement*, pp. 20-25. The case readings were judged according to criteria specially developed for the study, which are set forth in full in Sister Mary Paul, *Criteria for Foster Placement and Alternatives to Foster Care* (New York: New York State Board of Social Welfare, May 1975).

[7]For children 0-3, 28 percent of the placements were described as inappropriate; for children 3-9, 38 percent; for children 9-12, 44 percent; for children 12-15, 50 percent; and for children 15-18, 51 percent. The fact that just over half of the children 12-18 were judged to be inappropriately placed is especially significant when related to the fact that in 1974, 42 percent of the 28,000 children in out-of-home care in New York City were 12 or over. Bernstein, Snider, and Meezan, *Foster Care Needs and Alternatives to Placement*, pp. 7, 22. While these data cannot be generalized beyond New York City, the CDF survey indicated that 50 percent of the children who were reported to be in out-of-home care under child welfare auspices were 12 or older. See Appendix C.

[8]Accurate data on the institutionalization of children are difficult to obtain. A comparison of data from the 1960 and 1970 national censuses of the population does not reflect a significant increase in the total number of institutionalized persons under 18 years of age. However, closer analysis shows an uneven picture. While there were decreases in the numbers of children in institutions for dependent and neglected children and for the physically handicapped, there was a 90 percent increase in the number of children in mental hospitals and residential treatment centers. Similarly, there was a 24 percent increase in the number of children reported to be in prisons and reformatories, local jails and workhouses, chronic disease hospitals, and homes for the aged and dependent. Over 16,000 of the 238,000 children institutionalized in 1970 were in such facilities. U.S. Bureau of the Census, Census of Population: 1960, *Inmates of Institutions*, Subject Report PC(2)-8A (Washington, D.C.: U.S. Government Printing Office, 1963), Tables 3-11; and U.S. Bureau of the Census, Census of Population: 1970, *Persons in Institutions and Other Group Quarters*, Tables 3-10.

home after the father deserted the family. The child was learning to walk with braces and maneuver a wheelchair. But no one had thought of moving the child to a less restrictive setting such as a specialized foster home.

- In Massachusetts, the Commissioner of the Division of Youth Services reported he had been forced to abandon the preventive services program and place children in inappropriate out-of-home care because of budget cuts. He commented, "Unfortunately diagnostic factors become irrelevant in a time of fiscal crunch."

- In South Dakota, Indian children were sent to jails because there were no alternative facilities on the reservations. The state institutions would not admit Indian children because of jurisdictional problems. Suicide attempts in the jails were so frequent that the Bureau of Indian Affairs regional office reportedly issued an order that it was "against the regulations to commit suicide."

- In South Carolina, the Commissioner of Social Services asked local child welfare offices how many children had been placed in jails or other correctional facilities. The answer: 18 counties placed 53 children in jails between October 1974 and September 1975.[10] Jails in South Carolina are no place for children. In 1974, CDF brought suit against the state on behalf of black and white youths placed in adult jails.[11] The black children were placed in segregated jails with black adults, the white children with white adults. All the children had been sodomized and brutally beaten.

Inappropriate Care

It is not enough to know where a child is placed. It is also necessary to know something about the quality of care the child is receiving—how the daily schedule goes; what kind of discipline is permitted; what attention is paid to the child's health and education; who speaks for the child; and how many times the child has had to readjust to new surroundings.

Our study did not investigate in detail the quality of care for children in specific foster family homes.[12] But we did examine the patterns of movement of children from one out-of-home—frequently one foster home—setting to another. There is no clearer way to get a sense of the lack of continuity and stability in the lives of so many children who are the responsibility of public agencies.

The following excerpt was taken from a story in the *Washington Post*.[13]

Dennis Smith is in his 17th year and his 16th foster home. "It's like a scar on your brain," he says. "I want people to realize what's happening to foster children," he adds. And he has filed an unusual lawsuit with that purpose in mind.[14]

The suit, filed in Alameda County Superior Court. . .asks damages of $500,000 from the county social service agency and officials of the public school system there.

Smith claims the agency told his mother he would be placed for adoption but sent him instead to one foster home after another. He says the schools accepted what he called a mistaken diagnosis that he was mentally retarded and put him in classes for the handicapped.

"If I had known I was going to spend the first 16 years of my life this way, I'd rather have been dead. I'd have wished my mother could have aborted me," said Dennis. . . .

The *Tucson Daily Citizen* reported another example:[15]

Seven-year-old twins, moved from one foster home to another since they were babies, were dropped off at their latest foster home with this request by a caseworker: "Try to keep them as long as you can. They usually last only three months."

The cavalier treatment of Dennis and the twins are perhaps extreme examples. But, in fact, the practice of moving children from place to place has been long

---

[10]South Carolina Department of Social Services, Follow-up report on data collected as a result of Memorandum 75-86, March 2, 1976. (Mimeographed.)

[11]*Larry W.* v. *Stone*, C.A. No. 74-986 (D. S.C.). This action was for individual damages and class injunctive relief. The damage claims of the individual plaintiffs were settled. However, the District Court thereafter dismissed the plaintiffs' class claims for injunctive relief against the incarceration of children in adult county jails on grounds of mootness. Because of technical problems it was decided not to appeal.

[12]For a study that focuses only on foster family care, see G. Thomas, et al., *Supply and Demand for Child Foster Family Care in the Southeast* (Athens, Ga.: Regional Institute of Social Welfare Research, Inc., 1977).

[13]"Youth Sues Over Foster Homes," *Washington Post,* 17 November 1976, p. A3.

[14]*Smith* v. *Alameda County Social Services Agency, et al.,* No. 488366-5 (Alameda County, California, Super. Ct., filed November 15, 1976). On April 15, 1977, the Court granted defendant's motion to strike the complaint in this case, and the matter is currently on appeal. The case was brought by the Youth Law Center in San Francisco, California.

[15]R.S. Vonier, G.P. Merrell, and C. Graham, "Children Adrift—An Arizona Crisis," *Tucson Daily Citizen,* 6 April 1977.

identified as an evil of the child care systems.[16] It is an evil that continues. In our own survey of child welfare offices in 140 counties, officials reported 18 percent of the children out of their homes had been moved three or more times. An analysis of statewide California data showed that 29.6 percent of the children placed by the child welfare system had moved three or more times, 9.6 percent five or more times.[17] A New Jersey study relating the length of time in care for children in institutional settings to the number of moves found that children in care for five to ten years had an average of 4.5 moves. For children in care over ten years, the average was 5.8 moves.[18]

Behind these percentages are children: children who must repeatedly cope with new authority figures, new expectations, often new schools, and above all new stresses. Sometimes children are moved for arbitrary and capricious reasons—for example, because a caseworker feels a child is becoming "too attached" to foster parents.[19] Sometimes foster parents initiate the removal because they like younger children but do not want the adolescents they turn into. Sometimes the fiscal and psychological demands of caring for a child with special needs become overwhelming for foster parents who receive little money, training or support. And sometimes the child becomes too troublesome in the eyes of a group home or residential treatment program: running away, for instance, is often a reason for kicking a child out of a facility.

In our meetings with state placement officials and with those who place children directly, we found few who had developed specific strategies to reduce the movement of children from place to place.[20] In New Jersey, there was an administrative case review system programmed to flag children who had been in care two years or less and had already moved three or more times.[21] California too required a special administrative review of children who had been moved three times.[22] But these efforts were often not carried out in practice.

We also looked at the quality of care provided to children placed in private or public group care facilities at public expense.[23] We visited one or two such facilities in each state, and talked with state licensing officials, lawyers, and caseworkers from our study states and other states who do visit facilities frequently.[24] Reports were

---

[16]Numerous studies have documented the movement of children from placement to placement. A review of data from studies of foster care in four states (Arizona, California, Iowa and Massachusetts) revealed that approximately 50 percent of the foster children studied experienced at least two foster home placements and between 10 and 15 percent of the children in care had been moved four or more times. S. Vasaly, *Foster Care in Five States: A Synthesis and Analysis of Studies from Arizona, California, Iowa, Massachusetts and Vermont* (Washington, D.C.: Office of Human Development, HEW, 1976), pp. 55-57. Two studies of children in foster care in New York City reported that almost 30 percent of the children studied had been in three or more placements. D. Fanshel, "Status Changes of Children in Foster Care: Final Results of the Columbia University Longitudinal Study," *Child Welfare* 55 (March 1976): 163-168; and New York City Comptroller's Office, *The Children Are Waiting* (New York: Institute of Public Affairs, 1977), pp. 10-11. Several of these studies also reported a correlation between the number of placements a child experienced and the severity and frequency of emotional disturbance in the child.

[17]For children in out-of-home care who were the responsibility of other systems, 17.8 percent had been moved three or more times, 5.3 percent five or more times. However, there was no information for 33.6 percent of the children for whom the other agencies was responsible as compared with 3.6 percent of the children for whom child welfare agencies were responsible. California Department of Health, Center for Health Statistics, "Children in Foster Care," p. 13.

[18]New Jersey Department of Institutions and Agencies, Division of Youth and Family Services, Case Review Unit, "Summary of Case Review Reports," New Jersey, April 7, 1976. (Mimeographed.)

[19]Historically, foster parents frequently were cautioned against any expression of interest in adoption. Even in 1974, a nationwide survey of foster placement agreement forms used by state foster care divisions revealed that references to adoption were infrequent and in all cases but one, were negative. See T.B. Festinger, "Placement Agreements with Boarding Homes: A Survey," *Child Welfare* 53 (December 1974): 643-652.

[20]A number of states have legislation requiring notification of foster parents and/or natural parents concerning plans to change a child's placement. The statutes vary significantly in the manner in which the notice is to be given, to whom notice is to be given, and the time and manner in which a hearing on the proposed removal is to be held. Compare, for example, D.C. Code §16-2320(g) (as amended by Act No. 2-53, §407(d)), New York Social Services Law §400, and Wisconsin Children's Code §48.64. The issue of the constitutional adequacy of the New York State and New York City procedures governing the removal of foster children from foster homes was before the U.S. Supreme Court in *Smith* v. *Organization of Foster Families for Equality and Reform*, 431 U.S. 816 (1977).

[21]This is discussed more fully in Chapter 4.

[22]Since the time of our study, Arizona has started a special Foster Care Demonstration Unit, the purpose of which is to find permanent families for the children in care. In that unit, which serves approximately 450 children, children cannot be moved from one foster placement to another without a meeting involving the caseworker, the caseworker's supervisor, the local Social Services supervisor, the foster parents, the natural parents and, if over 12, the child. R. S. Vonier, G. P. Merrell, and C. Graham, "Children Adrift—An Arizona Crisis," *Tucson Daily Citizen*, 7 April 1977.

[23]We focused more attention on the quality of care to children in group settings than in foster family care for two reasons: (1) foster parents often act as advocates for the children in their care, while children in group settings often lack such advocates; and (2) without case readings, it is more difficult to determine inadequacies. We are well aware, however, that there are also examples of inadequate foster homes, where discipline is excessive and children fail to get the health, education and social services they need.

[24]We are particularly grateful to the staff of OCHAMPUS (Office of Civilian Health and Medical Program of the Uniformed Services) in Denver, Colorado, who shared with us their knowledge of institutional facilities for emotionally disturbed children—knowledge based on extensive and intensive site visits to facilities receiving CHAMPUS reimbursement.

CHAMPUS, administered through the Department of Defense, provides financial assistance for the medical care of dependents of military personnel, including emotionally disturbed children and adolescents. In 1974, Congressional hearings revealed dreadful abuses in the program—for instance, children placed in facilities in which, as punishment, mock burials of the children were held—with no oversight by the CHAMPUS officials. As a result of those hearings, there have been efforts to improve the program, including the establishment of rigorous standards, with which compliance is required for approval of a facility for CHAMPUS reimbursement. We did not, in our study, try to evaluate the CHAMPUS program as it now exists. At the time of our visit CHAMPUS estimated that 900 emotionally disturbed children were in out-of-home care, but that countless more were in facilities for the retarded which had not been inspected by the CHAMPUS staff. See Chapter 5 for further discussion of the CHAMPUS program.

also given to us in confidence.[25] A sample of the conditions we learned of follows.

- A private midwestern facility, which operated for 26 years without a license, was recently licensed under a "grandfather"[26] clause although it failed to meet health, fire and sanitation standards. When one child who lived in the facility was asked where his toothbrush was, he smiled and said he didn't need any. . .he had no teeth. Further checks revealed this twelve-year-old had never received any dental care. Despite frequent complaints about this facility by professionals in the community, it continues to thrive.

- In a private "intensive care facility for adjudicated youths," inspection revealed open garbage pails, defecation of animals, a program manager with two years of college as a math/physics major, and a day supervisor with seven years experience—as a business secretary. The counseling coordinator in charge of staff supervision and group and individual therapy was a high school graduate with no training in individual or group counseling theory or techniques. The adolescent youth in this "program" spent an average of 21 minutes per day in an academic class.

- A private eastern psychiatric facility had a psychiatrist on the payroll who said he neither evaluated nor treated children nor reviewed treatment plans. He was "available" to anyone who wished to see him when he was there. Children in this facility had been referred for severe abuse or depression. There was no evidence that they were receiving any help at all. Moreover, the physical facilities were deteriorated. But the facility was licensed because, in the words of the state representative, "the standards are concerned with numbers, not quality."

- A licensed private psychiatric treatment facility in a southern state had a seclusion room made of cement blocks, no opening in the door for staff to make sure a secluded child did not harm himself, and no light in the cell. Any staff member, without prior approval, could place a child in this room. This same facility assigned "a child advocate" to the children to ensure their physical needs were met and grievances attended to. Yet no one had challenged the seclusion practice.

- A private residential facility in the southwest disciplined its residents by placing them on "underwear restriction"—that is, taking away all their clothes and forcing them to lie on a bed in only underwear. According to the staff, underwear restriction was limited to three days. Yet one teenager had been without clothes for over 30 days.

- The director of a southern facility for the retarded not only gave staff permission to hit the children, she paved the way, hitting the children with her hand and a soup ladle. She did, however, caution the staff not to leave bruises on the children and when parents visited, to untie the children from their beds and dress them.

These examples of excessive and humiliating discipline and of inadequate or nonexistent attention to the health and mental health needs of children in group care facilities are not isolated horror stories.[27] They reflect a widespread pattern. The problem of the neglect and institutional abuse of children in group facilities is an increasingly serious one. Growing numbers of children, often adolescents, are placed in such facilities,[28] and states are not carrying out their responsibility to protect them.[29]

The Reasons For Public Neglect

The causes of public neglect of children are complex and varied. They are sometimes rooted in local practices, sometimes in policy and funding patterns.

No Time to Know the Children

Theoretically, caseworkers are supposed to get to know the children for whom they are responsible. But for far too many children, caseworkers change so quickly or have so many cases that they do not get to know the children at all.

---

[25]We have not quoted directly from these reports and do not, for the most part, identify particular facilities, although our records indicate their names and locations. Our purpose in this chapter is not to single out facilities we happened to learn about, but to show the extent to which children in institutions and residential treatment centers are subject to inadequate—sometimes overtly dangerous or abusive—conditions.

[26]A "grandfather" clause exempts facilities existing prior to the passage of a law or regulation from having to meet the new requirements.

[27]For further discussion of the institutional abuse of children, see K. Wooden, *Weeping in the Playtime of Others* (New York: McGraw-Hill Book Co., 1976).

[28]Arizona, for example, reports that in 1971, the Department of Economic Security was paying for 283 dependent and delinquent children in 27 institutional settings. In 1975, over 1,000 children were in 53 institutional settings. R. S. Vonier, G. P. Merrell, and C. Graham, "Children Adrift—An Arizona Crisis," *Tucson Daily Citizen*, 5 April 1977.

[29]The problem of institutional abuse is slowly beginning to receive more attention. For example, the San Francisco Child Abuse Council is conducting a demonstration project in six counties designed specifically to prevent neglect and abuse of children in out-of-home placement by providing specialized training to foster parents and institutional staff.

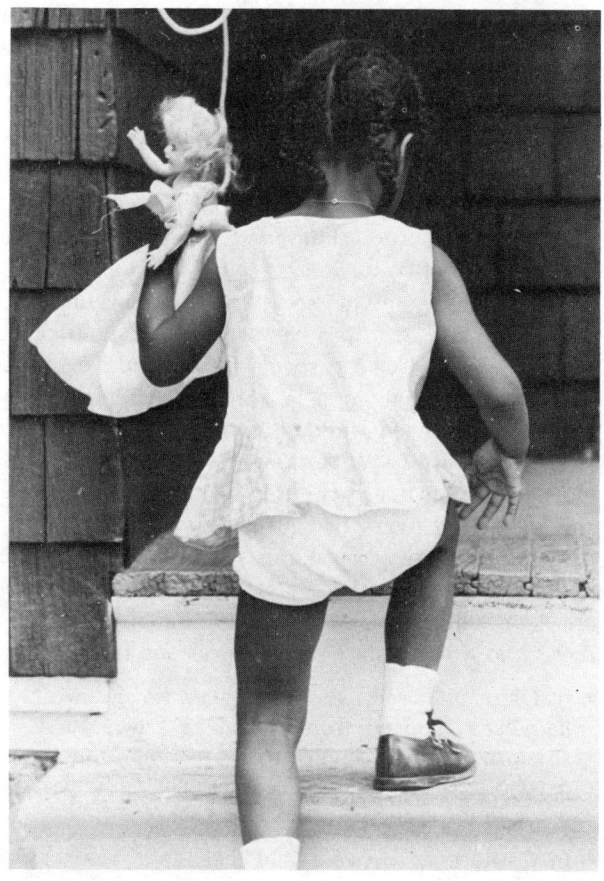

seen once every three months. Typically, there was no time for the child to visit a foster home or facility before moving in. With both foster parents or child care staff and child unprepared, the likelihood of a smooth adjustment was reduced. The replacement rate in that county was estimated at 50 percent, costly to the county and the children. The staff morale was desperate.

- On paper, the Ohio Youth Commission (OYC) assigned one caseworker and one youth worker to each committed child. The caseworker worked with the child in the OYC facility; the youth worker helped to plan for the child's release and to provide liaison work with the child's family, school and community. In reality, the youth workers considered themselves lucky if they saw a child once before discharge.

For some children, there are no caseworkers at all. In an eastern city we learned of a ten-year-old child who had lived with the same foster family for five years. The family had been trying to adopt him for two years. Finally, the caseworker told them that their home study would begin. But then she resigned. The case was not reassigned and another two years passed with no plans made for the child's adoption. This is not atypical. In the study of foster care in Massachusetts referred to earlier, 32 percent of the 5900 cases surveyed had no caseworkers assigned to them.[32]

- In South Carolina, in one county we visited, the annual caseworker turnover rate was 100 percent.[30]
- On an Indian reservation in Arizona, one Bureau of Indian Affairs child welfare worker had a caseload of 178 out-of-home children, in addition to 20 families with children still in the home who had been referred for abuse or neglect.[31]
- In an urban California county, the child welfare caseloads averaged 78.5 per worker. At best, children, foster parents, and natural parents could be

Excessive paperwork also keeps on-the-line workers from knowing the children. According to many of those we interviewed, the burden has worsened considerably as a result of Title XX, the federal social services program.[33]

- In a rural Ohio county, the director of children's services estimated that about two out of every five working days for her direct service staff were spent filling out forms about cases, rather than seeing children and families.
- In a rural California county, the child welfare office was being reorganized simply to make the completion of forms more efficient. Its effect on services had not been considered.
- In that same county, the time spent by a probation officer writing a report on a child was considered

---

[30]Vasaly reports that in the Arizona study of children in out-of-home care, the average "life" of a child welfare worker in some districts was nine months. In the Massachusetts study, only 16 percent of the children had been with the same caseworkers for one to two years. Vasaly, *Foster Care in Five States*, pp. 84-85.

[31]The American Public Welfare Association recommends that caseloads of direct service workers not exceed a maximum of 35 foster children and their families. *Standards for Foster Family Services Systems* (Washington, D.C.: APWA, March 1975), p. 36. Arizona BIA officials reported that their staff had remained at the same level for nine years while the caseload was ten times larger. San Mateo County, California, in its 1974-75 annual report noted that while staff positions in the Children's Protective Service Unit remained stable since 1973, the referrals had increased by 64 percent.

---

[32]Vasaly, *Foster Care in Five States*, p. 83.
[33]For a fuller discussion of the Title XX Program, see Chapter 5.

more important for his career advancement than time spent taking a child to a new placement.

- In Massachusetts, if a child was moved from one foster setting to another, we were told the paperwork was manageable. If a child was discharged, the paperwork was "monumental."

Unfortunately, there seems to be little evidence that the paperwork burden, presumably related to more effective accountability and management systems, makes a difference in the lives of children. Few efforts have been made to assess the forms being completed to ensure that required paperwork actually results in meaningful case documentation. Indeed, it is sobering to note that when the accuracy of aggregate data reports have been questioned, they very often turn out to be grossly inaccurate, and that individual case records often lack crucial information about children.[34] Despite the volume, there is too little attention to the quality of the data required.

Inadequate Training and Qualifications of Staff

The irony of the paperwork burden is compounded by the fact that often the only in-service training received by those who work directly with children and families in public agencies deals with how to fill out forms correctly. Substantive training by the counties and the states we visited was virtually nonexistent. Other evidence suggests this is not atypical[35] despite recognized needs for such training. Over and over again, we were told that children, particularly adolescents, were entering care with more problems than ever before.[36] Many workers find status offenders who are being moved out of the juvenile correctional system and into the child welfare system difficult to handle. Other workers are resistant to carrying out procedures to ensure children permanence, and need concrete help in "how to do it."

The failure to provide specialized training for those who must make decisions having life-long significance for children, and who carry on the difficult, demanding work of trying to help children and families is tragic. Well-trained workers are the core of an effective helping effort. Without such training, many who must work with these children and their families are simply not able to respond adequately to them.

Not only has there been a massive failure to provide in-service training, there also appears to be an increasing willingness to lower the qualifications of those who work directly with children and families.[37]

- In Ohio, civil service requirements for caseworkers had been reduced from a college education to a seventh grade education, with one course in psychology or one month's experience and a passing grade in the civil service exam.

- In California, we were told that there was serious talk of no longer requiring the child welfare staff to have masters' degrees in social work.

- In Massachusetts, the requirement that supervisors have an advanced degree in social work or a related clinical field, one year of experience in providing direct service to children, and a knowledge of services and placements to prevent family breakdown was ignored in the offices we visited.

While formal degrees are no guarantee of compe-

---

[34] In a recent review of 172 case records of children in out-of-home care in New York City, information reported to a computerized information system differed from information in agencies' case records. New York City Comptroller's Office, *The Children Are Waiting*, pp. 36-37. A New Jersey study found a similar pattern of discrepancies. W. E. Claburn and S. Magura, "Foster Care Review in New Jersey: An Evaluation of Its Implementation and Effects," New Jersey, 1977. (Mimeographed.) In Massachusetts, a review of the Foster Family Program cited extensive gaps in case records of children and concluded that the Department of Public Welfare was out of compliance with the state regulations. Similar non-compliance was cited in the review of the records of the group care unit. Office for Children, "Approval Study Report: Department of Public Welfare's Foster Care Services, Part I," Massachusetts, 1975. (Mimeographed.) A review of case records of New York City children in long-term foster care found only half of the case folders had the appropriate referral forms, including information on a child's current functioning. Specialized evaluations were present in only one-fourth of the cases. B. McGowan, J. Knitzer, and M. Nishi, "Special Services for Children Case Reading Study," New York, Memorandum to New York Civil Liberties Union, July 1, 1976.

[35] A review and assessment of child welfare service delivery systems in 25 selected states revealed that most states considered staff training and development inadequate. The need for training was particularly critical for staff dealing with children with special needs. U.S. Department of Health, Education and Welfare, Office of Human Development, Children's Bureau, *Child Welfare in 25 States—An Overview* (Washington, D.C.: HEW, 1976), pp. 72-74, 107-108.

[36] Although hard to document, this is widely believed and therefore an extremely significant psychological reality that shapes the expectations of those who work with the children. It may merely be a reflection of a widespread sense of staff helplessness and inadequacy. It may be that child welfare systems are increasingly receiving children previously cared for by the mental health and juvenile justice systems. Others have suggested it may reflect the failure of socialization vehicles: the family, the schools, and the like. But clearly, the child caring systems are not generally structured to respond adequately to the phenomenon.

[37] The National Association of Social Workers has been particularly concerned about the trend to drop requirements from social work job classifications without prior efforts to justify the changes. It has recommended that such changes be preceded by a validation study of the social work skills needed for particular jobs. For a further description of their work in this area, see "Validation Studies Regarding Declassification Trend," *NASW News*, November 1977, p. 8.

tence, the lowering of qualifications reflects a growing "anyone can work with children" mentality that is simplistic and destructive.[38]

Inadequate Procedures to Limit Inappropriate Placements

Even if a child has a caseworker with a reasonable caseload, adequate training and minimal paperwork, the placement process is still a "catch-as-catch-can" effort. Workers rarely have sufficient, if any, information about placement alternatives. This is particularly true when the need is for residential treatment centers, special schools, and institutions.

In almost every county we visited, neither probation officers nor caseworkers had time to visit a facility before placing a child in it. Workers had to rely for information on promotional—sometimes misleading—brochures, informal grapevines, reports from children, personal solicitations by agency owners, and to a startlingly lesser extent, on formal evaluations by the state. If facilities were found to be inadequate, there were few formal mechanisms to transmit such information from one worker to another, one agency to another, or one county to another. Enforceable procedures to guard against inappropriate placements, particularly the excessive use of institutional facilities, were either nonexistent or ignored. As a result, the institutionalization of children—a very serious step—was often a haphazard process.

- In one state, we learned of two adolescent boys who were transferred from a detention facility to a state mental hospital. They were committed by a musicologist with a doctorate, not a medical doctor.

- In another state, we learned of ten-year-old twins who were almost committed to a mental hospital for 30 days because no one in an urban area supposedly rich in placement alternatives could decide what to do with them. The parents had petitioned the court on the advice of a caseworker, and a judge declared the children incorrigible (status offenders). The caseworker did not think the children were incorrigible at all, but did think the parents *might* be neglecting the children. To *protect* these children from their *possibly* neglecting parents, he encouraged the parents to initiate court action. They did. The judge, not sure how to handle the disposition of the children, ordered them to a psychiatric facility for 30 days for diagnosis (at a cost of $505 per day for each, or $30,300 per month). The case was heard on a Friday but the hospital refused to admit the twins until the following Monday. The court thus requested the Youth Service Bureau to find an emergency shelter for them. At that point, a youth service worker voluntarily offered to find a more permanent home for the children, questioning the need for hospitalization. The judge then willingly modified his order.

In this case, no one challenged the coercive quality of the allegedly voluntary initial removal of the children. Further, when the decision for placement was made, no serious effort was made to place the children in the least restrictive setting. That happened by chance.

The problem of the inappropriate institutionalization of children is now beginning to receive more careful scrutiny. There have been legal cases challenging the procedures by which children are "voluntarily" committed to mental institutions by parents, and there are cases challenging the confinement of status offenders in training schools.[39] But abuses continue to be extensive.

Difficulty of Developing Appropriate Alternatives

Deinstitutionalization,[40] proposed as an alternative to the inappropriate placement of children in institutional settings, refers to specific efforts to keep or get children out of institutions, and to enable them to remain in less restrictive family and community settings. The juvenile justice system has been particularly vocal in calling for deinstitutionalization, especially

---

[38]Indeed, of our study states, only South Dakota provided a liberal tuition and leave policy.

[39]See, for example, *Bartley* v. *Kremens*, 402 F. Supp. 1039 (E.D. Pa. 1975), *vacated on other grounds*, 431 U.S. 119 (1977), *on remand*, Civ. No. 72-2272 (May 25, 1978), *prob. juris. noted, sub nom. Secretary of Public Welfare* v. *Kevin S.*, 46 LW 3776; (June 19, 1978) (No. 77-1715); *J.L. and J.R.* v. *Parham*, 412 F. Supp. 112 (M.D. Ga. 1976), *prob. juris. noted*, 97 S. Ct. 2647 (1977) (No. 75-1690), reargument scheduled, 98 S. Ct. 761 (1978), and *Poe* v. *Califano*, C.A. No. 74-1800 (D.D.C., filed December 9, 1974). See also *In Re Ellery*, C. 32 N.Y. 2d at 591 (1973) and *Blondheim* v. *State*, 84 Washington 2d 874, 529 P. 2d 1096 (1975).

[40]Deinstitutionalization of children is part of a broader movement that includes the mentally disabled of all ages, the elderly and persons processed through the criminal justice system, especially juveniles. For a discouraging overview of the impact of federal programs on deinstitutionalization for the mentally disabled, see General Accounting Office, *Returning the Mentally Disabled to the Community: Government Needs to do More* (Washington, D.C.: GAO, January 7, 1977).

for status offenders.[41]

Deinstitutionalization requires the availability of a range of placement options within a community. Some efforts at deinstitutionalization for children have been successful, but in general, progress has been slow. Specialized foster homes, often necessary for children with handicapping conditions, rarely exist. Nor are there day treatment or homemaker services available which would allow a parent or foster parent caring for a handicapped child occasional relief. Thus, often children who could be in their own or specialized foster homes are instead institutionalized.[42]

Attempts to develop community-based facilities[43] have been beset by legal and fiscal difficulties.[44] Very often communities try to block efforts to establish group homes through legal tactics, political action and harassment, primarily because they do not want any "troublemakers" around. Zoning regulations are often restrictive. Courts have generally upheld the group home efforts, but at times the cost is high in terms of ultimate community acceptance. Further, start-up monies—either for building renovations or staffing—are often not available either from the local community, the state or the federal government. Nor are reimbursement formulas structured to encourage the development of community-based alternatives.[45]

Once operational, community-based facilities have not always lived up to their promise. Instead of offering a less restrictive alternative, they sometimes turn out to be nothing more than mini-institutions. In some states, group homes have been located on the grounds of large institutions.[46] Moreover, even if located in the community, some group homes continue to isolate children from family contacts and community activities. A recent study of group homes in New York City, where the number of homes increased from 158 in 1973 to 253 in 1977, found that few group homes saw their role as facilitating child-family contact.[47]

---

[41] For an overview of issues relating to the deinstitutionalization of status offenders as well as a discussion of some of the resources available for them, see W. L. Hickey, "Status Offenses and the Juvenile Court," *Criminal Justice Abstracts* (March 1977): 91-122.

Massachusetts provides a particularly dramatic example of a state effort to deinstitutionalize. In 1971, the state closed its major juvenile correctional institutions and placed the youth in community programs. The results have been uneven, and the experiment plagued with problems of developing new purchased services and monitoring contracts. See, for example, M. Serrill, "Juvenile Corrections in Massachusetts," *Corrections Magazine* 2 (November-December 1975): 3-12, 17-20, and C. Holden, "Massachusetts Juvenile Justice: Deinstitutionalization on Trial," *Science* 192 (April 1976): 447-451.

A national study estimated that on any given day in 1974, 28,000 adolescents were in correctional facilities, compared with 5,600 in community-based programs. The report also estimated states spent over $300 million on institutions, compared with $30 million on community-based residential programs. R. Vinter, G. Downs, and J. Hall, *Juvenile Corrections in the States: Residential Programs and Deinstitutionalization; A Preliminary Report* (Michigan: National Assessment of Juvenile Corrections, 1975).

There may also be a backlash against deinstitutionalization within the juvenile justice system. For example, a bill was introduced during the 1977 legislative session in California which would have undercut a statute enacted in 1976 prohibiting the detention of status offenders in juvenile halls and their commitment to correctional institutions. The bill, which did not pass, would have allowed the limited detention of status offenders in secure facilities. Recent amendments to the federal juvenile justice statute give the states an additional two years to comply with deinstitutionalization requirements as a condition for eligibility for federal funds. See Chapter 5 for a further discussion of the Juvenile Justice and Delinquency Prevention Act.

[42] A study of foster family care in eight southeastern states in 1976 concluded that "specialized foster family care is virtually nonexistent in the Southeast." All but two of the states, Tennessee and Georgia, did not even issue licenses for, or have standards for establishing and monitoring, specialized foster family homes. Little organized emphasis was placed upon recruiting foster family homes for children with special needs. And none of the states had information on the extent to which local agencies were using foster homes to serve children with special needs. G. Thomas, et al., *Supply and Demand for Child Foster Family Care in the Southeast* (Atlanta: Regional Institute of Social Welfare Research, Inc., 1977), pp. 44-45.

An overview of child welfare service delivery systems in 25 states also identified the lack of foster family homes for "seriously acting out" children, the multiply-handicapped and other children with special needs as a significant problem. (U.S. Department of Health, Education and Welfare, *Child Welfare in 25 States—An Overview*, p. 68.)

After finding that almost 40 percent of the children in foster family care in Massachusetts in 1971 were handicapped, a further study was conducted of a sample of 96 handicapped children (the majority with cerebral palsy, mental retardation or epilepsy) to determine the problems foster parents experienced in trying to care for them. The problems cited included the lack of available treatment facilities, difficulties securing services from hospitals and other institutions, monetary problems including the lack of funds and over-restrictive use of funds, and the reluctance of professionals to share information about the child's condition and needs with the foster parents. Other problems were related to the limited assistance received from social workers. For a further discussion, see A. R. Gruber, *Children in Foster Care: Destitute, Neglected...Betrayed* (New York: Human Sciences Press, 1978), pp. 73-129.

[43] For a national directory of existing halfway houses and group homes, including eligibility and cost data, see R. Rachin, ed., *Directory of Halfway Houses and Group Homes for Troubled Children* (Tallahassee, Florida: Journal of Drug Issues, Inc., 1977).

[44] Recent fiscal pressures have further escalated the difficulty of making appropriate out-of-home placements, as the already minimal range of alternatives is further reduced. For example, when CDF staff visited Ohio, we were told the Cuyahoga County Court had used up the county funds allocated for the purchase of a range of placement services for court-involved children. Consequently, since March 1975, it had had to refer all children needing placement to the state juvenile correctional agency so that the state, not the county, would assume the cost.

[45] In the course of our study, we did learn that at least one state is trying a fiscal incentive approach. In Pennsylvania, Act No. 148, which was passed by the legislature in 1976 and went into effect January 1, 1978, tries to encourage deinstitutionalization by providing a higher rate of state reimbursement to counties when they make placements in Department of Public Welfare-approved community residential programs rather than in institutions. See also, New York Temporary State Commission on Child Welfare, "Foster Care Reimbursement: A New Approach," Albany, N. Y.: Temporary State Commission on Child Welfare, May 1978. More typical, however, was the comment of a Tennessee administrator to CDF staff, "We need more group homes, but we do not have the money to develop them."

[46] These are different from the institutions which house residents in cottage living arrangements.

[47] While it may be that this was appropriate in some cases, the anecdotal evidence suggests this is merely one more manifestation of the attitudinal problems of the caregivers identified in Chapter 1. The majority of staff interviewed viewed parental visits as an intrusion. Some permitted visits only in public rooms or insisted that a staff member be present. Citizens' Committee for Children of New York, *Group Homes for New York City Children* (New York: Citizens' Committee for Children of New York, Inc., December 1976), pp. 3, 33-34.

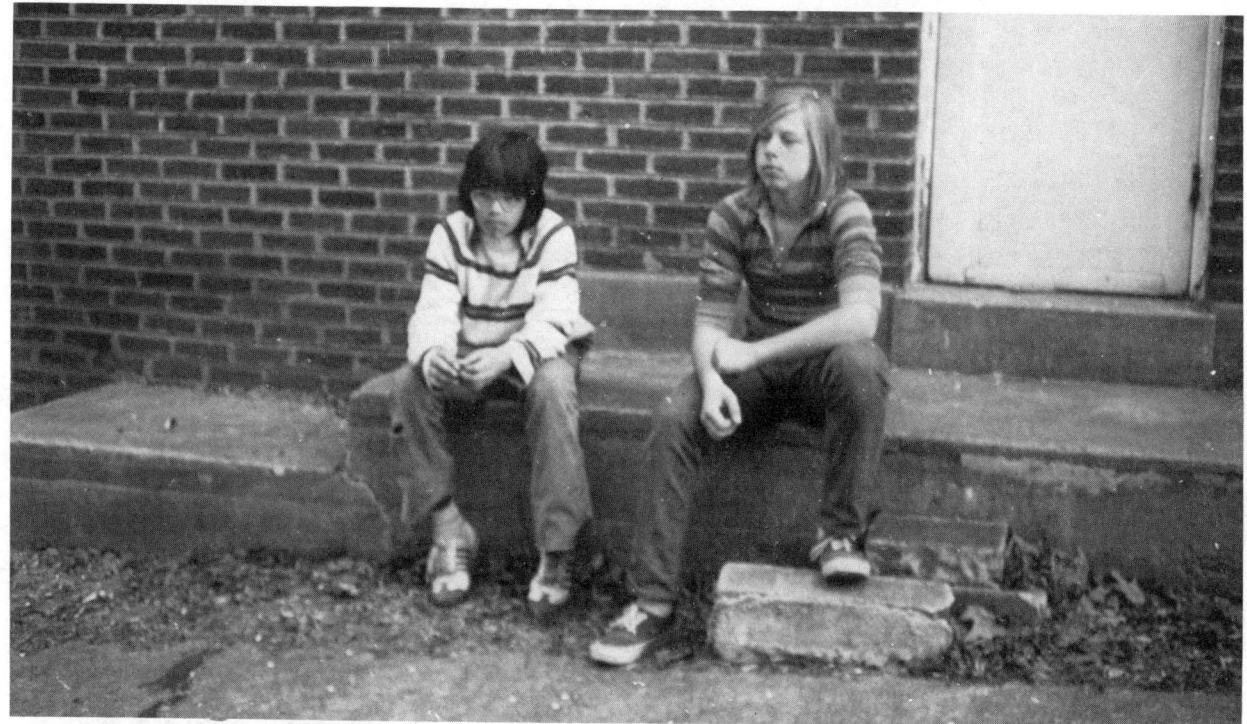

Sometimes, children within community-based facilities are subjected to institution-like abuse: humiliation therapies, physical abuse, and various intrusive behavior modification techniques. In a peculiar form of discrimination, children in group homes may be refused access to or suspended from local schools. Massachusetts also told us of age discrimination. Placement workers reported that some community-based facilities will not accept children between 12 and 15, because they prefer to work with children between 9 and 12 years old.

Purchased Services: An Unproven Strategy

During the past few years, there has been a tremendous growth in the purchase of human services.[48] These services are purchased from private and sometimes public providers by public agencies, often with funds supplied at least partly by the federal government.[49] Day care for children and residential treatment services for children and youth have been among the services most heavily purchased.[50]

Proponents of purchased services argue that contracting for services allows the state and local agencies with legal and fiscal responsibility for children more

---

[48]States vary considerably in the extent to which different public child care systems purchase services. Of our seven study states, Massachusetts has used the purchase-of-service mechanism most extensively, particularly in the juvenile justice network, but also for the provision of homemaker and day care services. In fact, a recent Massachusetts study has concluded that the shift from public agencies providing services directly to contracting out for them marks a fundamental shift in the state human service network. D. Sheehan, *The Children's Puzzle* (Massachusetts: Institute for Governmental Services, University of Massachusetts, February 1977), p. 1. Ohio, in contrast, uses few public funds for the purchase of service. In California, the extent of purchase of service varies by county.

[49]Authority for purchase of services from private sources was first included in the Social Security Act Amendments of 1967. It was preceded by legislation five years earlier authorizing state public assistance agencies to purchase services from other state agencies. The original intent of the concept was to enable state welfare agencies to expand services available to public assistance recipients. For a further discussion of the development of the purchase of service concept, see M. Derthick, *Uncontrollable Spending for Social Services Grants* (Washington, D.C.: The Brookings Institution, 1975).

[50]The first national data on purchased services were released by HEW in December 1977 in a report on social services expenditures under Titles XX, IV-B and IV-C of the Social Security Act for the period April through June 1976. These data indicate that, for that three-month period, approximately 47 percent of the expenditures were used to purchase services from public and private vendors and that purchases from private vendors were nearly twice that of purchases from public agencies—31 percent contrasted with 16 percent.

Twenty-seven of the 48 states supplying data reported that over 50 percent of their services expenditures were for purchased services; and in 20 of these states the majority of purchased services were from private rather than public vendors. For the 48 states reporting, purchased services accounted for 68 and 56 percent, respectively, of the expenditures for day care and foster care services for children, but only 15 and 10 percent, respectively, of expenditures for adoption services and protective services for children. U.S. Department of Health, Education and Welfare, Office of Human Development Services, Administration for Public Services, *Social Services U.S.A. (April-June 1976)* (Washington, D.C.: HEW, December 1977), pp. 70-78.

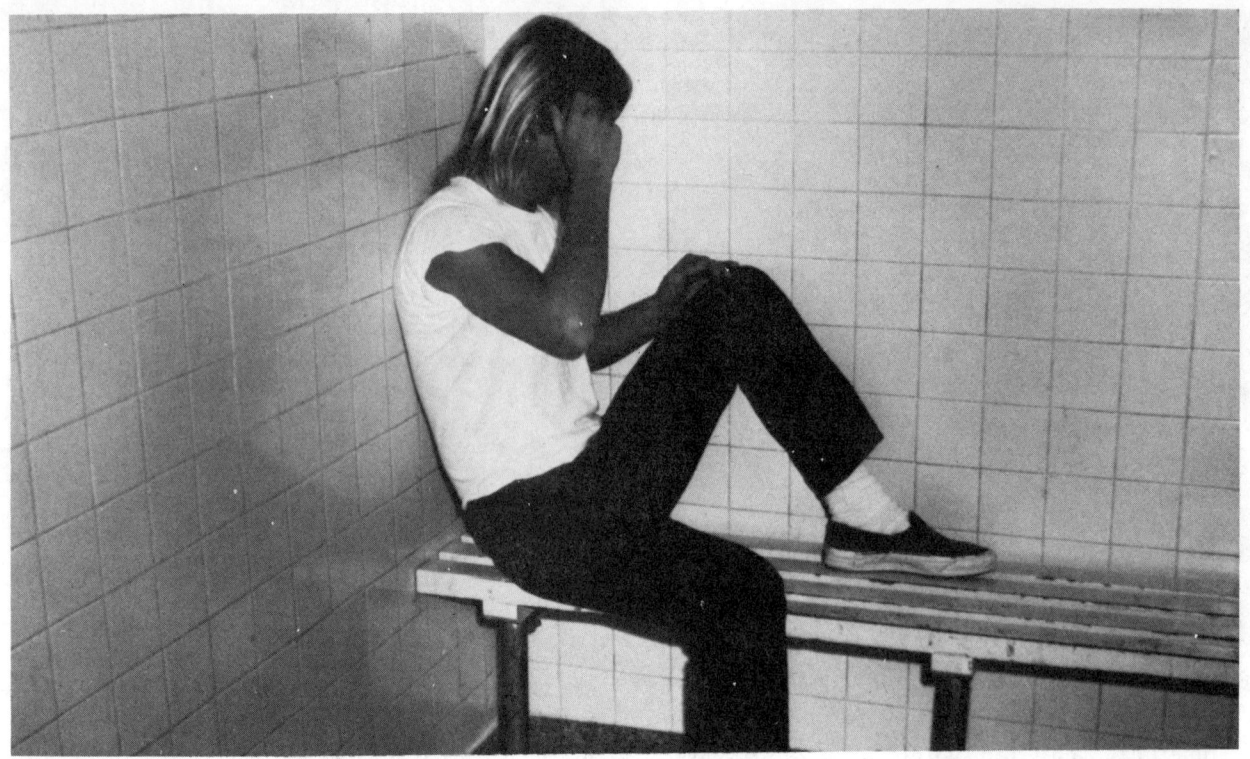

flexibility in obtaining innovative, cost-effective and appropriate services than they would have if all services were administered and delivered by the public agencies. But there has been no careful analysis of the impact of the increased use of purchased services either nationally or locally. And so, we do not know to what extent, if any, this method of providing services has led to new kinds of children's programs, more services, or improved services to children and their families. Nor are there any data on the cost-effectiveness of the strategy.

We have, however, seen evidence of serious and continuing abuses to children by the providers of services. Many of the private institutions cited earlier for their inadequate care of children provided "purchased services" to public agencies. In the absence of a careful study, it is impossible to determine how widespread these abuses are, but we know they exist, particularly in residential facilities.

We also heard scattered reports of fiscal abuses under purchased services, although we did not examine these in detail. For example, in December 1976, the *New York Times* reported that a realty company leasing group homes to New York City for foster care tripled its investment in the homes. The investors denied the charge.[51] CHAMPUS also told us of suspected instances of double billing. Further, in an investigation of private, nonprofit residential facilities caring for children paid for by federal foster care funds, the General Accounting Office found such problems as missing fiscal records and the claiming of personal expenses as institutional costs.[52] At one facility, for example, personal expenditures for appliances, clothing and entertainment were all billed as child care costs.

The unmonitored use of purchased services also carries with it the risk of developing a seller's market. Despite the fact that private facilities frequently receive extensive funds from public sources, many are highly selective in accepting children. There may be legitimate reasons for a group facility, for example, to include some, but not too many, children with specific problems. However, there is strong evidence that many private facilities simply refuse, for arbitrary reasons, to

---

[51] N. Sheppard, "Owners of Foster Care Homes Reportedly Triple Investments," *New York Times*, 17 December 1976.

[52] General Accounting Office, *Children in Foster Care Institutions–Steps Government Can Take to Improve Their Care* (Washington, D.C.: GAO, February 22, 1977), pp. 16-21. The report also found in several cases that the reported costs were inaccurate, unsubstantiated, not allowed or, in the view of the GAO, unreasonable.

serve certain children who need the kind of care the facility is supposed to provide. Such practices only increase the pool of children whom no one will serve.

The energy and emotional investment required to find facilities that will accept adolescent children who are not models of sedate behavior is often exhausting. Even a request for a temporary placement can require multiple referrals. One caseworker we spoke with told us about contacting 17 separate facilities in order to find temporary shelter for an adolescent boy whom caseworkers described as "likeable and warm." The responsible public agency is faced in these circumstances with choosing the politically difficult route of challenging the private facilities, developing sanctions for inappropriate refusals to serve children, and setting up alternatives; or continuing to make inappropriate placements. Unfortunately, the latter route is most frequently taken.

Two caveats. In the first place, the fact that there have been abuses in purchased services should not obscure the fact that there are abuses in publicly provided services, ranging from inadequate staff and poor or nonexistent programming to habitual conditions bespeaking cruel and unusual punishment. Secondly, while there are philosophical arguments regarding whether private agencies providing human services should be "for profit" or nonprofit, fiscal and program abuses have occurred in both types, just as both types have provided a high quality of care.[53]

The significant point is that adequate monitoring mechanisms to ensure public accountability do not exist.[54] Thus, there are numerous opportunities for the provision of inadequate services by those seeking a quick profit at the expense of children. If contracting is to be a major function of public agencies, the contracting procedures must be strengthened to ensure not just fiscal accountability but programmatic accountability and the protection of the child's right to decent care and treatment. The power of the purse should be used to enforce this right.

Special Burdens of Minority Children

Minority children are especially vulnerable to inappropriate placements and inadequate care. Often, they are over-represented in child care systems, and they may receive differential treatment.[55]

Discrimination in the Child Welfare System[56]

There is evidence that discrimination within the child welfare system takes several forms. First, on the basis of available data, minority children are clearly over-represented[57] (see Figure 2). But in some parts of the country, particularly rural areas, minority children, regardless of their needs, may be under-represented. They do not become part of a formal system, either because their families fear the consequences, or because the system ignores their needs. As child welfare officials told us: "Their families will take care of them." There is, of course, a certain irony to this situation: these children are obviously able to remain with relatives, whereas many of the children who formally enter the child welfare system may not by virtue of official policy. On the other hand, the children and the relatives

---

[53]In an effort to counter the growing "image" problem of residential treatment centers and to protect quality programs from inappropriate criticism, the California Association of Children's Residential Centers is seeking to develop a peer review system, and to limit membership to nonprofit agencies that meet the standards. A national membership organization of non-profit residential group care agencies, the National Association of Homes for Children, was formed in 1975. Since its formation, the Association has formulated standards for its membership, effective July 1978.

[54]The Code of Federal Regulations (45 CFR 74) does set forth principles for determining costs applicable to activities assisted by HEW grants awarded to state or local governments, institutions of higher education, hospitals and other nonprofit organizations. The regulations address allowable and unallowable costs and activities.

[55]The following discussion focuses on the special burdens of ethnic and racial minority children. However, within the child welfare system, children with handicapping conditions and adolescents are also particularly likely to be subject to abuses. They too are especially vulnerable to inappropriate placements and are frequently left to linger indefinitely in care.

[56]Many states and localities do not even maintain aggregate data by race for children in the child welfare system. In the CDF survey, responding child welfare officials could not provide data on the race of 54 percent of the children reported to be in out-of-home care. A national survey of state departments of social welfare conducted by the Interagency Adoption Project of the National Urban League in early 1977 to gather statistical data on black children in foster care and adoption revealed great gaps in the information available at the state level. A preliminary report on the results of the survey indicated that of the 28 states responding by that time only 19 reported any data at all about foster care. Only 12 of these states reported figures on the number of black children in foster care and even fewer provided any data by race on the length of time in care or number of placements the children had experienced. Although 20 of the states reported the number of black children placed for adoption by public agencies, only nine of these also reported figures on the total number of black children in foster care. National Urban League, "Preliminary Report for IAP Nationwide Survey on Adoption and Foster Care and the Black Child," New York, Fall 1977. (Unpublished.)

[57]As we indicated in Chapter 1, children whose families are in poverty are more likely to be at risk of foster care placement, as a result of both the financial and psychological stresses poverty imposes. Minority families are disproportionately poor.

who care for them informally may not receive the financial help or services which they need and to which they are entitled.[58]

For those minority children who do enter the formal child welfare system, there is also evidence that they receive differential treatment particularly in where they are placed[59] and in the efforts made to ensure their return home or adoption.[60] The discriminatory treatment of minority children within the child welfare system, in fact, has been the subject of at least two major class action lawsuits.[61]

In *Player* v. *Alabama*,[62] the plaintiffs charged that the state engaged in segregated referrals to child care institutions; provided foster care in segregated settings; failed to ensure that the child care institutions it licensed operated on a nondiscriminatory basis; and failed to provide adequate foster homes for black children. Evidence was introduced at the time the suit was filed showing that only about five percent of the 800 Alabama children in group homes or institutions were black. Instead, black children needing out-of-home care were frequently placed with inadequate foster parents, including feeble or incapacitated great aunts and great grandmothers on pensions.[63] Finding these practices to be unconstitutional, the court ordered the state to cease all referrals to institutions and group homes unless the facilities agreed to accept referrals without regard to race or color; monitor the facilities and referral practices of county offices; ensure that facilities used had nondiscriminatory policies; and provide to black children the same opportunities for group and institutional care as were provided to white children.

In *Wilder* v. *Sugarman*,[64] the plaintiffs charged that New York City and the private, nonprofit child-placing agencies engaged in referral practices which resulted in the discriminatory treatment of minority children, particularly black Protestant children. Further, they claimed that minority children disproportionately ended up in public rather than in private facilities; and that within the private nonprofit agencies, placement according to religion[65] produced further discriminatory patterns.

Such discrepancies were generally defended on grounds that minority children are allegedly "harder to place and have more emotional and behavioral difficulties" than non-minority children. However, in a special study of case records conducted at the request of the New York Civil Liberties Union, there was no evidence that black Protestant children were described in case records as having significantly more problems in terms of health, school performance, relationships with others or intelligence. Since a private facility's decision to accept or reject a child was supposedly made on the basis of the case record information provided by the City, these findings suggest other factors were operating.[66]

There is also scattered evidence that in some jurisdictions minority children remain in care longer and are treated differently by adoption units. South Carolina, for example, conducted special studies two years in a row, and found that black children spend longer periods in out-of-home care than white children.[67]

---

[58]For further discussion of informal placements, see R. B. Hill, *Informal Adoptions Among Black Families* (Washington, D.C.: National Urban League, 1977).

[59]In the Bernstein study referred to earlier which analyzed the appropriateness of placements in New York City, 29.5 percent of the white children were judged to have been inappropriately placed, compared with 46.6 percent of the Hispanic children and 46.1 percent of the black and other minority children. Bernstein, Snider, and Meezan, *Foster Care Needs and Alternatives to Placement*, p. 22.

[60]For an historical account of discrimination against black children within the child welfare system, see A. Billingsley and J. Giovannoni, *Children of the Storm: Black Children and American Child Welfare* (New York: Harcourt, Brace and Jovanovich, Inc., 1972).

[61]It should also be noted that in *Gary W.*, cited earlier, black Louisiana children were disproportionately at risk of placement in Texas. While the entire caseload of the responsible public agency was 73 percent white and 27 percent black, 49 percent of the children placed in private facilities in Texas under child welfare auspices were black, as were 54 percent of the children placed by the unit responsible for exceptional children. Ninety-four percent of the children who received agency assistance but were not placed either out of home or out of state were white, six percent black. See Plaintiffs' Proposed Findings of Fact, and Transcripts of Depositions on file at CDF and the U. S. Department of Justice.

[62]400 F. Supp. 249 (M.D. Ala. 1975), aff'd, 536 F. 2d 1385 (5th Cir. 1976).

[63]In Chapter 1, we recommend that preference be given to placement of children with willing and interested relatives. This is not to encourage placements with relatives who are not given adequate resources to care for the children or who, for other reasons, are not able to assume responsibility for the children. Dumping children with relatives without attention to the additional responsibility involved or their concern for the children benefits no one.

[64]No. 73 Civ. 2644 (S.D.N.Y.). The case was filed on June 14, 1973, and on February 28, 1978, plaintiffs filed a motion for voluntary dismissal. Similar claims were subsequently alleged in *Parker, et al.* v. *Bernstein, et al.*, No. 78 Civ. 957 (S.D.N.Y., filed on March 3, 1978).

[65]In New York City, to a greater extent than elsewhere in the country, the voluntary agencies are organized by religion. Religious matching, if possible, is required by state statute.

[66]McGowan, Knitzer, and Nishi, "Special Services for Children Case Reading Study."

[67]The study found that 40 percent of the children in care over six months were white, 52 percent were black and 12 percent were "other." Sixty-five percent of the total South Carolina population is white, 35 percent black. South Carolina Department of Social Services, "Final Report on Schedules of Termination of Parental Rights," Columbia, South Carolina, November 25, 1975. (Mimeographed.)

	Total Population[2]		Children In Foster Care			Percentage Breakdown of Non-White Children in Foster Care			
	Percent White	Percent Non-White	Percent White	Percent Non-White	Unknown	Black	Spanish Speaking	Native American	Other
Arizona[3]	90.8	9.2	41.0	53.7	5.2	11.9	19.8	22.0	—
California[4]	88.0	12.0	56.0	43.4	—	19.5	12.6	1.2	10.1
Massachusetts[5]	96.4	3.6	77.3	22.3	.4	14.8	1.8	.5	5.2
New Jersey[6]	87.1	12.9	44.0	55.0	—	51	3	—	1
Ohio	90.4	9.6	NA	NA	—				
South Carolina	69.2	30.8	NA	NA	—				
South Dakota[7]	94.2	5.8	44	55	—	—	—	55	—
CDF Survey[8]	85.1	14.9	48	52	—	32	13	1	6

Figure 2. Percentage of Children in Foster Care Under Child Welfare Auspices by Race and Ethnicity[1]

[1]This table represents data drawn from sources indicated below in the study states and the CDF survey. We found no published breakdowns for Ohio or South Carolina. The South Carolina annual report of 1975 provides adoption and protective service information on children by race, but not on children in foster care.
[2]U.S. Bureau of the Census, *Statistical Abstract of the United States: 1977* (Washington, D.C.: Government Printing Office, 1977), Table 35. Population, By Race-States: 1960-1975.
[3]Vasaly, *Foster Care in Five States: A Synthesis and Analysis of Studies From Arizona, California, Iowa, Massachusetts and Vermont* (Washington, D.C.: Office of Human Development, U.S. Department of Health, Education and Welfare, 1976), p. 45. These figures are based on a case review of a random sample of 462 foster children out of 1,808 in foster care in Arizona. The study was reported in 1974.
[4]California Department of Health, Center for Health Statistics, "Children in Foster Care," (Sacramento: Data Matters, Topical Reports, September 1974), p. 9.
[5]Vasaly, *Foster Care in States,* p. 45. These figures are based on a review of all children in foster care in 1971.
[6]New Jersey Department of Institutions and Agencies, Division for Youth and Family Services, "Administrative Review of Children in Out-of-Home Placements" (Mimeographed), dated April 7, 1976. These figures represent approximately 8,400 children entering care between November 1, 1974 and May 31, 1975.
[7]South Dakota Department of Social Services, Office on Children and Youth, Foster Family Care Recommendations for Change, December 14, 1976: Plate I.
[8]See Appendix C for a description of the survey findings.

Efforts to ensure the adoption of minority children have also, at times, been hindered by debate about whether transracial adoptions are appropriate. For example, a Massachusetts study of state adoption practices found that a *de facto* policy against transracial adoptions was preventing some minority children from being adopted.[68] The issue of transracial adoptions is a complex one. We support the idea that where possible, adoptive children and parents should be of the same racial background and believe there should be vigorous recruitment efforts to identify minority adoptive parents. However, if the alternative is growing up in foster care without a permanent family, then we believe transracial adoptions are preferable. In fact, there have been a number of successful projects designed to increase the adoption of minority children either by adoptive parents of the same or different racial or ethnic backgrounds. One in New York City increased the adoption of black children from 239 in 1969, to 411 in 1974.[69] Other communities have established projects to promote the adoption of black children in long-term foster care who cannot be returned home by focusing on more effective agency outreach to black families, increased public education about the need for adoptive homes, and efforts to alter current agency practices and

[68]Massachusetts Office for Children, "Approval Study Report of the Department of Public Welfare's Adoption Placement Services," Massachusetts, 1975, p. 2. (Mimeographed.)

[69]Lash and Sigal, *State of the Child*, pp. 72-73.

procedures which obstruct the adoption of black children.[70]

Discrimination in the Other Child-Placing Systems

It is not only the child welfare system, however, that reflects discriminatory patterns. Minority children also tend to be over-represented in out-of-home care under the auspices of the juvenile justice and the mental health systems. A recent study surveyed a sample of juvenile correctional facilities in 16 states, including three of our study states, Massachusetts, California and Ohio. It found 45 percent of the youth in institutions, group homes and day treatment programs were white, and 55 percent were non-white (33 percent black, eight percent American Indian, four percent Spanish-speaking, and ten percent other).[71] According to the 1970 Census, in 21 states over 30 percent of the youth population in facilities for delinquent children were black; in ten states the percentage of black youths was 50 percent or higher.[72] New Jersey reported that since the passage of the "Jins" (Juveniles in Need of Supervision) law requiring the deinstitutionalization of status offenders, there had been a 16 percent decrease in the commitments of white youths and a 38 percent decrease in commitments of black youths.[73]

There are very limited racial data available on children served by mental health and developmental disabilities systems. However, a special survey recently conducted by the National Institute of Mental Health found that white children under 14 were twice as likely to have had treatment prior to psychiatric hospitalization as non-white children. Moreover, non-white children under 14 were two and one-half times more likely to be admitted to mental hospitals than were white children.[74]

American Indian Children

American Indian children appear to bear a particularly heavy burden in the child-placing and particularly child welfare systems.[75] Historically and by most current accounts, Indian children have been removed from their homes and culture at a much higher rate than non-Indian children.[76] Often they have been placed with white families for adoption, resulting in severe identity conflicts.[77]

Further, many Indian children are placed in special boarding schools and dormitories run by the Bureau of Indian Affairs (BIA). In 1975-76, approximately 25,000 Indian children were housed, often at great distances from their families, in 74 federal boarding

---

[70]For example, the Interagency Adoption Project of the National Urban League is attempting to design a model for improving adoption services for black children and black families, and has demonstration efforts underway in Illinois, South Carolina and Texas. The NAACP also operated a Tri-State Adoption Project in Florida, Georgia and Tennessee, and is currently establishing a Southern regional adoption exchange. Agency efforts have been undertaken too in San Diego, California, Chicago, Illinois, and Detroit, Michigan.

[71]R. C. Vinter, ed., *Time Out: A National Study of Juvenile Correctional Programs* (Michigan: National Assessment of Juvenile Corrections, June 1976), p. 25. There were some interesting variations by program. The authors found 46 percent of the institutionalized youth were white and 54 percent non-white (30 percent black, 24 percent other non-white). In the group homes, 54 percent of the youth were white and 46 percent non-white (24 percent black, 22 percent other non-white). In day treatment programs, 34 percent of the sample was white and 66 percent non-white (55 percent black, and 11 percent other non-white), p. 19.

[72]U.S. Bureau of the Census, Census of Population: 1970, *Persons in Institutions and Other Group Quarters*, Table 40.

[73]Interview with Ann Klein, Commissioner of the Department of Institutions and Agencies, New Jersey, February 1976.

[74]National Institute of Mental Health, Division of Biometry and Epidemiology, Survey and Reports Branch, "Tabular Material Prepared on Children, Adolescents and Young Adults Under Care in Mental Health Treatment Facilities/Services," Washington, D.C., 1977.

[75]Problems of jurisdiction among reservations, local counties and states make this issue an exceedingly complex one, which we only explored peripherally in our study. For further analysis of the problems, see U. S. Department of Health, Education and Welfare, Office of Human Development, Children's Bureau, *Indian Child Welfare: A State-of-the-Field Study* (Washington, D.C.: HEW, 1976); S. Unger, ed., *The Destruction of American Indian Families* (New York: Association on American Indian Affairs, 1977), and Center for Social Research and Development, *Legal and Jurisdictional Problems in the Delivery of SRS Child Welfare Services on Indian Reservations* (Denver: Denver Research Institute, University of Denver, October 1975), pp. 25-70.

[76]In 1976, the Association on American Indian Affairs conducted a special survey on the out-of-home placement of Indian children. While some of the statistical assumptions they made are questionable, it is clear that Indian children are placed at proportionately far greater rates than non-Indian children, and the vast majority are placed with non-Indian families. For the results of their survey, see Association on American Indian Affairs, "Indian Child Welfare Statistical Survey, July 1976," printed as Appendix B in Task Force on Federal, State and Tribal Jurisdiction, *Report on Federal, State and Tribal Jurisdiction—Final Report to the American Indian Policy Review Commission* (Washington, D.C.: U.S. Government Printing Office, 1976). The Arizona Governor's Committee reported that in 1972, the BIA was responsible for 384 children in out-of-home care, yet only 63 of these children, or 16 percent, were in Indian foster family homes; 268, or 70 percent, were in non-Indian off-reservation homes; 53, or 14 percent, in non-Indian homes on the reservation. Arizona Governor's Committee on Community Coordinated Child Care, *Arizona's Children: Problems Unique to Minority Children*, October 1975, p. 18.

[77]When we visited the Yakima reservation outside of Seattle, we were told that Indian adolescents raised in white homes are increasingly returning to the reservation in search of their cultural roots. In an article in *The Destruction of American Indian Families*, a psychiatrist examines how social agencies exacerbate the problems of Indian families. He presents case studies of eight Indian families whose children were in his view needlessly placed in foster care at the time of a family crisis (a familiar pattern for many foster care children) and argues that the removal of the children led to the further destruction and disintegration of the families. J. Westermeyer, "The Ravage of Indian Families in Crisis," in Unger, *The Destruction of American Indian Families*.

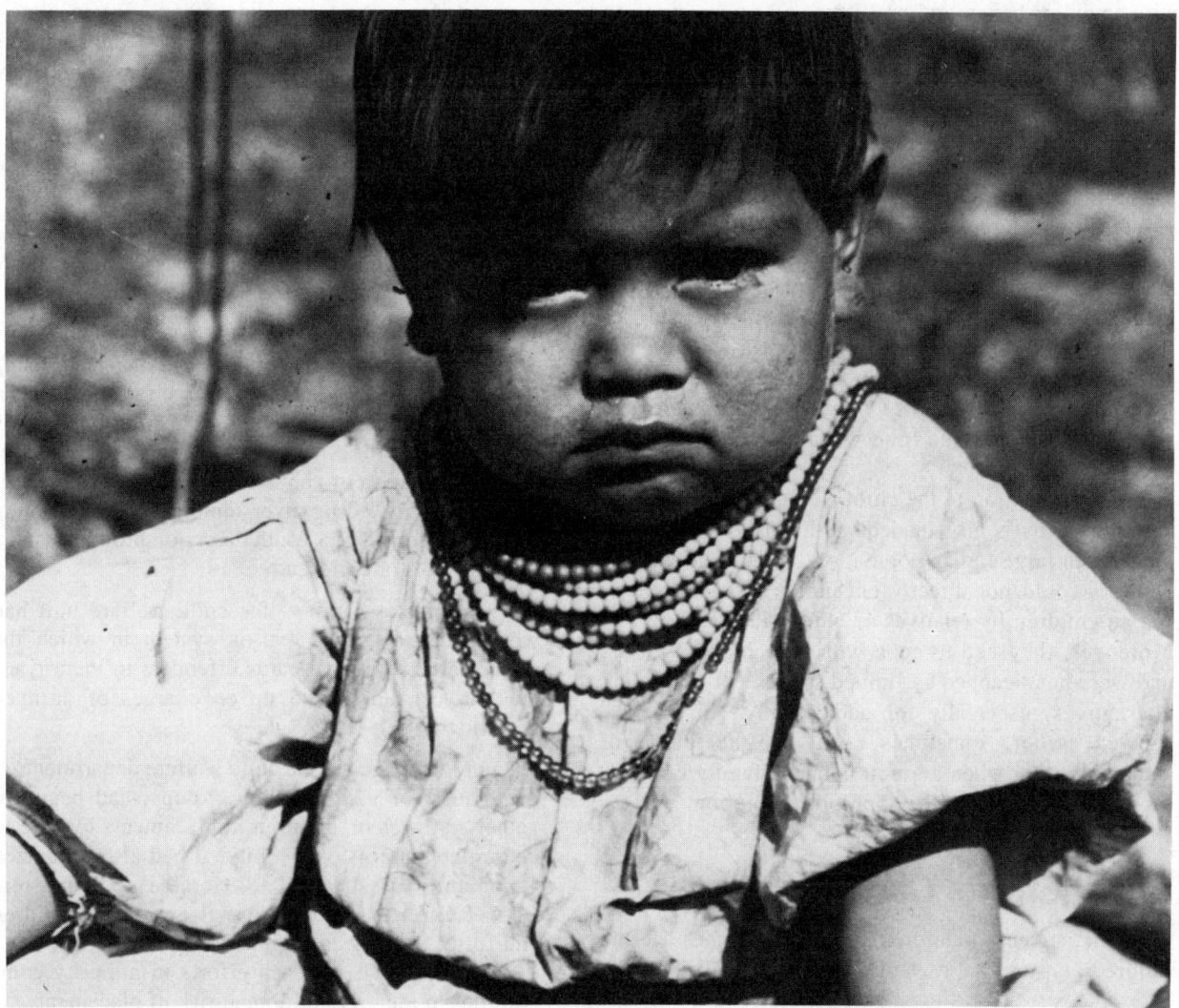

schools operated by the Bureau of Indian Affairs.[78] These BIA schools are in effect an alternative form of foster care, with large proportions of the students enrolled for social, not educational reasons.[79] For example, a survey conducted in the fall of 1973 by the North American Indian Women's Association, under contract from the BIA, found that approximately 76 percent of the children enrolled in boarding schools were there for non-educational or economic reasons.[80] A more recent study which received responses from 15 BIA boarding schools, reported that an average of 67 percent of the children at these schools were there for social rather than educational reasons. Nevertheless, five of these schools reportedly had no programs to deal

[78]U.S. Department of Interior, BIA, Office of Indian Education Programs, Fiscal Year 1976, *Statistics Concerning Indian Education* (Lawrence, Kansas: Publications Service, Haskell Indian Jr. College, 1977), pp. 12-15.

[79]According to BIA guidelines students who meet the criteria are those who: (1) are rejected or neglected, and for whom no suitable plan can be made; (2) belong to large families with no suitable home and whose separation from each other is undesirable; (3) have behavior problems too difficult for solution by their families or through existing community facilities and who can benefit from the controlled environment of a boarding school without harming other children; and (4) by virtue of the illness of other household members cannot be cared for. 62 IAM 2.5.2B. Placement in a federal boarding school is listed in the BIA Social Services Manual as one of the ways foster care may be provided for a child who requires it. 62 IAM 3.2.6B(2) (Draft #4).

[80]North American Indian Women's Association, Inc., *Project Report for Development of Prototype Program for Indian Children With Special Needs* (Washington, D.C.: U.S. Government Printing Office, 1973), p. 72.

with social or behavioral problems and saw no need to make changes in their programs.[81] This and other evidence suggest that students in these schools often get little education and little help with special needs.[82]

State and local agencies in jurisdictions with large Indian populations often do little to respond to the special cultural traditions of the Indian family. Of the 17 states with large Indian populations surveyed for a state-of-the-field study, only four included special information about Indian child welfare in state plans or manuals. And only the State of Washington had developed specific policies regarding Indian children and families.[83] Washington required workers to place Indian children with families of their own or a related tribe, and to notify the tribe when the state placed an Indian child.

Federal attention to the child welfare needs of reservation Indians is also inadequate.[84] In both our study states with large Indian populations, BIA child welfare workers could not directly encourage the adoption of Indian children by relatives or other tribal members.[85] Moreover, they had to cope with very high caseloads and were handicapped by limited services or placement alternatives, especially for adolescents. This, as we showed earlier, sometimes results in the jailing of Indian children when a group home or family counseling program would be the appropriate solution.

Local Efforts Can Work

Public neglect of children out of their homes and the failure to ensure that each child receives quality care in an appropriate setting are widespread. But in almost every community we visited, we found people working within both public and private agencies who were angered and concerned about what happens to children. We also found, although less frequently, responsive local efforts on behalf of children who are at risk of or are in out-of-home care.

- In an Ohio county, when the county children's home was demolished to build a new road, the child welfare director insisted that four small group homes replace the one institution.

- A number of small rural counties had managed, using limited funds effectively, to set up a range of special programs designed to prevent the institutionalization of children. In rural Pike County, Ohio, for instance, with a population of about 19,000, there was a foster home program, a drug diversion program, an evening recreation program, a youth diversion program, and a night school for children.

- In Los Angeles County, the child welfare unit had worked out a special liaison system in which the police referred young status offenders to them (i.e., the ten-year-old picked up on charges of drunken behavior).

- Also in Los Angeles, the child welfare department, at the request of various ethnic groups, had begun to gather statistics on children in placements by race to determine patterns of inequity. It had also organized Community Assistance to Homeless Youngsters (C.A.T.H.Y) to conduct special events for children and foster parents; to recruit for the department; and to initiate special outreach efforts in minority communities to identify children at risk of placement.

- In another California county a special unit was set up within the child welfare office to attend to the needs of developmentally disabled children. (The unit was developed because the state agency program mandated to deal primarily with developmentally disabled persons was so ineffective.)

Commitment, leadership and some imaginative use of admittedly too scarce resources clearly can make a difference. In general, however, we can only conclude that the majority of local officials charged with responsibility for children out of their own homes fail to provide anything but the most perfunctory attention to the children in their care.

---

[81] Department of Health, Education and Welfare, *Indian Child Welfare: A State-of-the-Field Study*, pp. 21-22.

[82] Congressional hearings have elaborated on the abusive conditions in Indian boarding schools and their failure as educational institutions.

[83] Department of Health, Education and Welfare, *Indian Child Welfare: A State-of-the-Field Study*, pp. 3-8, 14-19.

[84] Legislation passed in the 95th Congress, however, establishes legislative standards to govern the placement of Indian children in foster care and adoptive homes. It gives first preference to placement with the child's extended family, and then to Indian homes on reservations or tribally licensed homes. The bill would also address the respective jurisdiction of state and tribal governments in matters relating to child placements. See P.L. 95-608, approved November 8, 1978).

[85] The BIA is not an authorized adoption agency and must refer children to state child welfare agencies. Indian law gives the tribal council the authority to determine whether adoption shall be permitted on the reservation, but in many states the authority of the tribal court is not recognized by the state agency.

What Can Be Done?

In later chapters, we will outline specific changes needed at the state and federal level to reverse the harmful practices and policies that result in public neglect of children. But local officials and advocates can also act independently for change. Our recommendations follow.

1. Procedures should be developed and enforced to ensure placement in the least restrictive setting, with relatives if possible, and within reasonable proximity to the child's family consistent with any special needs of the child.

2. Procedures should be developed and enforced to reduce the number of placements a child experiences, including an early warning system for children who seem especially vulnerable to transfers.

3. Substantive interdisciplinary training should be provided for those who work with children and families, drawing on such resources as local professional associations and universities.

4. Local advocacy teams of parents, lawyers and other community representatives should be established to visit and monitor local facilities housing children.

5. Provisions for reporting, exposing to public view, and correcting institutional abuse of children and inadequate care practices should be implemented and enforced.

6. Assurances should be provided that children and youth in the community and in institutions, as well as their families, are aware of their rights and of procedures for redress of grievances.

7. A critical examination of existing services and facilities should be conducted. Plans should be developed and implemented for generating community support and the resources necessary for creating alternative services.

8. A special advocacy effort should be made in areas with minority children to ensure their nondiscriminatory treatment by public and private agencies and to correct any inequities identified.

9. If purchase-of-service contracts are negotiated locally, procedures should be established to ensure that reimbursement is contingent on tough standards of performance and nondiscrimination.

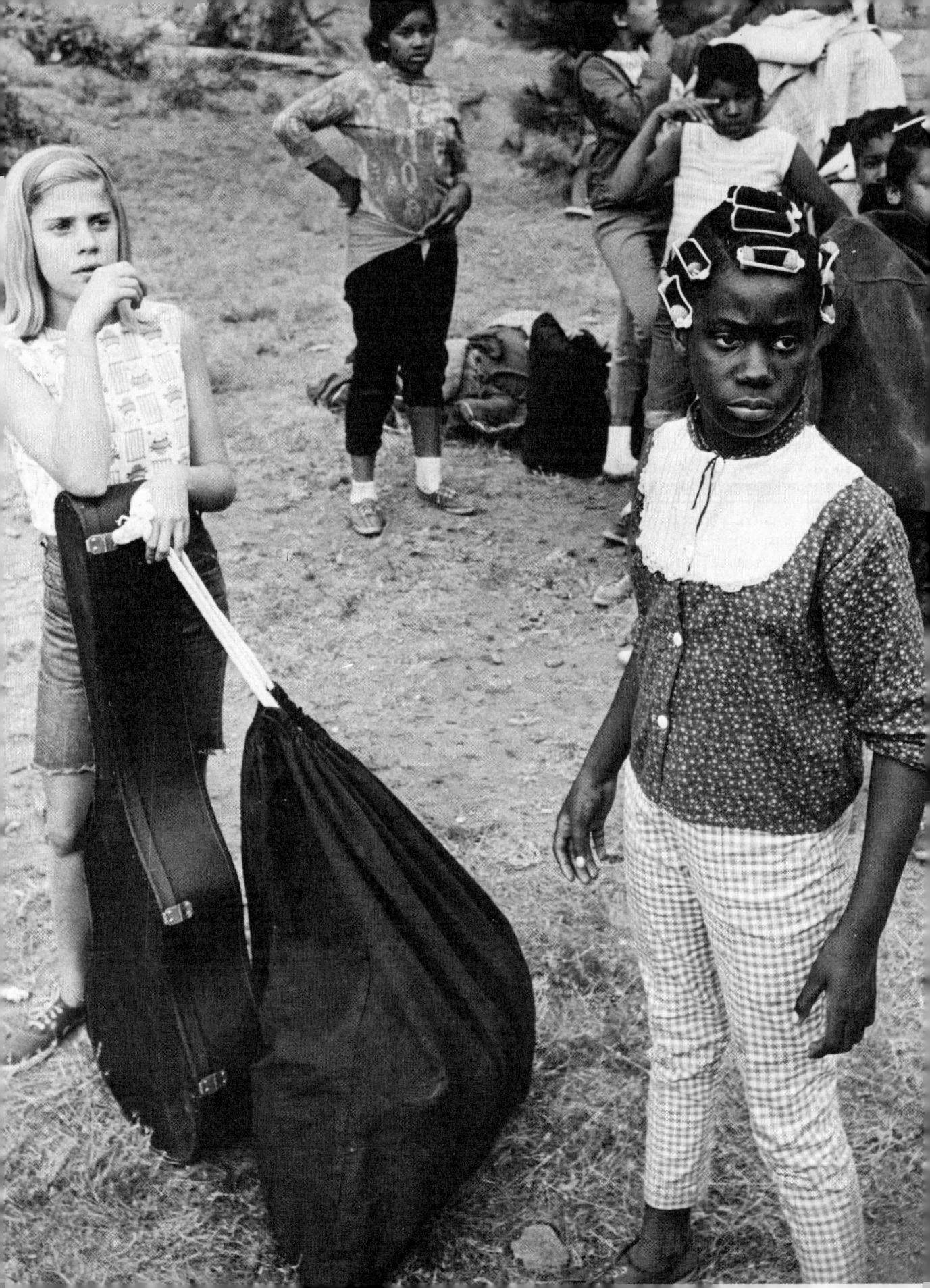

3 Children Placed Out of State

Public Neglect Compounded

Jimmy is a 15-year-old status offender who was declared "incorrigible" by the court. He was to be removed from the children's shelter and sent by the State of Michigan to Caribe Vista Youth Safari in Haiti. Only quick action by a legal aid lawyer prevented his exportation.[1] *At the Safari, Jimmy would have received what the owner called "culture shock therapy." Culture shock therapy is based on the theory that if a child is removed from his home environment and exposed to a punitive living situation in a foreign country, then his behavior is likely to improve.*

Paul is also an adolescent. He was hospitalized in a psychiatric facility in an eastern state for four years. After three years, the hospital said he could be discharged. But it took hospital officials an additional year to find a new home for him—1,500 miles away in Texas. His Texas placement prevents him from maintaining contact with an older sister in his home state who cannot care for him but wanted to be close to him.

The inappropriate placement and care of children does not end at the state's boundaries. For far too many children, it is an interstate phenomenon with children sent great distances from their homes—from Oregon to Maine, from California to Florida, from Washington to Texas, from New York to Idaho. As we began our study of children without homes, we found there was very little systematic information available about such placements.[2] Accordingly, we decided to take a special look at what happens to children who are so dramatically cut off from families, communities and their own homes.

Between October 1975 and April 1976, we conducted a telephone survey of state child welfare administrators identified in the *1975 Public Welfare Directory* as responsible for interstate placements. We sought to discover: whether they knew how many children were out of state; where the children were sent; and what mechanisms existed to monitor the progress of the children and the quality of the programs. We sought information only about children in residential facilities and not about children placed across state lines in adoptive or

---

[1] "Jailed Boy Saved from Torture Camp," *Detroit Free Press*, 16 September 1974. We later learned the Safari was abruptly moved to the Dominican Republic when the residents were arrested for the use of drugs and, along with the owner and his son, deported from Haiti. A 1977 article reported that Illinois children were still being sent to the facility in the Dominican Republic. "Illinois Delinquents Being Sent to Caribbean Camp," *The Chicago Sun Times*, 20 June 1977.

[2] For examples of the information that was available, see P.A. Keenan, *An Illinois Tragedy: An Analysis of the Placement of Illinois Wards in the State of Texas*, Report to State of Illinois Department of Children and Family Services, August 1973; E. Back, "The Case of the Banished Child," *New Orleans Courier*, 16-22 May 1974; and S. Kantor, "Interstate Business: Troubled Youngsters," *The Washington Post*, 21 September 1975. Since our study was done, the New York State Council of Voluntary Child Care Agencies has also conducted a national survey. New York State Council of Voluntary Child Care Agencies, *"Where Are The Children?" Report of National Survey of Out of State Placement Arrangements* (New York: 1978).

foster homes. Additionally, we surveyed state juvenile justice and mental health officials with responsibility for interstate placements, to assess the extent to which the out-of-state placement of children is a cross-system phenomenon. Finally, we tried to understand the role of relevant "interstate compacts"[3] and other regulatory mechanisms in protecting out-of-state children against institutional abuse and state neglect.[4]

It should be noted that out-of-state placements are not always inappropriate. For children with specialized needs, particularly those living in small states, there may be no other way of getting appropriate treatment except placement in a distant facility. Indeed, often such children must be placed far from their own homes within their own states. Other children are technically placed out of state, but are actually in nearby facilities located just over a state border, or within a metropolitan area covering two states. But reports from relatives of children like Jimmy and Paul and from state officials willing to speak out persuaded us that often out-of-state placements are used without evidence that they can meet the particular needs of individual children and that closer, appropriate placements are unavailable.

How Many Children Are Out Of State?

The Child Welfare System

We surveyed child welfare officials in 49 states, and the District of Columbia.[5] Data from Louisiana were taken from information gathered for a lawsuit in which CDF was a party.[6] In addition, we met with New York City officials. Alabama and Mississippi provided information on policies related to out-of-state placements, but refused to provide statistics. Hawaii and North Dakota did not respond at all. We received partial or complete information from all the other states.

California, Florida, Georgia, Ohio, Missouri, Pennsylvania, Texas and the District of Columbia reported that they did not know how many children were in out-of-state residential facilities. Maine and Oklahoma reported no children were placed out of state at the time we asked. The remaining 37 states reported that in the spring of 1976, a total of 4,049 children were out of state under child welfare auspices. Most of the administrators were also able to give some idea of the states to which the children were sent.

The data revealed tremendous variation from state to state in reliance on out-of-state placements. Several states accounted for large numbers of children, while others sent only a few children out of state. At the time of our survey, the responding states sending the largest numbers of children out of state through the child welfare system were: New Jersey (735), Louisiana (715), Virginia (436), Indiana (329) and Iowa (207).

Information on children entering other states was virtually nonexistent. Only nine state officials were even able to estimate the numbers of children coming into their states. Among these, we found many inconsistencies.

- Delaware reported that they did not have out-of-state children because their resources were limited, but both Virginia and New Jersey reported sending children to Delaware.

- Idaho reported that 58 children from 20 states were in one facility, Edgemeade, yet only seven states reported sending children to Idaho.

- Oklahoma reported that only two out-of-state children were placed in their facilities, but four states reported sending children to Oklahoma.

- Pennsylvania reported that they knew of only three out-of-state children placed in the state, but 13 states reported sending children to Pennsylvania.

- Utah reported that only three children, all from Idaho, were placed in the state, but three states reported sending children to Utah.

- Wisconsin reported that 100 to 150 out-of-state children were placed in eight of their facilities, but they could not give an exact count or say where the children came from. Twelve states reported sending children to Wisconsin.

- Florida conducted a special survey in response to our question about children coming into the state and found 287 children from 18 states. However, 22 states reported sending children to Florida.

---

[3] Interstate compacts are legal agreements between states establishing jurisdictional obligations and responsibilities in specific areas. They must be approved by each state legislature. See further discussion of relevant state compacts at pp. 70–73 infra.

[4] For a fuller description of our methodology, see Appendix A.

[5] The majority of these officials were contacted by telephone, although in several of our study states we personally interviewed the appropriate staff. See Appendix H. for a summary of the type of contact and the information gathered.

[6] *Gary W.* v. *Cherry*, sub nom. *Gary W.* v. *State of Louisiana*, 437 F. Supp. 1209 (E. D. La. 1976).

The Mental Health and Juvenile Justice Systems

To determine the extent of out-of-state placements under mental health and juvenile justice auspices, we surveyed 49 states and the District of Columbia by mail.[7] We received responses from 31 mental health administrators and 31 juvenile justice administrators.

Within the mental health system:

- Twelve states reported no children were placed out of state under mental health auspices.
- Eight states reported all out-of-state placements of children in the mental health system were through child welfare.
- Five states did not know how many children were out of state as a result of mental health agency action.
- Six states reported a total of 136 children out of state. Rhode Island accounted for 95 of these children, Tennessee for 30.

Within the juvenile justice system:

- Fourteen states[8] reported a total of 306 children in out-of-state placements under juvenile justice auspices. Of the states reporting out-of-state children: Maryland reported 111 children, Connecticut 58, Idaho 44, and Virginia 30. The remaining states reported 20 or fewer children placed out of state under juvenile justice auspices.
- Five states did not know how many children had been placed out of state under juvenile justice auspices.
- Twelve states reported no such placements.

These figures suggest that although the child welfare system is responsible for the majority of out-of-state placements, other systems in particular states also send many children out of state.

The Children Not Counted

The combined total estimate of children placed out of state at any one time in 1975-1976 as reported by surveyed state officials was 4,491. While this figure represents a significant number of children, there are

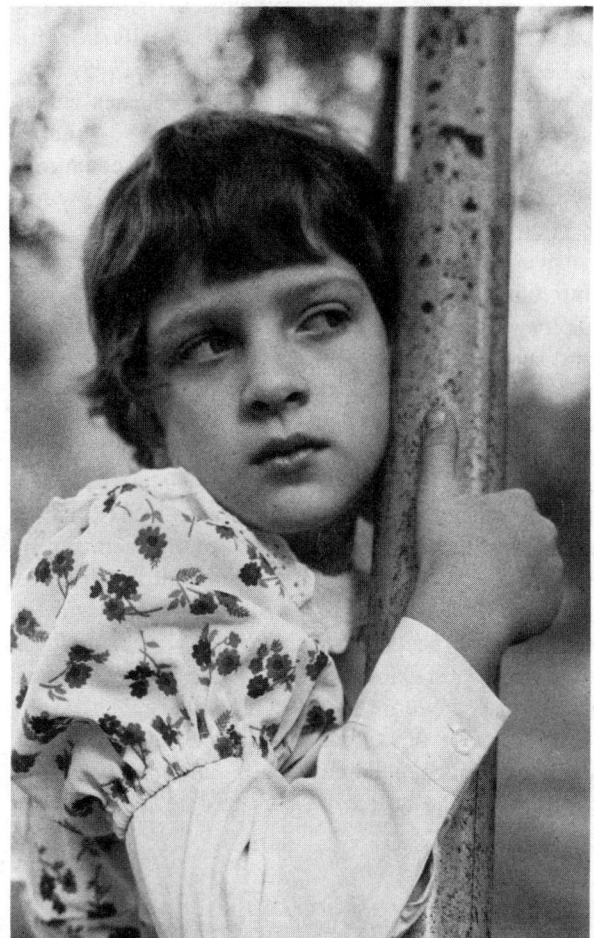

compelling reasons to suggest it is a very conservative estimate, and that the actual figure may be at least 10,000.

What are the reasons? First, juvenile court judges in many states have the authority to place children out of state directly without making any referral through a state agency. These children are therefore not accounted for in our survey. As state child welfare officials told us, the juvenile court judges may bypass their offices, ignoring any regulation to notify state officials.

Second, in states with county-administered welfare departments, the responsible state agencies claimed they had little authority to demand that out-of-state placements be arranged through or reported to state officials. In California and Ohio, two of our study states with county-administered child welfare systems, the officials responsible for out-of-state placements said they had no way of even knowing the number of such placements.

---

[7]We did not contact Louisiana because we were a party to *Gary W.* v. *Cherry* cited earlier.
[8]Although Idaho responded, it included children placed under juvenile justice auspices in its child welfare data.

Even in state-administered systems, the slippage between children reported and children actually affected can be of absurd proportions. In the fall of 1975, New York State, for example, reported four children out of state, while New York City alone reported 197 children out of state during the same period.[9] A study conducted shortly after our inquiry by the New York State Division for Youth revealed a dramatically different picture from what was reported to us. It found 804 New York State children in 70 facilities in 21 states.[10]

Third, private placement agencies may also fail to report out-of-state placements to a central state authority. The Child Welfare League of America conducted a survey of 202 voluntary agency members and associates regarding out-of-state placements from 1970 to 1974. Forty-eight percent of the respondents reported making such placements in at least one of these years, and 58 percent reported receiving out-of-state placements at least once. Yet only about three-quarters of the agencies reported that consent was required from a public body in the sending or receiving state for such placements.[11] It is likely, therefore, that our survey missed a number of children placed out of state by voluntary agencies.

Finally, our estimate does not include the number of mentally retarded children placed out of state under non-child welfare auspices,[12] or children placed under special education auspices.[13] Nor does it take into account the out-of-state placement of Indian children or children with special needs in military families. The former are at great risk of being sent far from their reservations to BIA boarding schools for "social reasons";[14] the latter of being sent from military bases to residential placements anywhere in the country.[15]

Since our data were gathered, some states may have increased and others decreased the use of out-of-state placements, particularly if the issue has attracted public attention. For example, a few years ago Illinois had over 800 children in out-of-state facilities—over 600 in Texas alone. By June of 1976, after a major exposé about the conditions in which those children were placed, Illinois had reduced that number to 164 children.[16] However, it is startling to note that, based on our survey, every state placed some children in out-of-state residential placements.[17] Twelve states reported sending children to ten or more states—six of these to 15 or more. And 11 states reported receiving children from ten or more states—three of these from 15 or more states.[18]

---

[9] Since that time the number of New York City children placed out of state has substantially increased. By the fall of 1976, the city reported 340 children placed out of state. W. Creighton, "The Placement of New York State Children Out-of-State for Treatment," New York: New York State Division for Youth, February 25, 1977, pp. 2-3. (Mimeographed.)

[10] The special survey found that of the 804 children, 395 were placed by the Department of Social Services and 409 by the Department of Education. There were at least 54 children placed out of state by the Department of Mental Hygiene. These 54 were not counted in the 804, as an undetermined number of them might also have been counted in the Social Services figure. Creighton, "Placement of New York State Children Out-of-State," pp. 2-3.

[11] Child Welfare League of America, Memo to Executives of Member Agencies and Associates from Research Center Regarding Inter-state Placements, November 3, 1975. The placements surveyed included adoptive and foster home placements, as well as institutional placements.

[12] The Council of State Governments has conducted a national study of the problems of developmentally disabled individuals (adults and children) placed in out-of-state facilities. A report of their findings includes data on practices in the ten states in which there were ten or more out-of-state placements and more detailed case studies of Alabama, Maryland, and New Jersey regarding out-of-state placement patterns. They too found the out-of-state placement problem to be part of the larger problem of inappropriate placements, and recommended that "[f]uture inquiries into the problem of out-of-state placement should only be incidental to the larger issues of institutional placement, where the best developmental interests of the individual should be vigilantly reviewed in any decisions made by public agencies about private individuals." For a further discussion of their findings and recommendations, see Council of State Governments, *Final Report - A National Study of the Problems of Developmentally Disabled Individuals Placed in Out-of-State Facilities* (Lexington, Kentucky: Council of State Governments, November 1977).

[13] For instance, in Massachusetts in September 1975, 340 of the 772 children placed by the Department of Special Education in private residential facilities were placed out of state. Massachusetts Department of Education, Division of Special Education, Communication to Children's Defense Fund.

[14] For example, Intermountain, a Bureau of Indian Affairs' school which used to have children primarily from the Navaho reservation, now has children from all over the country. Several years ago, by a tribal resolution, the Navaho reservation refused to send any more children to Intermountain. Consequently, Intermountain is now recruiting elsewhere. It has been charged that children at Intermountain are disciplined harshly, receive no mental health services, and are over-medicated. Interview with staff of the Indian Youth Council, 31 October 1975. See also further discussion of boarding school placements in Chapter 2.

[15] Funds for these placements are provided through the federal CHAMPUS program (see Chapter 5). In the winter of 1976, CHAMPUS estimated that a total of 900 emotionally disturbed children were in the program but could not give us estimates of the number of mentally retarded children.

[16] In September 1975, 215 Illinois children were out of state. By June 1976, this number was reduced to 164. Illinois Department of Children and Family Services, "Report of Out-of-State Placements in Residential Care Facilities for DCFS's Wards," December 16, 1975. (Internal Memorandum.) Michigan reported that four years prior to our survey there were over 100 out-of-state children. By the time of our survey, that number had been reduced to 14. We know too of reductions in out-of-state placements in Louisiana, New Jersey, and Virginia.

[17] While administrators in Maine and Oklahoma reported no children were currently out of state, other states reported facilities in their states had children from Maine and Oklahoma.

[18] See Appendix I. for a state-by-state analysis of the pattern of receiving and sending states.

STATES EXCHANGING CHILDREN

Alaska—Washington
Arizona—Nebraska
Arizona—New Mexico
California—Nevada
California—Nebraska
California—Washington
Colorado—Iowa
Colorado—New Mexico
Colorado—Utah
Colorado—Washington
Connecticut—Massachusetts
Connecticut—New Jersey
Connecticut—New York
Connecticut—Rhode Island
Delaware—New Jersey
Florida—Georgia
Florida—Massachusetts
Idaho—Montana
Illinois—Indiana
Illinois—Iowa
Illinois—Wisconsin
Indiana—Ohio
Iowa—Minnesota
Iowa—Nebraska
Iowa—Washington
Kansas—Minnesota
Maine—Massachusetts
Maine—New Jersey
Maine—Rhode Island
Maryland—New Jersey
Maryland—New York
Maryland—Virginia
Massachusetts—New York
Massachusetts—Rhode Island
Massachusetts—Vermont
Michigan—Nebraska
Michigan—Wisconsin
Minnesota—Wisconsin
Missouri—Nebraska
Nebraska—Ohio
Nebraska—Oklahoma
Nebraska—Texas
Nebraska—Wisconsin
Nevada—Utah
New Jersey—New York
New Jersey—Virginia
New Mexico—Utah
New York—Rhode Island
New York—Vermont
New York—Virginia
North Carolina—Virginia
Oklahoma—Texas
Oregon—Washington
Texas—Utah
Texas—Washington

Which Children Are Sent Out Of State?

Joey was almost three years old when he was separated from his mother because she was in the process of a divorce and could not get money from public assistance for several months. Mrs. B placed Joey voluntarily for what she thought would be a brief period. He did not return home again for ten years.

From ages two to four Joey lived in three different foster homes in Louisiana. The only stable figure in his world was his mother, who visited him repeatedly. But he began to develop signs of stress, temper tantrums and other difficult behavior. In response, Louisiana placed him in a facility in New York State, where he lived for five years. While he was in New York, his mother could not afford to visit. His father, who was living in New Jersey, tried but was refused permission by the child welfare officials.

After three years the New York facility urged his return to his mother. Lousiana officials claimed they could not locate Joey's mother. When Joey's mother sent him a birthday card, with a return address on it, the New York facility sent the address to the Louisiana officials. The officials still did not contact her. She also requested in writing information about her son and sought to have him returned–all to no avail. Two years later, the state of Louisiana sent him to another institution, this one in Texas. Finally as a result of a lawsuit, Joey is now home with his mother and attending public school.

Joey is one of the 591 children who as of 1975 had been placed by the State of Louisiana in Texas facilities. Unlike Joey, many of these children were seriously handicapped. All were plaintiffs in a class action lawsuit, *Gary W.* v. *Cherry*, brought on behalf of Louisiana children sent to Texas.[19] The testimony in the *Gary W.* trial confirmed that state neglect and abuse were even more likely for children placed out of state than those placed in the state. It showed that Louisiana parents were forced to agree to out-of-state placements; offered no options; and told if they did not accept this "help" they would receive no help at all. The state provided no funds for parents to visit the facilities,

---
[19]This case was brought by Rittenberg and Wilkes of Louisiana and the Children's Defense Fund. The United States Department of Justice, initially requested to join the case on behalf of Louisiana, also joined the case on the side of the plaintiffs.

Interstate Placement of Children

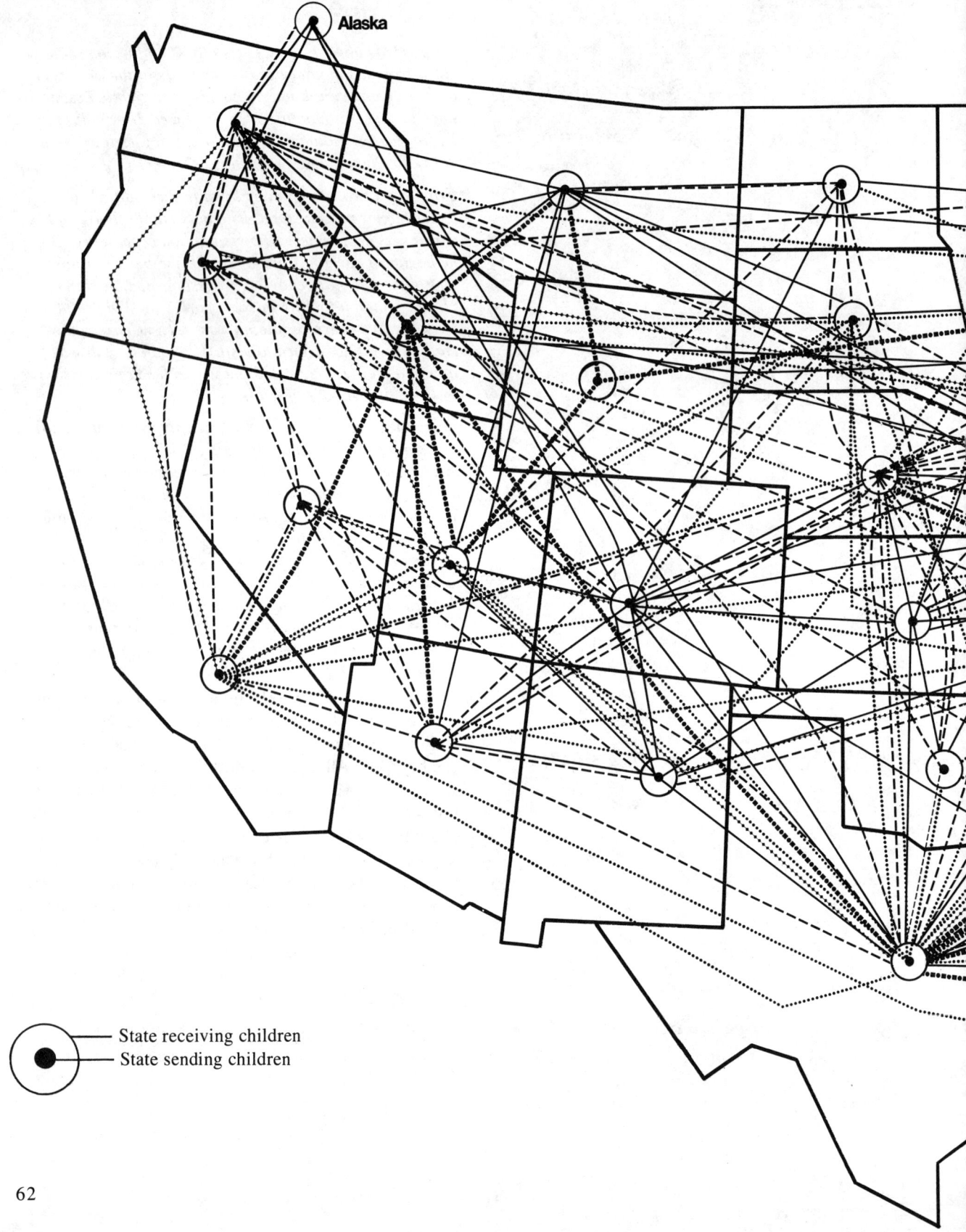

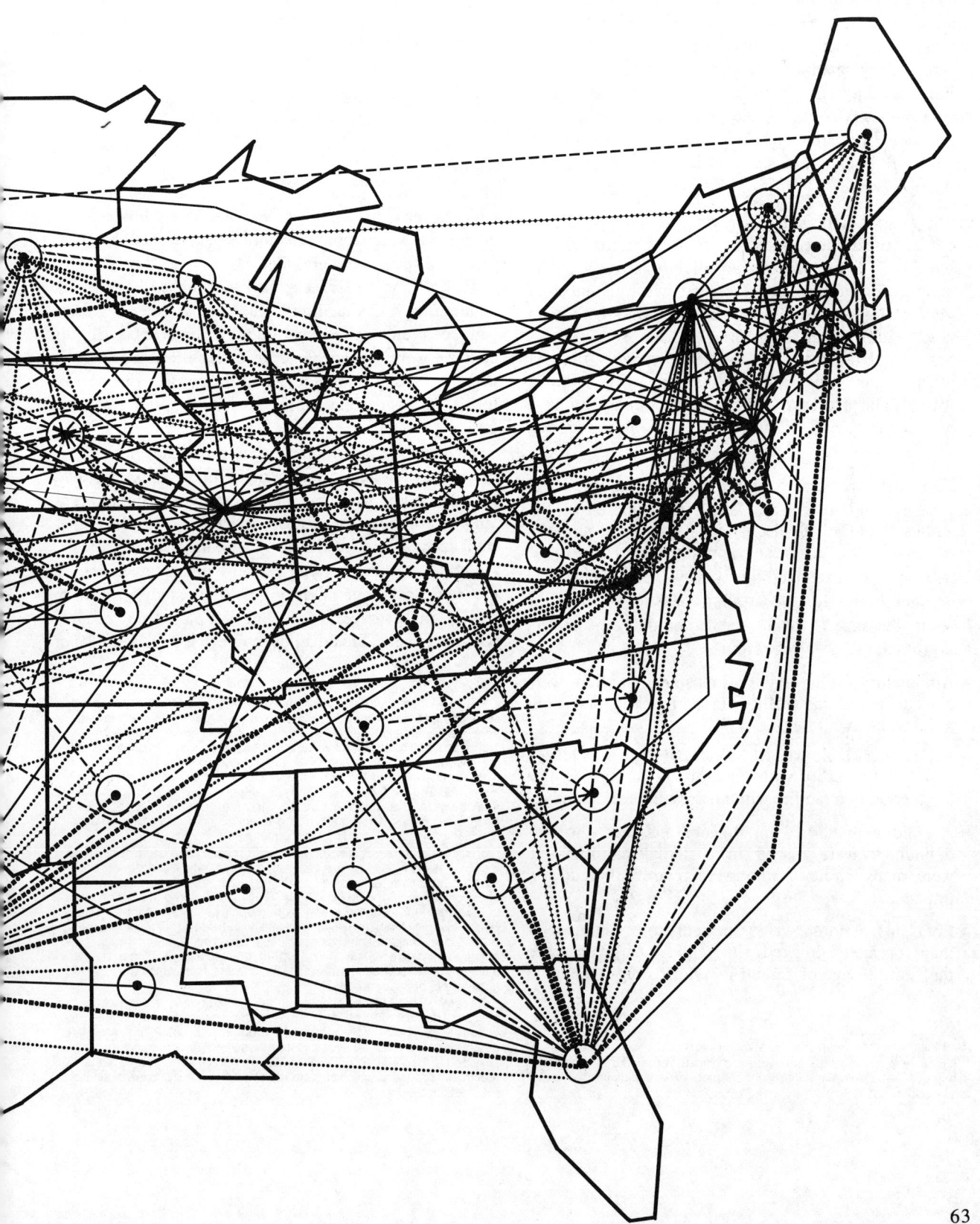

either before or after their child's placement. Indeed, some parents were misled about the types of programs available within in-state and out-of-state facilities. Few parents received any information about their children's progress. Joey's mother was no exception.

For the children, according to poignant testimony during the *Gary W.* trial, the placements were lonely. They were "literally starved for contact with someone from home." One Louisiana official who visited the children reported:

> The yearning for home—or whatever they conceive of as their home—is ever present in all of them. . . . Some accept their plight passively, others simply run away. . . . Our visit was undoubtedly very meaningful to the children with whom we were able to talk. That they may not have ever seen us before did not matter. . . . They invariably did ask about home: "Did we know the name of their home town? Their address? . . . How long would they have to remain here? Would we come back to see them?". . .[20]

This visit was an exception. In general, the state made no effort to find out about the children or the facilities.[21] Indeed, Louisiana officials were required to visit in-state facilities, but not out-of-state facilities. Yet, when the Texas facilities were visited by experts at the request of the U.S. Department of Justice as part of the lawsuit, the experts found repeated evidence of neglect and gross abuse of the children.

- Ambulatory, toilet-trained Louisiana children were placed in a Texas facility for non-ambulatory, non-toilet-trained children.

- A Louisiana child who was deaf and mute was placed in a Texas facility with no program for the deaf; a blind child in a facility with no program for the blind.

- A child with normal intelligence and one who was delinquent were placed in custodial facilities—so were many children who were retarded but clearly trainable.

- Louisiana children were repeatedly over drugged or inappropriately drugged. One child was given twice the adult dosage of an anti-psychotic drug. One child was given a drug for seizures—although he had never had seizures. Another child was given repeated dosages of a drug whose safety for use with children had not been established—a fact indicated on the drug bottle by the manufacturer.

Perhaps most tragic, once the children were placed, the state made no effort to bring them back to Louisiana or ensure their placement in the least restrictive setting. Until required by court order, Louisiana initiated no efforts to train foster parents to care for handicapped children, establish small, specialized group homes,[22] or determine which children could be returned home if special services were provided.[23]

Gary W. v. *Cherry* exposed the plight of Louisiana children in Texas facilities. But prior to *Gary W.* there had been an expose charging that over 600 Illinois children were in inadequate Texas facilities. Despite the negative publicity about Texas institutions, our survey found 32 states continuing to send children into the state.

Two types of children appear to be the most likely candidates for out-of-state placements: adolescents who are retarded or who have behavioral or emotional problems and multiply handicapped children needing specialized treatment resources. They are also likely to be children who have been rejected by in-state agencies. In the New York State Division for Youth study referred to earlier, the average age of children placed out of state was 15.5 years. Most had been rejected by at least 10 or

---

[20]Plaintiff's Exhibit 94, p. 2, in *Gary W.* v. *Cherry*.

[21]Even when such visits were made and officials reported that conditions in many of the facilities were totally unacceptable, the reports produced no action or response.

[22]This failure to generate appropriate resources is particularly shocking since private agencies testified that the state would not provide them with equivalent funds to those being spent to send children out of state. They indicated that if funds were available they would be willing to serve the children. New Jersey, which tried to stimulate the development of new resources, encountered a different response from private providers. There, in an early effort to reduce out-of-state placements, the state tried to encourage private facilities to expand their programs to serve the types of children being sent out of state. At that time, no incentive, not even capital construction monies, was enough. The facilities refused.

[23]The Court in *Gary W.* ruled that every Louisiana child placed in a Texas facility "has the right to care, education, medical and personal treatment suited to his characteristics and needs regardless of his age, degree of retardation or handicapping conditions." The Court ordered that the children in Texas be returned to Louisiana for thorough evaluations by the Louisiana State University Medical Center, and that an individual treatment plan be prepared and implemented for each child, taking into account the least restrictive alternative for that child. It further required that all children be permanently removed from certain of the Texas institutions which were proved at the trial to be inadequate.

As of May 31, 1978, final recommendations had been provided by the evaluation team for 293 children returned from Texas. These recommendations specified both the placement and program necessary for appropriate treatment of the child in the least restrictive setting. According to figures provided to the Court and CDF as of May 31, 185 children were in placements and programs which conformed, at least generally, to the evaluation recommendations.

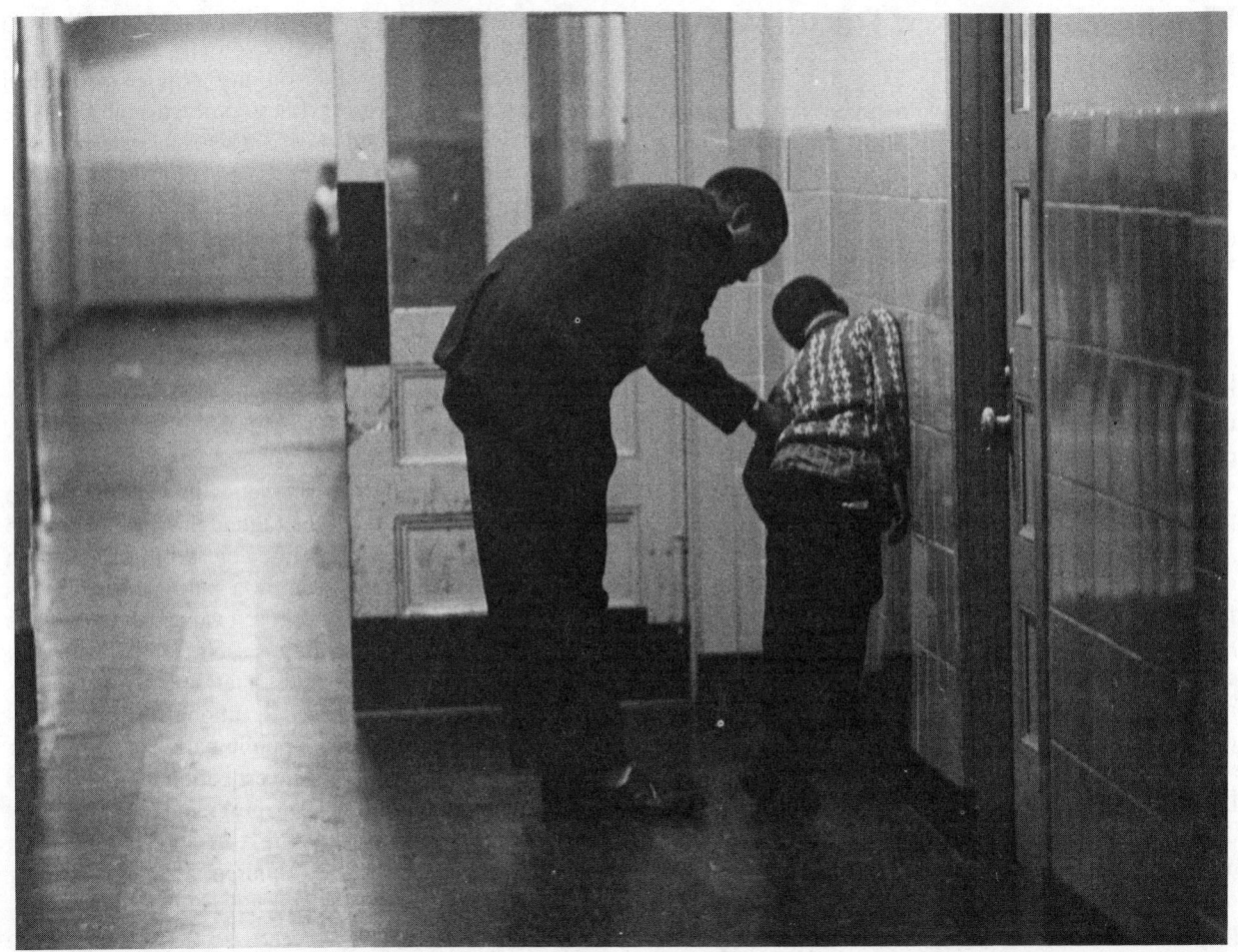

12 facilities. Illinois also reported that many of its out-of-state children had been rejected by in-state agencies.[24] A special analysis by the New York City Office of Special Services for Children of 72 cases of children placed out of state indicated that 15 percent of the children were diagnosed as emotionally disturbed, 25 percent as schizophrenic, 42 percent as mentally retarded, and 18 percent as multiply handicapped.[25]

Our own data, however, revealed some puzzling patterns. One would expect, for instance, that children with special needs might be particularly difficult to place in small states likely to lack specialized resources. However, we found no relationship between the size of a state and the number of children sent out of state. In fact, some of the states with small populations—such as Maine, Delaware and Montana—reported sending relatively few children out of state. Many larger states, however, which could justify the development of specialized facilities—for example New York, Illinois and New Jersey—reported sending large numbers of children out of state. Further, many states seemed to be exchanging children. Thirty-six states, including neighboring states like New York and New Jersey, received children from states to which they sent children. It also appeared that some private facilities accepted children from out of state, but rejected children with similar problems from their own state.[26]

---

[24]Keenan, *An Illinois Tragedy*.

[25]L. Emmerth, "NCIB Cases," New York City Office of Special Services for Children, 1976. (Unpublished report.)

[26]We were not able to examine the rate structures but obviously where there are differentials between states, a facility has an incentive to accept a child from the state paying the highest reimbursement rate. Documentation of differential rate structures would provide important data on the forces motivating out-of-state placements.

The Inadequacy of Regulatory Efforts

Theoretically, there are two regulatory mechanisms to protect children placed out of state: the sending state's own procedures for ensuring the child adequate care and nurturance, and interstate compacts.[27] Neither is effective.

The State Effort

Licensing

In the CDF survey of child welfare administrators, 46 reported that prior to approving an out-of-state placement, they determined whether the facility to which the child was to be sent was licensed or approved by the state in which it was located. How rigorously this procedure was followed varied.

Arizona was the only state to report that it would not reimburse a facility unless it was licensed. Two jurisdictions—the District of Columbia and Illinois—indicated they required but could not always obtain, a copy of the facility's license. No state required that the out-of-state facility meet its own licensing standards; it merely accepted whatever standards the other state set. Frequently, these were inadequate. For example, Louisiana officials had been repeatedly informed that under Texas licensing laws the fact that a facility had been licensed did not mean that it had a treatment program or that, if it did, the state had evaluated the program's adequacy.[28]

On-Site Visits

Only ten states reported the use of on-site visits to facilities in other states. Only five states tried to apply the same program review procedures to both in and out-of-state facilities, and in at least two of these, the actual implementation of the evaluations was subject to budgetary restrictions. Three of the five states identified by the surveys as then sending the largest numbers of children out of state—Virginia, Indiana and Iowa—reported no special facility review mechanisms. New Jersey had a new evaluation system but it was not specifically oriented toward out-of-state placements.[29]

[27]Interstate compacts are legal agreements between states establishing jurisdictional obligations and responsibilities in specific areas. They must be approved by each state legislature. See further discussion of relevant state compacts at pp. 70-73, infra.

[28]For a fuller discussion of general licensing problems, see Chapter 4.

[29]Since the time of our survey, under pressure from legal and citizen advocates, New Jersey has developed a more rigorous policy to guard against inappropriate out-of-state placements. See p. 70 , infra, for a fuller description of their efforts.

Conducting an adequate on-site program review is at best a difficult task. The methodologies are not precise and the outcome depends on the skill of individual reviewers. As in licensing, these problems apply inside and outside state boundaries. But with in-state reviews, the knowledge about facilities is generally cumulative. Reviews, coupled with knowledge of the front line workers who visit facilities or get reports from the children in them, lead to general profiles of the facilities. Sometimes, such information results in the development of an informal "do not refer list" within a county or local office. But for children sent out of state, there is typically no such cumulative feedback. The views of the evaluation team, if there is one, prevail. The result is sometimes bizarre.

New York City, which theoretically requires on-site visits to out-of-state facilities (although New York State law does not), gave one facility a clean bill of health on the basis of a reported visit by a public official. The official had stated on a checklist evaluation form "the services offered to the children seem to be extensive, and the functional roles of the staff clearly defined." She noted under an item on recreational facilities "extensive: indoor and outdoor, public park and swimming pool in community." An investigation of this same facility by the CBS television program "60 Minutes" two years after this inspection revealed a different story: one playground for over 300 children, and no director of recreation. The same television investigation also spotlighted other inadequacies.

Interviewer: *... Why are so many of your kids on therapeutic drugs?*

Owner: *Because it makes them much easier to work with, and instead of putting them in chains.*

• • •

Interviewer: *... The Montanari catalog, ... [distributed] to state agencies around the country ... says "All schools benefit from auxiliary personnel in the fields of speech therapy, remedial reading, music therapy, arts and crafts and recreation."*[30]

But on screen, teachers reported the remedial reading program does not exist, there is no tutoring and the speech therapist had left.

[30]Reprinted with permission from CBS, "60 Minutes," 17 October 1976, "Interstate Commerce of Kids."

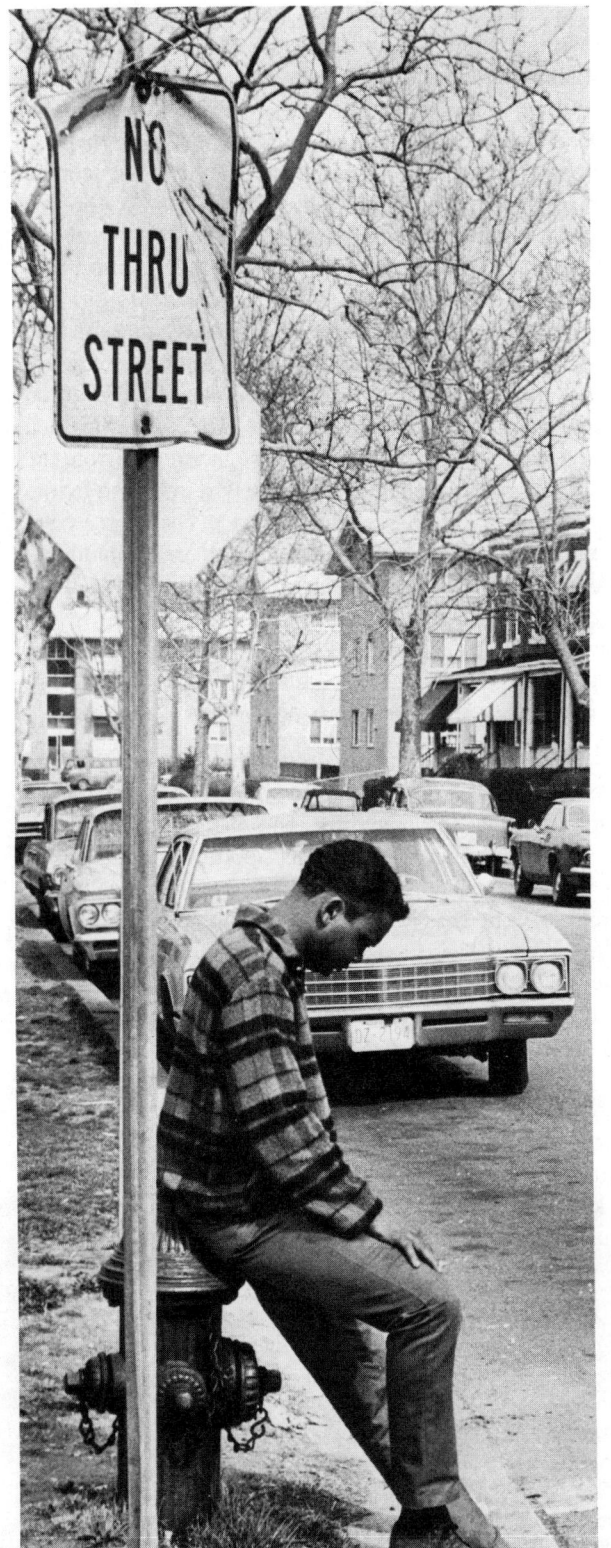

Monitoring Promotional Literature

In the television interview cited above, the owner of Montanari acknowledged that the literature sent to the states describing his program was inaccurate. He justified the discrepancy between the description and reality by saying it was necessary to say all these things to be accredited by states. He added "You know how much stuff there is there? If you did everything there is there . . . you'd go crazy."

Montanari is not an isolated case of a facility accepting many out-of-state children and failing to provide the level of services and care advertised. Similar allegations have been made about Edgemeade, a chain of facilities in Virginia, Maryland, Ohio and Idaho (with one scheduled to be opened in Texas), that accepts many out-of-state children. According to the Edgemeade brochure, each facility has a different program emphasis. Edgemeade recruits actively.[31] In the last year, for example, they have had booths at major mental health conventions. Their brochure entitled "A Place To Grow" promises, among other things: a tailored program for children with emotional problems, small classes, academic and vocational education, and casework services to parents and children.

Some of the Edgemeade facilities may indeed deliver what they promise, but official reports have been less than glowing. New Jersey has removed its children from the Maryland facility;[32] and Virginia, since 1973, has not placed its children in the Virginia facility.[33] In the fall of 1977, the Children's Rights Project of the New York Civil Liberties Union brought a class action suit challenging the policy and practice of sending New York City children out of state in violation of New York State laws, the state constitution and the Social Security Act.[34] The complaint alleges that one of the plaintiffs, a resident at Edgemeade, had been given

---

[31] Edgemeade is not alone. Eight out of 27 child welfare administrators responding to the question reported to us that owners and operators of state facilities had contacted them directly about placing children out of state.

[32] Interview with Robert Nicholas, Acting Chief, Bureau of Residential Facilities, New Jersey Division of Youth and Family Services, Department of Human Services, November 1975.

[33] Correspondence between Virginia licensing official and member of the New Jersey Public Advocate's Staff, June 11, 1976. Further, a program review by New Jersey officials in December 1975 concluded that the physical facilities were not well maintained; written treatment plans were lacking; and neither the educational program nor the services provided were comparable to those of the in-state New Jersey facilities. New Jersey Division of Youth and Family Services, Bureau of Residential Services, "Final Report, Edgemeade of Virginia," New Jersey, December 1975. (Mimeographed.)

[34] Carlos Sinhogar, et. al. v. Carol Parry, No. 14138/77 (N.Y. Sup. Ct., filed July 26, 1977).

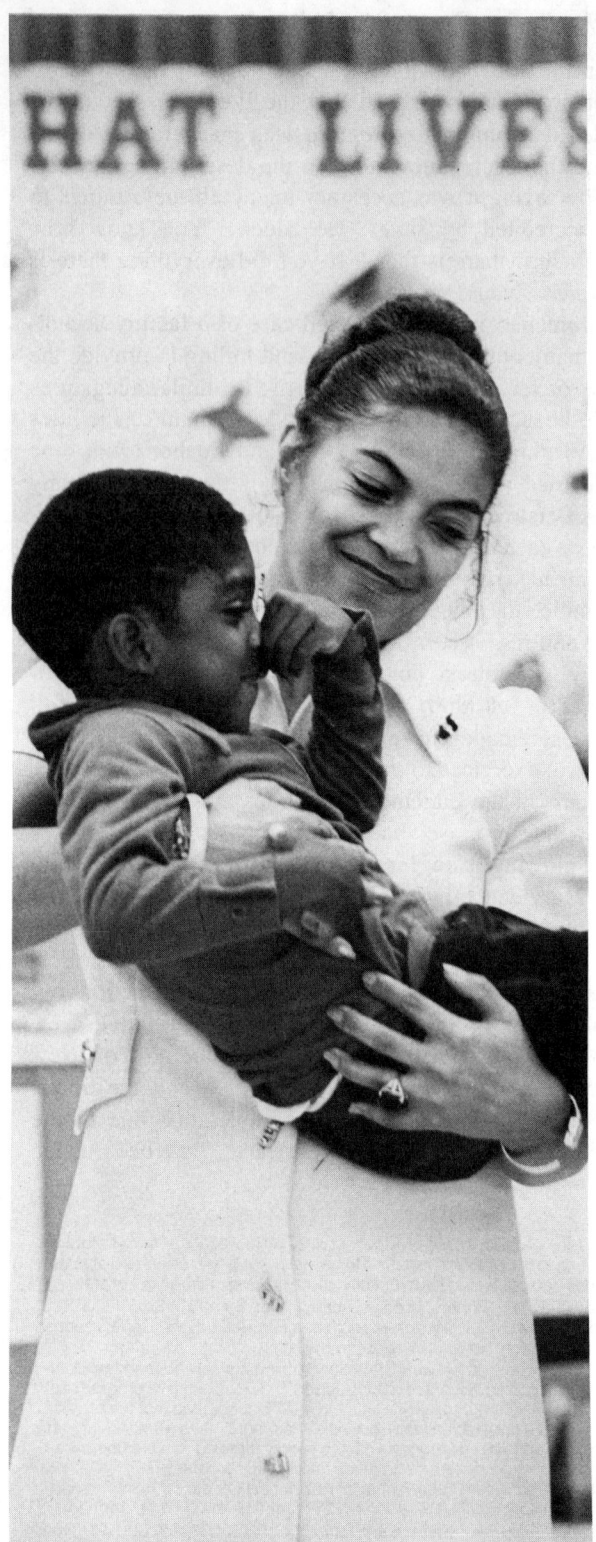

"powerful psychotropic drugs" without adequate medical supervision, had been frequently confined in an isolation room, and had been subjected to harsh and painful restraint and abuse.[35]

Reliance on promotional literature can also lead to serious mismatching of child and facility. We learned for instance of a child welfare worker who—on the basis of a facility's brochure—sent a bright 14-year-old to an out-of-state facility thousands of miles from her own home, only to learn a year later that the girl had been placed in a program for retarded children. The brochure had described programs for a range of exceptional children, but had not indicated that gifted children were not considered "exceptional." The worker learned of the tragic misplacement not through a report from the facility, which was being handsomely reimbursed by the sending state, but from the girl on a visit home. Yet many caseworkers have nothing but these promotional brochures to rely on in the absence of rigorous, regular site visits and monitoring by the responsible public agencies.

Ensuring Appropriate Placements

The state's failure to obtain detailed knowledge about the programs of out-of-state facilities is a serious abdication of state responsibility. But even more serious is the general failure to establish rigorous pre-placement approval procedures; or to monitor systematically the progress and care of individual children once placed out-of-state. There are two fundamental questions that the state should ask. First, does the child need to be placed out of state; and second, if the child is placed out of state, what kind of care and treatment does the child receive. States are not asking these questions.

Only six states, none of them among those reporting large numbers of children out of state at the time of our survey, stated that special administrative steps were taken to determine the appropriateness of an out-of-state placement when such placement was contemplated for a particular child.

- Idaho required the placing agency to prove to state officials that no in-state facilities were available.

---

[35]The complaint further alleges that he has not been visited by New York City social services officials, and has not received an individualized treatment plan. This placement costs New York approximately $15,000 a year. One of the other two plaintiffs is at Montanari, where the complaint alleges that, among other abuses, counselors make marijuana available to children in exchange for either money or sex.

- Illinois had developed a special profile sheet of a child needing placement that was circulated to all in-state facilities for a minimum of two weeks before out-of-state facilities could be considered.
- Iowa required the District Administrator to approve an out-of-state placement prior to negotiations with the out-of-state facility.
- Kansas required approval of an out-of-state placement by the district office and documentation of efforts to find the child a placement within the state.
- Michigan reported the development of a mandatory screening committee to consider all recommendations for out-of-state placements.
- South Dakota had developed the most comprehensive system to protect all children in placement from unnecessary removal to places far from home. A regional intra-state team reviewed the necessity for placing a child out of his own region. A state team composed of the commissioners of the departments of social service, special education, mental health and the division for youth services, then had to approve the placement of any child out of state.

We found that once children were placed out of state, the states generally made little effort to conduct either periodic administrative or on-site reviews. Five states—Colorado, Idaho, Massachusetts, New Hampshire and Vermont—reported that while visits to the children were theoretically required, in reality, implementation was dependent on cost and distance. Eleven states reported requiring written reports about the children.[36] Two states, Arizona and Missouri, reported court reviews of the cases: every six months in Missouri, annually in Arizona.[37] In the remaining states, administrative reviews for out-of-state children were either discretionary or nonexistent.

The failure of those charged with public responsibility to weigh continuously the costs of the psychological and geographic banishment of a particular child against the actual benefits of out-of-state placement is scandalous. The lack of concern was typified by the comment of a New Jersey official who said at a public meeting that he hoped that at the end of two years the state could review the cases of the out-of-state children. Two years may be a short time for administrators, but it is a long time in the life of a child, especially if that child is cut off from his home and community, is unhappy in a placement, or is subject to abusive conditions.

New Procedures

Since our survey, growing concern about the out-of-state placement of children has prompted a number of states to propose legislation or new policies restricting the practice and ensuring adequate monitoring of both children who are sent out of state and facilities in which they are placed. In July 1977, legislation was proposed in New York State to create an "out-of-state placement bureau."[38] The bureau would be required to approve all out-of-state placements to ensure they were necessary; in the least restrictive setting available; as close to the child's district as possible and reasonable; and in facilities which have been inspected by New York State officials and meet minimal New York State standards for child care facilities. The proposed legislation also required that the local social service agency pay for child-parent visits at least once a year. The bill, however, did not require periodic reviews of the children placed out of state, or on-site visits to the children by caseworkers.

Legislation to restrict out-of-state placements and require interagency monitoring and evaluation of out-of-state facilities was also introduced in Maryland in 1977.[39] However, by January 1978, neither of the proposed new statutes had become law. In Virginia, the House of Delegates and Senate both passed unanimous special resolutions in February 1977, declaring that out-of-state placement must be discouraged.[40]

---

[36]Colorado, Connecticut, Florida, Kansas, Michigan, Nevada, New Hampshire, New Mexico, Pennsylvania, South Dakota and Vermont.

[37]The Arizona review, as we show in Chapter 4, was clearly inadequate.

[38]Assembly Bill No. 9041.

[39]House Bill No. 1128 was introduced on February 9, 1977, but received an unfavorable report from the Judiciary Committee.

[40]The House of Delegates Resolution followed the release of a study on the placement and institutionalization of Virginia children in out-of-state and in-state facilities conducted by the Subcommittee on the Placement of Children of the House Committee on Health, Welfare and Institutions. See, Subcommittee on the Placement of Children, *Report of the House of Delegates Committee on Health, Welfare and Institutions*, House Document No. 16 (Richmond: Virginia Department of Purchases and Supply, January 12, 1977). In July 1977, the Virginia Department of Welfare also published revised regulations for the interstate placement of children which include detailed requirements for placement of youth in out-of-state residential facilities. Among other things, the regulations require interagency collaboration and documentation that "no other appropriate placement is within the state or available nearer to the child's community." See Virginia Department of Welfare, *Social Services Manual* (Richmond: Department of Welfare, July 1977), Section 5600.

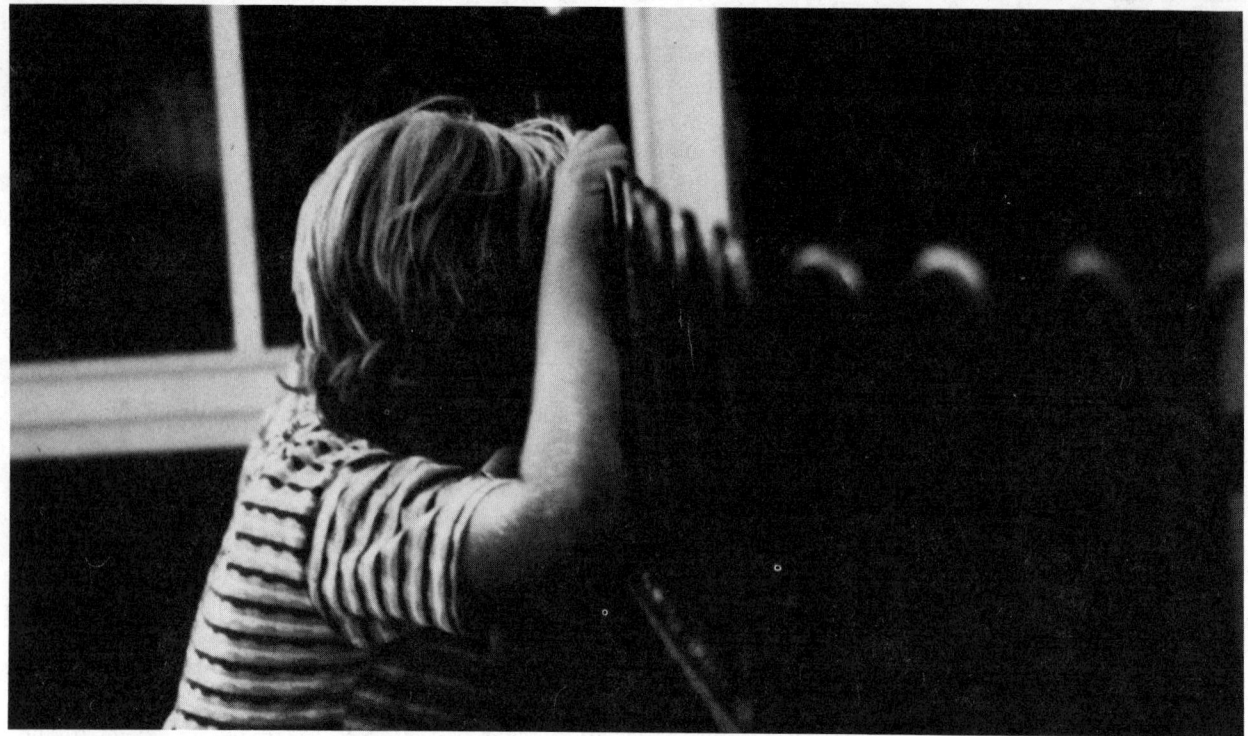

In New Jersey, as a result of continuing publicity and reports about the problem,[41] the state developed a comprehensive policy to reduce out-of-state placements. The new policy[42] requires: (a) prior to out-of-state placement, the rejection of a child by New Jersey agencies must be documented and out-of-state placements approved on a case-by-case basis by the central state administration; (b) the suspension of new referrals to all but two out-of-state facilities located more than 50 miles from New Jersey; (c) case reviews of all children currently placed beyond 50 miles of the New Jersey border; and (d) the expansion of placement resources within New Jersey. It is not yet clear, however, whether these and similar efforts will indeed result in more responsible use of out-of-state placement.

Interstate Compacts

Interstate compacts define jurisdictional responsibility across state lines. Three compacts are relevant for the out-of-state placement of children: The Interstate Compact on Mental Health, The Interstate Compact on Juveniles, and The Interstate Compact on the Placement of Children.[43]

The Interstate Compact on Mental Health applies to children and adults transferred by parental request from one public mental health or mental retardation system to another.[44] It is unclear whether it also applies to children transferred from psychiatric facilities to public child welfare agencies and then placed out of state by child welfare; or to children transferred by child welfare agencies to out-of-state psychiatric facilities.[45]

---

[41] See, for example, Office of Fiscal Affairs for the Joint Legislative Subcommittee on Children's Residential Facilities, "A Study of the Division of Youth and Family Services Out of State Placement Procedures," July 11, 1977, (Mimeographed); and The New Jersey Public Advocate, "A Report on the Placement of New Jersey Children in Out-of-State Residential Institutions," undated. (Mimeographed.)

[42] New Jersey Division of Youth and Family Services, "Plan to Address the Issue of the Placement of Children in Residential Facilities Outside of New Jersey," September 1, 1977, pp. 5-7. (Mimeographed.) This report notes that on May 31, 1977, 595 New Jersey children were still in out-of-state residential treatment facilities, 157 less than on May 31, 1976, p. 7.

[43] For citations to these and other interstate compacts, see Council of State Governments, *Interstate Compacts 1783-1977 (A Revised Compilation)* (Lexington, Kentucky: Council of State Governments, December 1977).

[44] As of October 1977, 44 states and the District of Columbia were members of the Interstate Compact on Mental Health. Arizona, California, Mississippi, Nevada, Utah and Virginia were not. The Council of State Governments and the National Association of State Mental Health Program Directors cooperatively serve the administrators of the Compact.

[45] A special study currently underway by the Office for Children and Youth in the New York State Department of Mental Hygiene is examining the applicability of the compact to New York children in such situations.

The Interstate Compact on Juveniles applies to delinquent children and runaways. For the former, it enables placement in public correctional programs in other states. For the latter, it provides a mechanism to return the runaway home. It also facilitates the supervision of youth on probation in a jurisdiction other than the one in which the adjudication occurred. First drafted in the 1950s, this Compact has since been ratified by all the states.[46]

The Interstate Compact on the Placement of Children[47] responds to a group of children that both overlaps with and is different from those covered by the Compact on Juveniles.[48] It applies to the out-of-state placement of adjudicated delinquents in private facilities, but it also applies to children placed in out-of-state adoptive and foster homes, as well as in group facilities or institutions where no adoption is contemplated.[49] It applies, in short, to many of the out-of-state children we have been describing.

According to Article III of the Compact, certain procedures must be followed by Compact members prior to the out-of-state placement of a child. The sending agency (note it does not say "state agency") must provide public authorities in the receiving state with: the child's name, date and place of birth; the names and addresses of parents or legal guardian; the name and address of the person, agency or institution with which the child is to be placed; and a statement of the reasons for placement. The Compact also provides that before accepting a child, a public official in the receiving state may request further information. There is no language requiring the public authority in the receiving state to furnish specific information to the sending state about the adequacy of the prospective placement setting.[50] However, prior to the placement, there must be written notification to the sending state by the receiving state that the placement "does not appear to be contrary to the interests of the child." The sending state retains jurisdiction over supervision, care, treatment and custody decisions affecting the child, as well as financial responsibility.

There is a further provision in the Compact on the Placement of Children that when a delinquent child is placed pursuant to the Compact there must be a court finding that "1. Equivalent facilities for the child are not available in the sending agency's jurisdiction; and 2. Institutional care in the other jurisdiction is in the best interest of the child and will not produce undue hardship."[51] However, for non-delinquent children—by far the majority covered under the Compact—there is no requirement that proximity to the child's home and community, placement in the least restrictive alternative, or hardship be considered prior to an out-of-state, Compact-sanctioned placement. Nor does the Compact specify the rights of children, once in out-of-home placement. There is, for instance, no provision to ensure continued monitoring of the child's program or progress while in placement.[52]

Our survey revealed that participation in the Compact appeared to have had little impact on the knowledge of state officials about children out of their own state, or on state efforts to protect such children more effectively. All but one of the states unable to provide data on numbers of children sent out of state were Compact members. Many Compact states could not tell us the numbers of children entering the state. Three of the six states requiring on-site reviews of the children were Compact members; three were not. Six of the ten states conducting some kind of on-site facility reviews were Compact members; four were not. Compact membership, in short, appears to have little effect on the extent of a state's effort to control out-of-state placements and monitor what happens to the children in them.

During the past several years, there has been a sys-

---

[46]The Criminal Justice Center at Sam Houston State University in Huntsville, Texas serves as the Secretariat for the Association of Juvenile Compact Administrators.

[47]As of December 1977, nine states—Alabama, Arkansas, Hawaii, Indiana, Michigan, Nevada, New Jersey, South Carolina, and Wisconsin—and the District of Columbia were not Compact members. For a further description, see American Public Welfare Association, *The Interstate Compact on the Placement of Children* (Washington, D.C.: APWA, undated); and B. Callanan and W. Mitchell, "The Interstate Compact on the Placement of Children," *Juvenile Justice* (May 1975): 41-46.

[48]A number of Compact administrators with whom we spoke could not explain the difference between this Compact and the Compact on Juveniles. In some states, both administrators worked closely together; in others they had no contact; and in some, the same person administered both Compacts.

[49]It does not include ". . . any institution caring for the mentally ill, mentally defective or epileptic or any institution primarily educational in character, and any hospital or other medical facility." (Article II. "Definitions.")

[50]Article I of the Compact, "Purpose and Policy," states that one of the Compact's purposes is to ensure that "The proper authorities of the state from which the placement is made may obtain the most complete information on the basis of which to evaluate a projected placement before it is made."

[51]Article VI, "Institutional Care of Delinquent Children."

[52]Compact supporters argue that such matters should not be addressed by an "interstate compact " because they belong in the domain of individual state action. Yet some states believe that by joining the Compact their children in out-of-state placements will be sufficiently protected, and that no further state action is necessary.

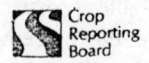
Crop Reporting Board
Statistical Reporting Service
U.S. Department of Agriculture
Washington, D.C.

MONTHLY HATCHERY REPORT
JANUARY 1978

Form Approved
O.M.B. Number 40-R1272
Approval Expires 12-31-90
C.E. 11-0001

Figure 1. Monthly Hatchery Report

Dear Reporter:

Your response to this survey will be appreciated but is not required by law. Your cooperation is important to insure more reliable chick estimates. Knowing the available number of broiler and egg-type chicks should help you with production and marketing decisions. Individual reports are kept confidential.

Please return your completed form in the postage paid envelope provided.

Thank you,

Bruce M. Graham, Chairman
Crop Reporting Board

CHICK OPERATIONS

(Please report "0" if answer is none)	Broiler-type Number	Egg-type Number
1. Chicken eggs in your incubators on February 1 (include custom set for others)		
2. Chicks hatched in your incubators during Jan. (include custom hatch for others)		
3. Of the chicks hatched in January, how many were:		
a. Placed for commercial broiler production		
b. Placed as:		
(1) Straight run chicks		
(2) Pullet chicks		
(3) Cockerel chicks (including any given away)		
c. Other disposition		

4. Of the chicks placed (Items 3a and 3b (1) and (2) how many were:	Broiler-Type Number	Egg-Type Straight Run Number	Egg-Type Pullets Number
Placed within this State			
Shipped to other States			
(State)			
(State)			
(State)			

5. Average cash price received per 100 for all chicks sold (based on actual sales):

	Broiler-Type	Egg-Type
a. Straight-run chicks	$	$
b. Pullets:		
(1) Pure breeds and cross breeds		$
(2) Others (including incrosses, incrossbreds, strain crosses and franchised breeds)		$
c. Cockerels		$

6. Average price per dozen paid to producers in your State for Broiler and Egg type hatching eggs (including any premium paid for hatchability) .... $

7. Total chicken egg incubator capacity (manufacturer's rating) including active capacity not now in operation .... Number _____

tematic effort to increase Compact membership. The federal government has provided substantial grants to the American Public Welfare Association (APWA) to provide technical assistance to states interested in enacting the Interstate Compact on the Placement of Children.[53] The number of Compact members has increased from 15 states in 1973, to 41 in December 1977. Our survey findings, however, lead us to question the value of a federal expenditure in excess of $800,000 for this purpose, and to ask whether individual children involved have in fact benefited.[54]

The federal government has no information on the extent of out-of-state placements and has made no effort to gather such information from the states. (It is interesting to note that the federal government does keep track of the number of chickens shipped out of state on a monthly basis. See Figure 1.) Nor has the federal government a specific regulatory role with respect to the interstate movement of children[55] although some interstate procedures, such as those pertaining to the transportation of goods, are regulated. The Federal Trade Commission Act prohibits unfair methods of competition and unfair or deceptive acts or practices in or affecting commerce, including deceptive and misleading advertising.[56] Thus, there is authority under this Act to challenge misleading advertising by child care institutions. To our knowledge, however, the Commission has not specifically monitored the promotional and explanatory materials used by states to authorize the purchase of care from various out-of-state facilities.

Other Accreditation Mechanisms

There are several additional mechanisms for regulating the quality of institutional care for children.[57] The Joint Commission on the Accreditation of Hospitals (JCAH) has developed standards and procedures for the accreditation of residential psychiatric facilities serving children and adolescents.[58] JCAH accredits psychiatric facilities for a two-year period, at which time the facility must reapply for an accreditation survey. Prior to accreditation, a facility may be reviewed (including site visits) several times before a final decision must be made. Each time a survey is conducted, the JCAH receives $750 a day for the visit. The survey visits are announced approximately six weeks in advance, and the accreditation manual further notes that accreditation need not require 100 percent compliance with every applicable item, but will be based on individual decisions.[59]

None of the relevant JCAH accreditation survey records or reports, other than a certificate of accreditation, are made available to the public without the facility's written authorization, unless state law requires otherwise. It is thus questionable, we believe, whether such accreditation can help families or public officials make a decision concerning different facilities. We were not able to examine in detail the role of the Joint Commission regarding residential facilities, but in the course of our study we learned of JCAH-accredited facilities that had, in the eyes of other observers, serious inadequacies.[60]

Institutions are also often required to meet certain federal standards to be eligible for federal reimbursement under such programs as Medicaid, SSI and CHAMPUS. These programs are discussed more fully in Chapter 5.

---

[53]Since Fiscal Year 1972, the APWA has been awarded $867,387 by the former Office of Child Development in the Department of Health, Education and Welfare. The federal grant for the project terminated on June 30, 1978. Figure compiled from individual "Notice of Grant Awarded" forms on file in the Grants Management Division, Office of Human Development Services, HEW.

[54]At the time of our survey, the project administrator at APWA could not provide any data or even estimate the numbers of children in Compact states who were in residential settings across state lines. He further stated that he saw no need to strengthen the Compact in any way. As of December 1977, figures on the number of children affected by the Compact were still not available.

[55]P.L. 95-225, the Protection of Children Against Sexual Exploitation Act of 1977, does address the problem of the use of children in pornographic materials and juvenile prostitution when children are transported or materials are transported or mailed in interstate commerce. More specifically, the Act amends Title 18 of the United States Code to make it a federal crime to cause any child under the age of 16 to engage in sexually explicit conduct for the purpose of producing materials which are to be mailed or transported in interstate commerce. It also prohibits the sale or distribution of any obscene materials that depict children engaging in sexually explicit conduct if such materials have been mailed or transported in interstate commerce; and prohibits the interstate transportation of children for the purpose of engaging in prostitution or other sexually explicit conduct for commercial purposes.

[56]15 U.S.C. §45.

[57]In July 1978, the Council on Accreditation of Services for Families and Children, the first independent accrediting body for agencies providing social services to families and children, also started accrediting, on a voluntary basis, both proprietary and nonproprietary agencies. The Council accredits agencies in 11 program areas, including day care, foster family care and child caring institutions.

[58]See, Joint Commission on Accreditation of Hospitals, *Accreditation Manual for Psychiatric Facilities Serving Children and Adolescents* (Chicago: Joint Commission on Accreditation of Hospitals, 1974).

[59]Joint Commission on Accreditation of Hospitals, *Psychiatric Facilities*, p. xiii.

[60]A thorough study of appropriate accreditation processes for children in residential treatment facilities is long overdue. It is particularly important that such a study inform the debate about how and under what conditions residential care for children should be reimbursed through national health insurance.

What Can Be Done?

The problems of children placed out of state are similar to those of children placed within their own states, but they are intensified by the distance separating children from their families and communities and from the public officials responsible for them. Finding solutions to the misuse of out-of-state placements will not be easy. Simply bringing the children now out of state back is not enough. In-state alternatives must be developed that will ensure more appropriate, less destructive care to the children now out of state, and to those children at risk of out-of-state placement in the future. In addition, specific procedural mechanisms to ensure against future inappropriate out-of-state placements and to ensure quality care to out-of-state children must be generated and closely monitored. These, in turn, should be linked to an overall effort to increase necessary services, placement options and review procedures for all children at risk of out-of-home placement. Our specific recommendations follow:

1. Each community should analyze the extent to which its children are sent to other states or to distant facilities within the state. How many are there? What are their needs? Where are they being sent? What fiscal resources are used? Are the facilities and children reviewed periodically?

2. Children inappropriately placed out of state must be returned and reunited with their own families, or provided with other appropriate placements within reasonable proximity to their own families.

3. Policies must be revised to ensure documentation of the need for out-of-state placement for individual children. There must be continuing contact with a caseworker from a private or public agency, including periodic visits to the facility and periodic reevaluations of the appropriateness of individual placements.

4. States must develop policies that encourage parent-child visiting for out-of-state children and inform parents and children of these policies in writing. Funds for the transportation costs of visiting must be provided.

5. No federal funds should be used for the out-of-state care of children unless there is clear documentation that the placement is in the least restrictive setting meeting the child's needs and within reasonable proximity to the child's home and family.

6. The Interstate Compact on the Placement of Children should be strengthened to include clear protections for children in out-of-state placements, such as documentation by a review committee or court that out-of-state placement will not be harmful to any child to whom the Compact applies. A delegate from the sending state should be required to visit periodically the child and facility. The Compact Secretariat should be responsible for maintaining national data on the extent of interstate placements.

7. Consumer groups and regulatory agencies, including the Bureau of Consumer Protection of the Federal Trade Commission, should monitor the promotional literature of private child-caring facilities, including residential treatment facilities, to uncover deceptive and misleading advertising practices.

Part II.
State and Federal Responsibility

Chapter 4
The Role of the State

Chapter 5
The Federal Role

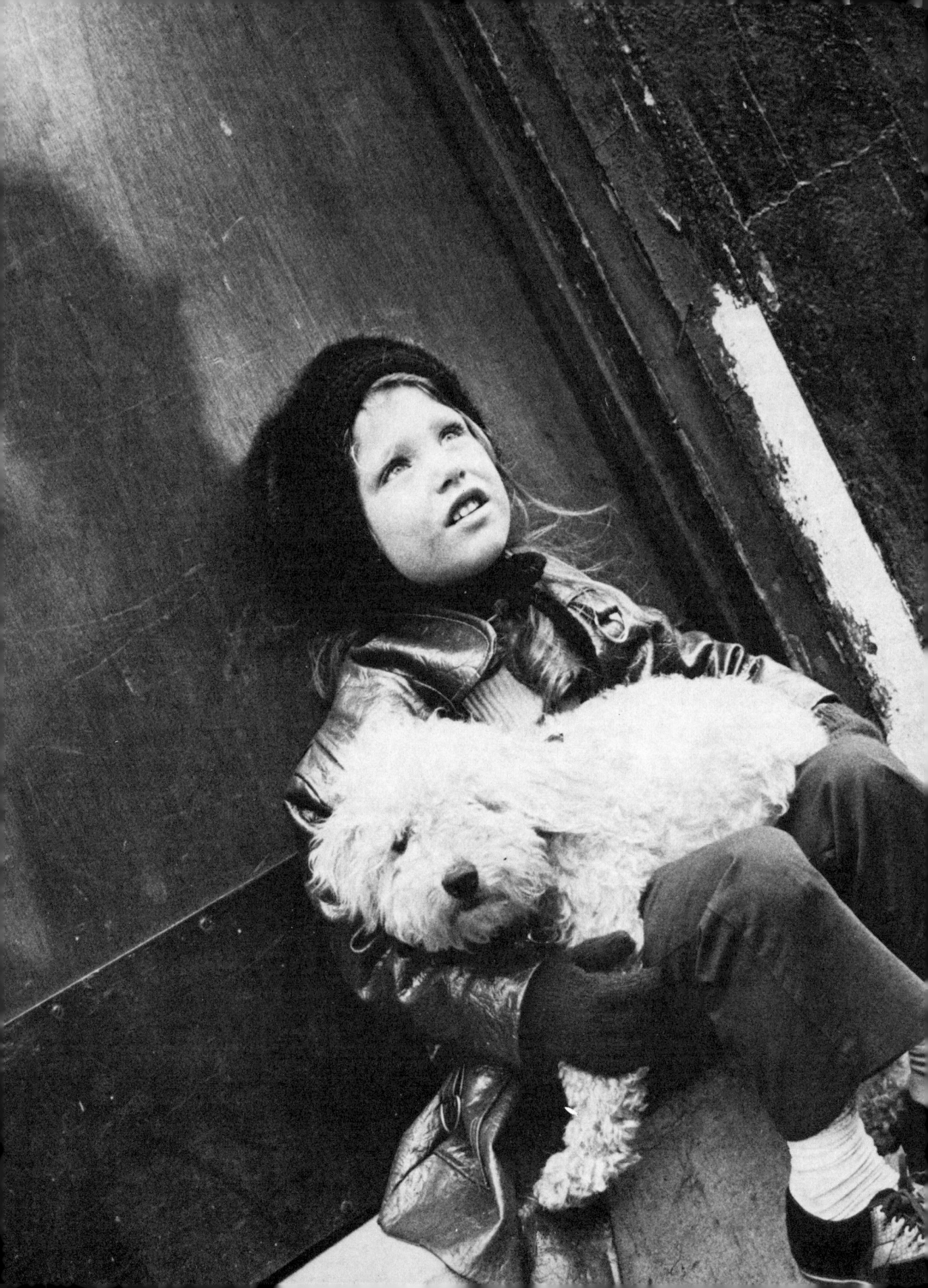

4 The Role of the State

Assessing Responsibility

The major responsibility for children without homes has historically rested with the individual state. Under the doctrine of *parens patriae* the state is empowered to intervene in families to protect children from harm. State statutes, as well as administrative guidelines and regulations, define the procedures, protections, and quality of services to which a family is entitled. State organizational structures reflect, in part, the priority and visibility given to children's services—and especially services to children at risk of removal or in out-of-home care.

Yet despite their far-reaching powers, the states have generally failed to play an active role in addressing the problems of children in out-of-home care. Too much of the state's attention has been focused on children at the point of removal from home—on just finding a place for them to live. Too little attention has been given to services that might eliminate the need for placement. Too little attention has been paid to the quality of care and services the children and their families receive. And too little attention has been given to defining who has ultimate responsibility for children out of their homes in the face of a complex delivery system that often involves courts,[1] one or more public agencies, private agencies from whom public agencies purchase services, and state and county political divisions.

The State's Responsibility

We believe that the state has eight fundamental obligations to individual children at risk of placement or in out-of-home care, and their families.

▶ To provide services that prevent family disruption and ensure that no child is unnecessarily removed from his natural family by default, coercion, or any other inappropriate means.

▶ To ensure due process rights and protections[2] to all

---

[1]The courts play a central role in the child placement process. Their jurisdiction encompasses many of the children at risk of out-of-home care and many public agencies responsible for the children. Juvenile or family courts (the name varies from state to state) may determine whether children are abused, neglected or dependent; adjudicate children as juvenile delinquents or status offenders; order out-of-home placement for certain abused, neglected or dependent children or children adjudicated juvenile delinquents or status offenders; rule on petitions to terminate parental rights; finalize the adoption of children; and depending upon the state, participate in reviewing the care received by children in out-of-home placements. Courts too may be involved in commitment procedures for mentally retarded or mentally ill children.

[2]At a minimum, we believe these due process protections must include notification prior to hearings or reviews, representation by counsel or other representative of choice, the opportunity to present evidence, to cross-examine witnesses, to attend hearings or reviews, to receive a record of a proceeding, and to have written findings concerning hearing or review dispositions.

children at risk of or in out-of-home care, regardless of which state system is responsible for them.
▶ To ensure appropriate placements, quality health care, education and mental health services, familial contact and permanence, consistent with the psychological and developmental needs of individual children out of their homes.
▶ To ensure basic due process rights and protections to the natural families of children at risk of or in out-of-home care and, where they exist, to the psychological families as well.
▶ To ensure nondiscriminatory treatment of minority children at risk of or in out-of-home care.
▶ To ensure that no child is denied permanence by state inaction regarding the provision of reunification services, or the initiation and completion of termination of parental rights and adoption proceedings when appropriate.
▶ To develop and maintain current data on both individual children and aggregate groups of children out of their homes covering how long they have been in care, provision of appropriate services, and implementation of plans for permanence.
▶ To develop and continuously evaluate the adequacy of systemwide, ongoing monitoring mechanisms for ensuring compliance with state and federal laws, court orders, regulations, and policies within all state and local systems that serve children at risk of removal or out of their own homes.

To learn more about the factors that contribute to the capacity of states to carry out these responsibilities, about state efforts to take corrective action where necessary, and about patterns of strengths and weaknesses, we studied seven states:[3] Arizona, California, Massachusetts, New Jersey, Ohio, South Carolina and South Dakota.[4] We reviewed:

1. Statutory and administrative protections addressing:
   — procedures for the removal of children from their homes;
   — periodic review procedures for children in out-of-home care;
   — procedures for the return of children to their own homes;
   — termination of parental rights and permanent planning provisions;
   — prevention of inappropriate institutionalization and/or out-of-state placements; and
   — prevention of institutional abuse.
2. Regulatory and enforcement procedures reflected in licensing standards, program reviews, complaint procedures and public reporting requirements;
3. The state administrative structure for delivering services to children;
4. The extent of state assistance to and oversight of local offices;
5. Coordination among different systems with responsibility for children out of their homes; and
6. The availability and accessibility of useful aggregate data.

This chapter summarizes our findings. Significant changes learned of since our visits are described in the footnotes.

The CDF Findings

Inadequate Statutory and Administrative Protections

Statutory and administrative protections afforded to children and families are often inadequate at all points in the placement process.

The Child Welfare System

Removal. Statutory criteria for the court's removal of a child from home are often vague and do not require that efforts be made to prevent the removal.

■ An Arizona statute, for example, defines a dependent child as: one who is adjudicated as "[d]estitute or who is not provided with the necessities of life."[5] Ohio's statutory definition of a dependent child is: one "[w]ho lacks proper parental care because of the faults or habits of his parents, guardian or custodian."[6] The relevant South Dakota statute considers a neglected or dependent child to be one "[w]ho is homeless, without proper care, or not domiciled with his parent, guardian or custodian through no fault of his parent, guardian or custodian."[7]

---

[3] See Appendices A. and J. for a description of our selection procedures, the methodology for the state study and a comparison of the study states on selected demographic variables.
[4] At the time of our visits there were, across systems, approximately 100,000 children in out-of-home placement in these seven states. See Appendix K.

[5] *Ariz. Rev. Stat.* §8–201(10)(b).
[6] *Ohio Rev. Code Ann.* §2151.03(B).
[7] *S.D. Comp. Laws Ann.* §26–8–6(5).

- No study state[8] requires that preventive services be provided to parents prior to the removal of a child in non-emergency situations.[9]

Voluntary Placements: Theoretically, a parent who voluntarily requests placement for a child is likely to see the placement as temporary. Yet, as we described earlier, some parents who place their children voluntarily in effect abandon them, either because they don't care, or, more typically, because agency policies discourage reunification. Still other parents request the return of their children but are told for a variety of arbitrary reasons they can't have them back. Our study states provide few statutory protections to children placed voluntarily,[10] or to their parents when the parents are victimized by the system.

- Only in Massachusetts is there a clear statutory reference to voluntary placements. The Massachusetts statute requires that the conditions of a voluntary placement must be agreed upon by both parent and state and may be terminated by either.[11] Statutes in New Jersey, Ohio, South Carolina and South Dakota do not even mention voluntary placements.[12]

Legal Representation. Provisions for legal representation for parents and children when children are removed from home as a result of a court hearing on a dependency, neglect or abuse petition are inadequate. Most state statutes include a general provision that children and parents have a right to counsel.[13] Few, however, *require* that the child have counsel and few specify whether or when the child shall have separate counsel, independent of both the parents and the agency providing care.[14] The study states are no exception.

- Only South Carolina requires that a neglected or abused child have both counsel and a guardian ad litem. It also requires that counsel for the child not be the same as counsel for the parent or agency.[15]

- New Jersey requires appointment of a "law guardian" to represent the child in neglect and abuse proceedings.[16]

- California, Massachusetts and Ohio statutes provide a general right to counsel for parents and child at all points in dependency and neglect proceedings, and include provisions for appointed counsel. Arizona provides that upon request, parents and children may have counsel, but does not specify notice must be provided. South Dakota has a general right to counsel, but provides for appointed counsel only if termination of parental rights is a possible disposition in a neglect proceeding.[17]

- No study state requires that counsel be appointed for parents. The New Jersey statute requires the court to inform parents of the availability of public defender services. Arizona, California, Ohio, Massachusetts and South Carolina specify the parents' right to court-appointed counsel if indigent and counsel is requested.[18]

Representation by counsel may be *pro forma*—lawyers may be either ill-prepared or over-worked. Yet

---

[8]Experimental California legislation, enacted in the spring of 1976, effective through June 30, 1981, stipulates that the court may order that services be provided to children in their own homes for up to six months as an alternative to filing a dependency or neglect petition. *Cal. Welf. & Inst. Code* §331.5. The original proposal required implementation of the legislation on a statewide basis, and allocated substantial funds for the cost of providing preventive and family reunification services. The legislation as passed permits the experiment in only two counties and provides limited funds.

[9]New York State, in 1973, also passed time-limited legislation to prevent unnecessary placements. *N.Y. Soc. Serv. Law* Ch. 911. Despite an evaluation suggesting the legislation was cost-effective, the provision has not been made permanent. However, the New York State Council on Families and Children has recently commissioned a survey of existing preventive programs in the state in order to propose administrative and legislative changes that would facilitate preventive programs. Part of the resistance to mandatory preventive services is linked to the fiscal disincentives built into federal programs. (See Chapter 5.)

[10]There must also be a clear means by which to protect the voluntarily placed child from lingering indefinitely in the system. For this reason it is crucial that independent reviews (see discussion, pp. 80-83 *infra*) apply to voluntary as well as court-ordered placements.

[11]*Mass. Gen. Laws Ann.* Ch. 119, 23 (A).

[12]The California Family Protection Act added a new detailed section on voluntary placements but it is applicable only in two demonstration counties. Among other things, it provides that a voluntarily placed minor be returned within 14 days upon parental request and within 24 hours if the request is made within the first three days of placement. *Cal. Welf. & Inst. Code* §16552. Other than this there is no mention of voluntary placements in the Code. In fact, we heard repeatedly in California that children placed voluntarily did not receive any reviews at all.

The Arizona statute says that voluntarily placed children may remain in receiving foster homes for only three weeks without a court review. *Ariz. Rev. Stat. Ann.* §8–515. The statutes say nothing about time limits for children placed in regular foster homes. (A receiving foster home is like an emergency shelter.) In practice, Arizona state officials told us they limited voluntary placements to three months.

[13]See Appendix E. for an analysis of statutory provisions for counsel in neglect proceedings in the 50 states and the District of Columbia.

[14]Frequently, when children are represented by separate counsel, that counsel is employed by the public agency in whose care they reside, regardless of the potential conflict between the child's and the agency's interests.

[15]*S.C. Code* §20–10–180.

[16]*N.J. Stat. Ann* §9:6–8:23.

[17]*Cal. Welf. & Inst. Code* §316; *Mass. Gen. Laws Ann.* Ch. 29; *Ohio Rev. Code Ann.* §2151.352; *Ariz. Rev. Stat.* §8–255 A; *S.D. Comp. Laws Ann.* §26–8–22.1,2.

[18]*N.J. Stat. Ann.* §9:6–8:43; *Ariz. Rev. Stat.* §8-225A; *Cal.Welf. & Inst. Code* §317; *Ohio Rev. Code Ann.* §2151.352; *Mass. Gen. Laws Ann.* Ch. 119 §29; *S.C. Code* §20–10–180. South Dakota, as indicated earlier, specifies the right to appointed counsel for parents only if termination is a possible disposition in a neglect proceeding.

the right to representation is a basic check on a system that has overused the placement of children. The failure of states to ensure children and parents a right to adequate counsel at the initial stages of the placement process sets the stage for many of the subsequent abuses we have identified.

Relatives. Financial barriers often prevent relatives who wish to and can otherwise adequately care for a child from doing so.

- In Arizona, New Jersey and South Dakota statutes specifically include placement with relatives as a placement option in neglect proceedings.[19] No study state prohibits such placements. Yet neither California nor New Jersey pay relatives foster care rates, and Ohio leaves the decision up to the counties.[20]

Appropriateness of Placement. The severing of parent-child ties often stems from placing the child at great distance from family and community, unnecessarily institutionalizing the child, or from failing to provide restorative services.

- None of the child welfare statutes in the study states requires that, consistent with a child's special needs, out-of-home placement be in close proximity to the child's family and in the least restrictive setting appropriate to the child's needs.[21]

- None of the child welfare statutes in the study states requires the provision of services to restore the family unit.[22]

Reviews. For a state to meet its responsibility to children, it should require individual periodic reviews for each child of the necessity of placement, the quality of current care, and the adequacy of future plans. It should also require that needed changes be carried out promptly.

- Only one study state, at the time of our visit, had established by statute a system of periodic independent reviews for children in foster care. South Carolina required that citizen boards review the cases of children in care for more than six months[23] to determine whether adequate efforts to ensure them permanence were being made.

- Although both Arizona and California[24] required annual court reviews, the reviews were unfocused and ineffective.[25]

The idea that a state is obligated to review the progress of individual children in out-of-home care is not a new one.[26] Yet, at the time of our visit there were serious inadequacies in the varied non-statutorily required review procedures in six of the seven study states. (These and subsequent changes are described in the box on pages 82-83.)

- Massachusetts did not even require a review by anyone not providing direct services.[27] New Jersey was implementing an internal administrative review system with no follow-up provision to ensure compliance.[28] The South Dakota review system focused only on the appropriateness of out-of-county and out-of-state placements.[29] Ohio, at the time of our visit, had no review mechanism.

---

[19]*Ariz. Rev. Stat.* §8–241; *N.J. Stat. Ann.* §9:6–8:54; *S.D. Comp. Laws Ann.* §26–8–35.

[20]The question of whether a state may deny AFDC–Foster Care payments to otherwise eligible children placed in the homes of relatives is currently before the Supreme Court, *Miller v. Youakim,* 431 F. Supp. 40 *(N.D. Ill. 1976),* 562 F. 2nd 483 (7th Cir. 1977), prob. jurisd. noted, 46 LW 3513, (No. 77–742).

[21]The Family Protection Act in California requires that in a demonstration county, if a placement is out of county, parents must receive written notice stating why such placement is necessary. If they object within seven days, the court must hold a hearing no later than five days after such objection is registered. *Cal. Welf. & Inst. Code* §361.5(c).

[22]There is a provision in the New Jersey statute that when there is a finding of abuse and neglect, the court may order the individual to accept evaluation for services including homemakers, group self-help programs and therapy programs if the court so requires. *N.J. Stat. Ann* §9:6–8, 58. The Family Protection Act also requires parents of children in placement to participate in counseling and requires that restorative services be provided for voluntarily placed children. *Cal. Welf. & Inst. Code* §362, §§1625–7; 16555.

[23]*S.C. Code* §43–13–10–70.

[24]*Ariz. Rev. Stat. Ann* §8–515(c); *Cal. Welf. & Inst. Code* §366.

[25]Two studies of the implementation of the judicial review procedure in two California counties concluded that the hearings were perfunctory and ineffective, with no planning or participation by caseworkers, natural parents or substitute caretakers. Wald, *State Intervention,* p. 683 and R. Mnookin, "Child Custody Adjudication: Judicial Functions in the Face of Indeterminacy," 39 *Law and Contemporary Problems* (1976): 226.

[26]Most public and private agencies, at least in theory, conduct administrative reviews. In fact, the standards for foster family care published by both the Child Welfare League of America and the America Public Welfare Association include provisions for such periodic administrative reviews of foster care cases. American Public Welfare Association, *Standards for Foster Family Services Systems* (Washington, D.C.: American Public Welfare Association, 1975), p. 25; Child Welfare League of America, *Standards for Foster Family Service* (New York: Child Welfare League of America, 1975), pp. 78–79.

[27]Administrative regulations required a review by the caseworker and supervisor, but in practice it rarely happened. In one office, we were actually told the reviews were done only if there was a new caseworker—as training, rather than to benefit the child. By statute, the court could review a case if petitioned to do so. *Mass. Gen. Laws Ann.* Ch. 119 §26.

[28]An evaluation of the New Jersey centralized administrative approach, comparing outcomes for children in care for 18 months before and after the review system was instituted, found no significant differences. Given the many structural and policy limitations of the administrative review, the findings are not surprising. That review has since been replaced by a statutorily mandated combined citizen and court review. W.E. Claburn, *Foster Care Case Review in New Jersey: An Evaluation of its Implementation and Effects* (New Jersey: Department of Institutions and Agencies, 1977).

[29]There was discussion at the time of our visit of expanding the review procedures to include all children.

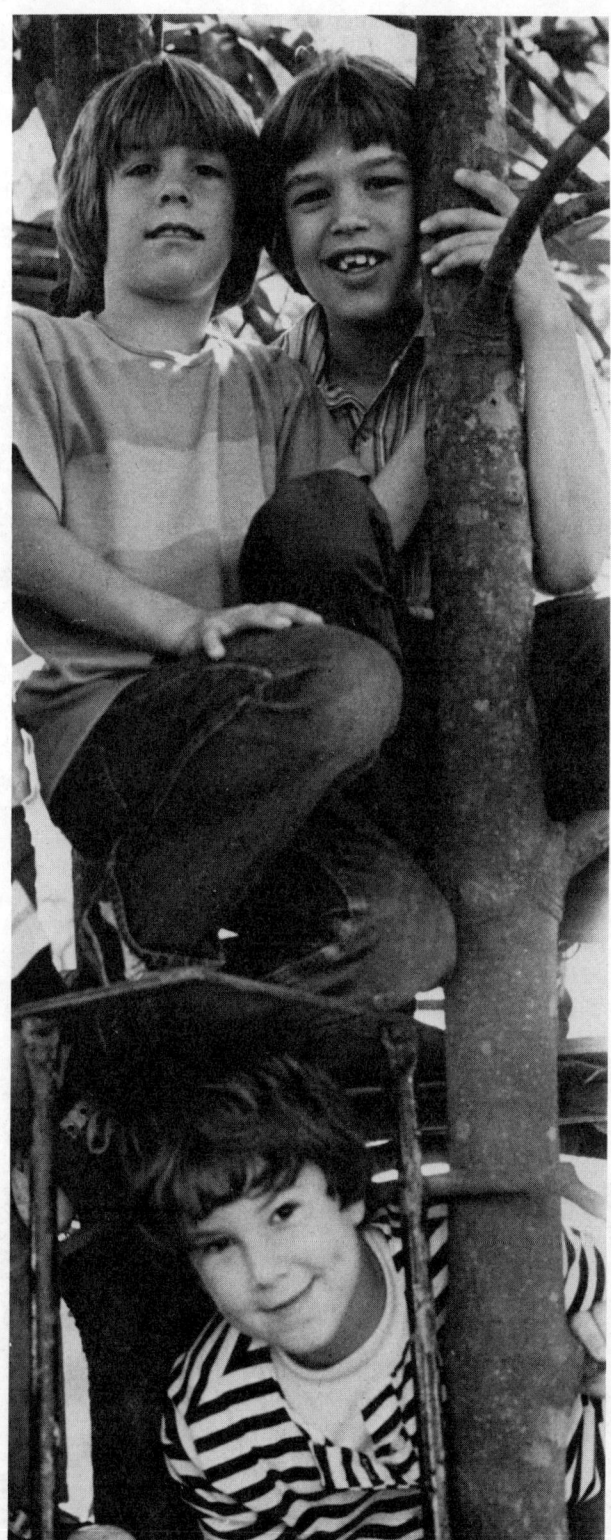

The lack of meaningful reviews for individual children out of their homes reflects a serious abdication of state responsibility.[30] It is, however, encouraging that within one month of our visit to Ohio,[31] and more recently in Arizona and New Jersey,[32] legislation mandating such independent reviews has been enacted. New review procedures in California are applicable only in two demonstration counties. We are not aware of any improvements in South Dakota or Massachusetts.

We recognize that independent statutory review mechanisms alone are not sufficient; that there must be adequate funds for implementation, provision for training of the reviewers, and continuous assessment of the effectiveness of the systems in improving outcomes for children. But the enactment of strong legislation provides a necessary starting point.

Termination. In view of the seriousness of the termination of parent-child relationships, the statutes should specify procedural and substantive protections for the child, the natural families, and where they exist, psychological families. At the very least the following types of questions should be addressed:

1. What are the grounds for severing all parental rights? Are they sufficiently specific?
2. Who has the authority to initiate termination proceedings?
3. Who has a right to counsel (child, parents, foster parents)? Do children and parents have a right to separate counsel?
4. Is the appointment of counsel for the child and for the parents, if indigent, discretionary or mandatory?
5. What procedural safeguards are provided to the child and parents at the hearing?
6. What evidence is required that efforts have been

---

[30]In the course of our study, we heard much discussion of the need at the state level for "tracking systems" for children in out-of-home care—computerized systems for recording what is happening to children and for making retrieval of this information more efficient. The establishment of such systems seems both sensible and timely—the technical expertise is readily available. But the presence of tracking systems and data collection systems does not ensure individual children will be protected. Information systems are important for other purposes, and they may be a useful tool in implementing periodic review mechanisms, but computers cannot make decisions about children.

[31]*Ohio Rev. Code Ann.* §5103.151. We visited in December 1975; the legislation passed in 1976 and became operational January 1, 1977. As of June 1, 1978, no data were available on the impact of reviews.

[32]Arizona Senate Bill 1261 (signed May 27, 1978), *N.J. Stat. Ann.* §30:4C–50.For a description of existing statutory review mechanisms in other states, see Appendix L.

CASE REVIEW MECHANISMS IN THE STUDY STATES AT THE TIME OF CDF VISITS AND AS OF MAY 1978[1]

Arizona
1976. Juvenile court required by statute to conduct an annual review to reaffirm or revise the dispositional order on each child in foster care.
1978. Local foster care review boards created by statute to review initial plans and subsequent progress reports of children in foster care every six months and to make recommendations to the court. Annual judicial review with notice to all parties required.

California
1976. Annual judicial hearings for children in court-ordered foster care required by statute with notice and right to counsel for interested parties. Probation officer required to prepare report of unspecified content.
1978. Experimental legislation, applicable to two counties, requires a court hearing every six months for children placed voluntarily or by court order in demonstration counties. Social worker or probation officer must file a report stating the services offered to the family, the progress made, the prognosis for the child and the worker's recommended disposition. Parents are guaranteed the right to be present, to be represented by counsel, and to have a copy of the report filed with the court. Judge may order any additional services to facilitate reunification.

Massachusetts
1976. Court, upon petition of interested party, required by statute to hold hearing on need for continued out-of-home care of children in court-ordered placements. Administrative regulations required review every six months by the caseworker but there were no provisions for participation by parties, reporting of decisions, appeals by interested parties, or required follow-through of decisions. The worker was charged to consider adoption after one year, and thereafter every six months if parents showed no signs of interest. No periodic review of all children in care was required by statute.
1978. No change.

New Jersey
1976. An administrative review required caseworkers to complete a pre-coded form on the status of children in care. A computer identified children for whom there appeared to be discrepancies or problems. For these children, a team from the central office (which did not include lawyers, citizen members or others independent of the agency) reviewed the actual case record and made recommendations to the regional director. The regional director was not required to accept or reject the recommendations or to report back on the actual resolution of the case. Parents, foster parents and children received no notice of the review and had no right to participate.
1978. A statute, effective October 1, 1978, requires the court to approve all placements within 15 days. It further provides for the establishment of child placement review boards in each county as an arm of the court. These boards are to review, within 45 days, and then annually, the progress of all children in placement, making recommendations, based on dispositional alternatives in the statute, to the court. The court may approve these or hold a hearing. All interested parties must receive notice of all board reviews and court hearings. An annual report on the implementation of the legislation to the governor, the supreme court and the legislature is required.

Ohio
1975. No review mechanism.
1978. A statute, effective January 1977, requires that for all children in placement a report be filed with the court within four months of placement, then annually. The judge or a board appointed by the judge must approve the report, or order it revised. No dispositional alternatives are defined in the statute, nor is there a requirement that parties receive notice that a case is being reviewed. A hearing is not required. The judge may terminate the agency's custody. Public reporting of the outcomes of the reviews is required.

[1] Citations to the statutes appear in Appendix L.

South Carolina

1976. The South Carolina review system, mandated by statute in 1974, relies on 16 citizen foster care review boards, each composed of five members appointed by the governor upon the recommendation of the county legislative delegations. The boards review cases of children in care for six months or more to determine what efforts have been made to ensure permanence for children. If an agency providing care does not intend to comply with the boards' advisory recommendations, it must notify the review boards within 21 days. All review board decisions may be reviewed judicially either upon the petition of any person questioning a board's recommendation or in instances when the board's recommendations have not been carried out.

The statute requires all public or private agencies to cooperate with local review boards in supplying information as a condition of continued licensure. Guidelines suggest that caseworkers, foster parents, biological parents, other interested parties and school-age children receive notice and be invited to attend reviews, but this is not mandated by statute.

1978. No change.

South Dakota

1976. The South Dakota review system was designed to guard against inappropriate out-of-county placements, not to provide a mechanism for continuing periodic and dispositional reviews. It was not mandated by statute. Intra-regional teams, composed of regional and local child welfare personnel and a foster parent, reviewed the necessity of the inter-county placement of children with special needs. These teams paralleled the state-level interagency team of Commissioners that reviewed out-of-state placements. While South Dakota was the only state to address so directly the geographical banishment of children, in other respects the review strategy was limited.

1978. No change.

CHARACTERISTICS OF A STRONG FOSTER CARE REVIEW SYSTEM

▶ Required by statute
▶ Applicable to all children in out-of-home care, those placed voluntarily as well as by court order
▶ Conducted independently of the public agency responsible for providing care and services to the child
▶ Conducted at specified periodic intervals
▶ Specified dispositional alternatives
▶ Time frame for a final disposition
▶ Written notice of the review and of available dispositional alternatives to interested parties including parents, foster parents, and children
▶ Right to participate afforded to interested parties
▶ Right of interested parties to bring a representative of their choice
▶ Right of appeal to a court if the independent review is conducted by a citizen review board or quasi-judicial body
▶ Provision for written record of the review, including recommended disposition
▶ Provision to ensure confidentiality of case information
▶ Provision to ensure cooperation of agencies providing services
▶ Provision to ensure training of reviewers
▶ Mandated follow-up to determine compliance with recommended disposition for each child
▶ Obligation of court or public agency to aggregate and make public data on the reviews and their outcomes
▶ Provision to ensure adequate funds to operate the review system

undertaken by the agency to strengthen the child's biological family? When can such evidence be waived?
7. What standing do foster parents have? Does their status change if they have continuously cared for a child for a significant period?
8. What consideration is given to the length of time the child has been out of the home?
9. What consideration is given to the child's wishes? At what age?
10. What, if any, procedures are defined to ensure that adoption proceedings, if appropriate upon termination, be initiated without delay?

None of the termination statutes in our study states address all, or even most, of these issues.

- Grounds for termination of parental rights are not specified at all in Ohio. Reference is simply made to permanent custody which vests in the county department of welfare all parental rights, duties and obligations including the right to adoption; and divests the natural or adoptive parents of any and all parental rights, privileges and obligations, including all residual rights and obligations.[33]
- Under the South Dakota statute the judge may, as a disposition in a neglect proceeding, terminate parental rights if the parents willfully abandoned the child for six months.[34]
- Like Ohio, Massachusetts has no termination statute, but it permits adoption without parental consent if in the best interest of the child.[35]

Only three study states direct the court to consider as grounds for termination the fact that the child has been lingering in foster care without evidence of parental interest in the child.

- The South Carolina statute provides that "if a dependent and neglected child has been in out-of-home care for six months, and the Department [of Social Services] or [private] agency has given consistent help to the parent to provide a suitable home, and the parent has made no effort to establish such a home or show concern for the child's welfare, or show that in the future that they would be sufficiently rehabilitated to do so, the court may order termination."[36]

- The California statute provides that termination may be ordered for a child who has been in foster care for two or more consecutive years and whose return to parents would be detrimental; or for one whose parents have failed, and are likely to continue to fail, to maintain an adequate relationship, provide a home, care or control.[37]
- Massachusetts provides that if a child has been in foster care for over one year, there shall be a presumption that the best interest of the child would be served by granting a petition for adoption.[38]

No study state requires that in termination proceedings the parent and the child each be represented by independent counsel.[39]

- The California statute specifies a general right of all parties to have counsel, requires the mandatory appointment of counsel for indigent parents unless they intelligently waive that right, and permits the appointment of counsel for children.[40]
- South Dakota provides for a general right of all parties to counsel, but requires mandatory counsel for indigent parents only if termination is a disposition in a neglect proceeding. There is no specific mention of counsel for the child.[41]
- Arizona provides that in termination proceedings a county attorney may represent the child. There is no requirement that counsel be appointed for parents, although a guardian ad litem is required if the mother or father is mentally ill.[42]
- The Massachusetts, New Jersey, Ohio and South Carolina statutes make no specific reference to due process protections regarding proceedings to terminate parental rights, although the general right to counsel specified in the neglect provisions apply. Administrative guidelines in the study states are also vague about when termination should be initiated, leaving workers and agencies to rely solely on their own opinions or prevailing local practices.

Grievance Procedures. Administrative grievance procedures for children and/or parents caught up in the child welfare system in the seven study states are either

---

[33]*Ohio Rev. Code Ann.* §2151.011(12).
[34]*S.D. Comp. Laws Ann.* §26–8–36.
[35]*Mass. Gen. Laws Ann.* Ch. 210 §3.
[36]*S.C. Code* §20–11–20(2)(a).

[37]*Cal. Civil Code* §232(7).
[38]*Mass. Gen. Laws Ann.* Ch. 210 §3.
[39]See Appendix E. for an analysis of statutory provisions for counsel in termination proceedings in the 50 states and the District of Columbia.
[40]*Cal. Civil Code* §237.5.
[41]*S.D. Comp. Laws Ann.* §26–8–22.1,2.
[42]*Ariz. Rev. Stat.* §8–535.

nonexistent or are merely paper mechanisms.[43]

- Five of the study states reported that they had no specific mechanisms through which parents or children could channel complaints about inadequate or inappropriate services or inequitable treatment. California outlined grievance procedures for foster care and adoptions,[44] but we found no evidence that families or those who work with them knew about the procedures. In Massachusetts there was a similar pattern of non-implementation of required grievance procedures by the adoption unit, as well as by the foster home and group care programs.[45]

The Other Child-Placing Systems

Juvenile Justice

As a result of a Supreme Court decision in 1967, all youths charged with delinquency must be advised of a right to counsel, and, if indigent, appointed counsel.[46] Beyond this, however, state statutes pertaining to children brought before the court as alleged juvenile delinquents or status offenders vary according to the definition of offenses,[47] due process protections provided, and dispositional options.

- Massachusetts requires the appointment of counsel for status offenders without any qualification. Ohio, South Dakota and California specify the child has a right to counsel although California permits the child to waive the right. The South Carolina statute makes no specific mention of counsel for status offenders, but its Family Court Rules require notice to parents or guardian of a right to counsel and for indigent parents, court-appointed counsel. Arizona requires the appointment of counsel upon request by parents, guardian or the child. The New Jersey statute requires appointed counsel if constitutionally required or if there may be an institutional commitment.[48]

- South Dakota prohibits the placement of children who have committed status offenses in training schools. Massachusetts and New Jersey prohibit their placement in facilities designated or operated for adjudicated delinquents, as well as training schools.[49] The other states do not have statutory prohibitions against such placements.

- Massachusetts limits the dispositional orders for children in need of services (that is, children involved in status offenses) to six months, although the statute provides for extensions after additional court hearings.[50] No other study state sets time limits on the dispositional orders for status offenders.[51]

- No study state requires that court-ordered placements for either status offenders or delinquents be in the least restrictive setting.[52]

Mental Health and Mental Retardation

Entry patterns within the mental health system are quite different from either the child welfare or the juvenile justice systems, as are the placement options. In general, placement within the mental health system is the result of a decision by parents or public officials responsible for children that the child's behavior or emotional state warrants hospitalization. The child is then, subject to approval by an admitting psychiatrist, voluntarily committed to a mental hospital. This kind of voluntary commitment permits the child no representa-

---

[43]In Chapter 6 we describe one effort to provide a grievance procedure for natural parents that is working.

[44]California Department of Health, Social Service Letter No. 74–17 and 74.4, May 22, 1974.

[45]Massachusetts Office for Children, "Approval Study Report, Department of Public Welfare's Foster Care Services, Part I," and "Approval Study Report on the Department of Public Welfare's Adoption Placement Services," Boston, Mass.: 1975.

[46]*In re Gault,* 387 U.S. 1 (1967).

[47]Massachusetts, for example, defines a status offender as a "Child in Need of Services"—"a child below the age of seventeen who persistently runs away from his parents or legal guardian, or persistently refuses to obey the lawful and reasonable commands of his parents or legal guardian—or a child between the age of six or sixteen who willfully fails to attend school or persistently violates the lawful and reasonable regulations of his school." *Mass. Gen. Laws Ann.* Ch. 119 –21. Arizona defines its "incorrigible child" in a similar way, but adds "who habitually so deports himself as to injure or endanger the morals or health of himself or others." *Ariz. Rev. Stat.* §8–201. In the California Code status offenses also include violations of any city, state or local ordinances; the New Jersey and Ohio codes include only violations of statutes or ordinances which are applicable to children. *Cal. Welf. & Inst. Code* §601; *N.J. Stat. Ann.* §2A:4–45; *Ohio Rev. Code Ann.* §2151.022.

[48]*Mass. Gen. Laws Ann.* Ch. 119 §39F; *Ohio Rev. Code Ann.* §2151.352; *S.D. Comp. Laws Ann.* §26–8–22-1; *Cal. Welf. & Inst. Code* §634; South Carolina, Rule 7; *Ariz. Rev. Stat.* §8–225(A); *N.J. Stat. Ann.* §2A:4–58.

[49]The Massachusetts statute permits placements of status offenders in group homes providing therapeutic care to adjudicated delinquents and referrals to the Department of Youth Services for placement in individual foster care. *Mass. Gen. Laws Ann.* Ch. 119 §39G; see also *S.D. Comp. Laws Ann.* §26–8–40.1 and *N.J. Stat. Ann.* §2A:4–62. Some states are limiting the institutionalization of status offenders administratively because of the mandate in the federal Juvenile Justice and Delinquency Prevention Act which conditions the state receipt of federal funds upon a state plan to deinstitutionalize status offenders. This is discussed more fully in Chapter 5.

[50]See *Mass. Gen. Laws Ann.* Ch. 119 §39G.

[51]New Jersey limits the commitment of a delinquent child to three years unless the offense involves a homicide. New Jersey, South Carolina and South Dakota set age limits upon the applicability of dispositional orders, although the age of children affected varies.

[52]While current federal law does not require such placement, the Juvenile Justice and Delinquency Prevention Act, as amended by P.L. 95–115, does require that states submit to the federal government annual reports on the progress made by the state to ensure that juveniles in placement are in facilities which "are the least restrictive alternatives appropriate to the needs of the child and the community" and "are in reasonable proximity to the family and home communities of such juveniles. . . ." 42 U.S.C. §5633(a)(12)(B).

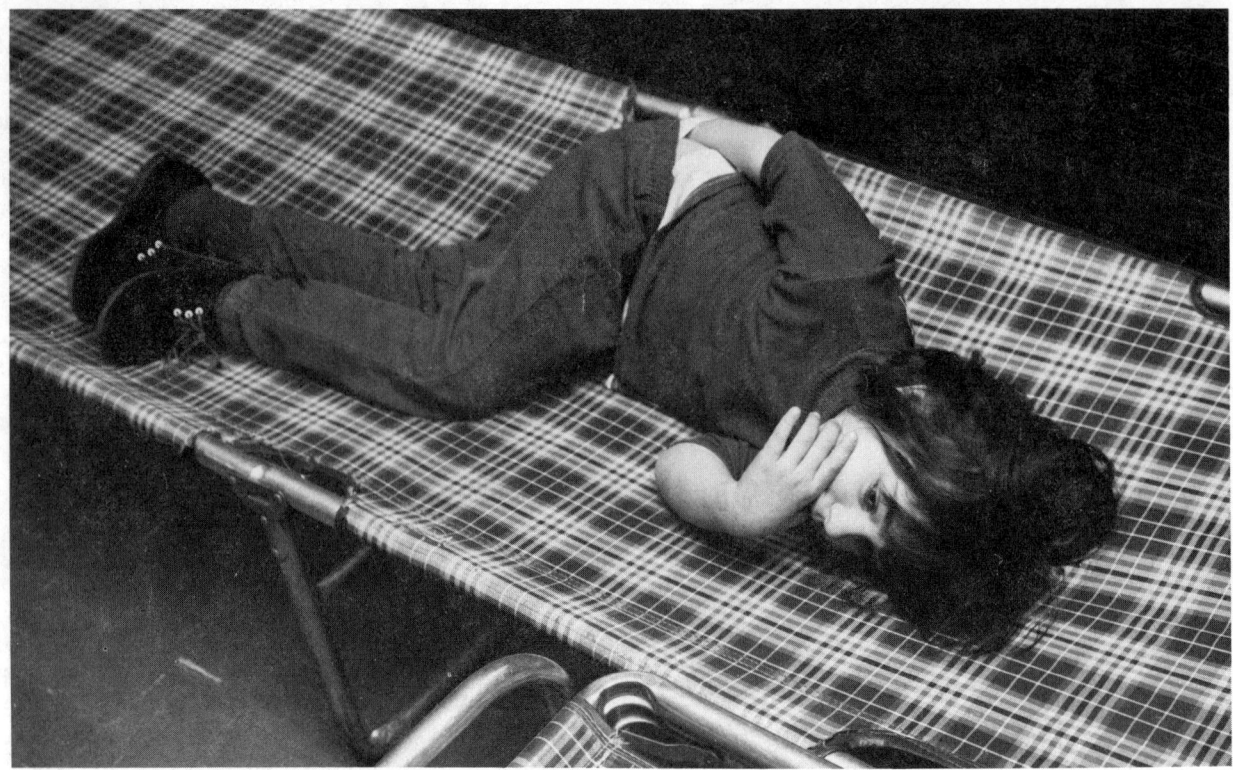

tion or other due process protections.[53] Indeed, because of evidence of abuses there have been both statutory reforms and legal challenges to the constitutionality of voluntary commitment procedures affecting children.[54]

In our seven study states, the protections afforded children against their inappropriate placement in mental hospitals varied markedly.

- In California and South Carolina a child may be voluntarily signed in by a parent or guardian with no procedural safeguards required by statute. Arizona provides that a child over 14 must co-sign the admission application.[55]

- Four study states provide voluntarily admitted minors with access to counsel. Ohio requires that, upon petition of the legal rights service, counsel, parent or relative, there be a court determination of whether hospitalization is in the best interest of a child admitted voluntarily to a mental hospital.[56] Massachusetts provides that the hospital superintendent afford the person applying for admission the opportunity for consultation with an attorney or person supervised by an attorney.[57] South Dakota outlines a specific procedure by which a voluntarily admitted minor, his counsel, or a county mental health board may object to his hospitalization. The statute further stipulates that the hospital must assist the minor in preparing an objection.[58] Under Administrative Rules of the Court, New Jersey requires that a minor have counsel and that there be a court hearing prior to a voluntary commitment.[59]

- No study state statute addresses protections for the admission of children in state custody to mental hospitals, for example, children referred by child welfare agencies for psychiatric commitment.

---

[53] This is not to be confused with involuntary commitment procedures, not addressed here, which often require a prior finding of dangerousness and afford some due process protections to the party involved.

[54] See, for example, *Bartley* v. *Kremens,* 402 F. Supp. 1039 (E.D. Pa. 1975), *vacated on other grounds,* 431 U.S. 119(1977), *on remand,* Civ. No. 72–2272 (May 25, 1978), *prob. juris. noted, sub nom. Secretary of Public Welfare* v. *Kevin S.,* 46 L.W. 3776; (June 19, 1978) (No. 77–1715); (*J.L. and J.R.* v. *Parham,* 412 F. Supp. 112 (M.D. Ga. 1976), *prob. juris. noted,* 97 S. Ct. 2647 (1977) (No. 75–1690); reargument scheduled 98 S. Ct. 761 (1978).

[55] *Ariz. Rev. Stat.* §36-518 (B).

[56] *Ohio Rev. Code Ann.* §5122.02.
[57] *Mass. Gen. Laws Ann.* Ch. 123 §10.
[58] *S.D. Comp. Laws Ann.* §27 A-8-4.
[59] *N.J. R.* 4:74-7.

- No study state statute requires that counsel or the admitting officer consider less restrictive alternatives prior to commitment.[60]

- Only the South Carolina and South Dakota statutes require clear notices to voluntarily committed patients of release procedures. Ohio requires the hospital head to make "reasonable means and arrangements" for informing patients.[61] Arizona, California, Massachusetts and New Jersey had no such requirements.

- Massachusetts provides for a periodic administrative review for both voluntarily and involuntarily committed patients specifying that alternatives to hospitalization be considered.[62]

- In New Jersey, court rules require that the court review a minor's commitment every three months until the minor is discharged or reaches majority.[63]

Only minimal attention has been given to protections for children committed to facilities for the retarded in the study state statutes.

- The South Dakota statute permits voluntary admission of a mentally retarded minor, but outlines procedures by which a person over 13 may object. Massachusetts requires the child or guardian be informed of a right to consultation with counsel. Ohio requires that upon petition by the legal rights service, the court shall determine whether voluntary admission or continued institutionalization is in the minor's best interest.[64] No other study state statute specifies procedures by which a minor may object to voluntary commitment in a facility for the retarded.

- The New Jersey statute requires that the state institution accepting a retarded person maintain contact with the person's parent or guardian.[65] No other study state imposes such an obligation.

- Only South Dakota provides for periodic annual reviews of voluntarily committed mentally retarded persons.[66] Massachusetts provides for periodic reviews and consideration of alternatives, but their frequency is unspecified.[67]

Special Education

The other system involved in the out-of-home placement of children is the special education system. Only two of our seven study states, New Jersey and Massachusetts, placed significant numbers of children through special education.

- New Jersey had no special statutory provisions protecting a child's right to appropriate placement or defining the parental role when out-of-home placement was required for educational reasons.[68]

- Massachusetts, in contrast, under Chapter 766 of its state laws, had mandated careful procedural and substantive requirements. Children with special educational needs must be identified, provided a full evaluation of those needs, and placed in the least restrictive educational program possible, with alternatives ranging from a modified school program to a residential school program. Parents are guaranteed the right to participate in educational decisions about their child, to an independent evaluation if they disagree with the school evaluation, and to due process and appeals procedures. Explicit procedures for periodic reviews are required. Parents may also bring an advocate with them to any meetings concerning their child.[69]

---

[60]The Arizona statute provides that for involuntary commitments, the court may order out-patient services prior to hospitalization. *Ariz. Rev. Stat.* §36-541. The New Jersey rules of the court provide that a minor may be admitted only if the patient is in need of intensive psychiatric therapy which cannot practically or feasibly be rendered in the home or in the community or on any outpatient basis. *R.* 4:74-7 (b).

[61]South Carolina requires that upon admission, and subsequently every six months, a voluntary patient and his guardian shall be informed and shall acknowledge receipt of such information. *S.C. Code* §44-17-340. South Dakota requires that the voluntary admission form contain such information in large type and simple language, and that such information be communicated orally to anyone 13 or over, and given in writing to the patient and other person. *S.D. Comp. Laws Ann.* §27A-8-3. *Ohio Rev. Code Ann.* §5122.03.

[62]*Mass. Gen. Laws Ann.* Ch. 123 §4. South Dakota provides for a 90-day and 11-month review, but no further reviews. *S.D. Comp. Laws Ann.* §A–12–17.

[63]*N.J. R.* 4:74-7 (f).

[64]*S.D. Comp. Laws Ann.* §27B-5-9; *Mass. Gen. Laws Ann.* Ch. 123 §10; *Ohio Rev. Code Ann.* §5123.69.

[65]*N.J. Stat. Ann.* §30:4-25.8.

[66]*S.D. Comp. Laws Ann.* §27 B-5-15. The Statute also protects in detail the personal rights of residents in a facility. *S.D. Comp. Laws Ann.* §27 B-8-2.

[67]*Mass. Gen. Laws Ann.* Ch. 123 §4.

[68]New Jersey does, however, have a statute addressing the funding of special education services for handicapped children. *N.J. Stat. Ann.* 18A:46–1.1 *et seq.*

[69]Public Law 94-142, the federal Education for All Handicapped Children Act passed in 1975 and subsequently amended, requires that by September 1978 *all* states provide procedural protections to handicapped children and their parents similar to those in Chapter 766. See, Children's Defense Fund, *94–142 and 504: Numbers that Add Up To Educational Rights For Handicapped Children* (Washington, D.C.: Children's Defense Fund, 1978).

The Limits of Statutory Reform

It is clear that the statutory protections provided to children and families involved with the child welfare and other child placement systems need to be strengthened in specific ways to define a clearer framework of state responsibility, and to provide grounds for systematically challenging implementation failures. In the past few years, there have been a number of efforts to define more explicit criteria for what happens to a child at various points in the placement process.[70] We support many of these efforts. But it is also important to recognize that although strong statutes are necessary, they alone are not a sufficient guarantee of quality care for children. Quality services and adequate fiscal resources are also essential. Reform efforts, therefore, must seek the difficult balance between improving the framework of protective rights and ensuring adequate services within the child serving networks.

Ineffective Licensing Standards and Program Reviews

Licensing standards often give inadequate attention to children's rights and the quality of programs and services in facilities for the out-of-home care of children. Information about licensing and program evaluations, when it exists, is not made available to those who place children.

Licensing Standards

The power to define and maintain minimum standards which agencies and facilities caring for children out of their homes must meet is a traditional state function. Licensing of facilities, in fact, is one of the most routinely accepted components of state responsibility to these children. To determine the specificity and scope of licensing provisions for out-of-home care in group settings in our study states,[71] we analyzed the licensing standards[72] and talked with officials, providers and advocates. Our discussion below is limited to the licensing of institutions under child welfare auspices in the study states.[73]

The content of the licensing requirements varies considerably in the study states.

- Program standards in South Carolina and South Dakota were vague. Ohio's licensing regulations did not even mention program standards for group homes. New Jersey, in contrast, under its program requirements included standards for admission, treatment plans, provision of child care, social, vocational and religious services, recreational, health and mental health care, education, administration of medication, participation in community life and aftercare services. The New Jersey regulations did not, however, specify a facility's obligation to the child's family.

- Only California and Massachusetts required that reports of licensing evaluations be available to the public. California required that an abbreviated form of the report be available, Massachusetts the entire report.

- No licensing regulations in the study states explicitly referred to institutional abuse, specified procedures for reporting abuse, or identified sanctions to be applied if children were abused in group settings.

- Grounds for suspension, denial or revocation of licenses varied greatly in specificity. For example, South Carolina cited only failure to maintain proper standards of care and service. Massachusetts included refusal to admit a representative of the licensing agency or to submit required reports. Arizona regulations specified as grounds misrepresentation by any employee or director regarding services to children or

---

[70]See, for example, the standards for children involved with the courts developed by the IJA-ABA Juvenile Justice Standards Project. Institute of Judicial Administration and American Bar Association Joint Commission on Juvenile Justice Standards, *Standards Relating to Abuse and Neglect* (Tentative Draft) (Cambridge: Ballinger Publishing Company, 1977).

[71]Approval, certification or licensing of foster homes is very often delegated to local jurisdictions, while the state carries out the task of licensing group facilities. We focused on the state role and group facilities because of our concern about the inappropriate use of such facilities, although we realize there are many difficulties in the licensing of foster homes.

[72]Our analyses are based on the following sources: *Arizona:* Group Care Agency Licensing Standards (Article 74, Revised 6–77); Group Foster Home Licensing Standards (Article 59, Revised 3–77). *California:* Laws and Regulations Relating to Licensing of Community Care Facilities. Excerpts from the California Health and Safety Code and the California Administrative Code, effective August 31, 1975. *Massachusetts:* Regulations for the Licensing or Approval of Agencies Placing Children Into Family Foster Care or Group Care, published October 31, 1974. *New Jersey:* Manual of Standards for Residential Child Care Facilities, New Jersey Division of Youth and Family Services. *Ohio:* Rules for Child Care Agencies and Boarding Homes. *South Carolina:* Basic Requirements for Licensing Child Caring Institutions and/or Agency Operated Group Homes. *South Dakota:* Standards for the Licensing of Group Homes for Minors.

[73]In general, children's mental retardation and mental health facilities are licensed by units with responsibility for all mental health and mental retardation facilities. Juvenile correction facilities are typically exempt from licensing but are supposed to be monitored by juvenile correctional personnel.

physical, sexual or emotional abuse, but they did not cite actual abuse of children. The California Code required that personnel be instructed in the detection and reporting of suspected physical abuse while a resident was away from a facility. None of the regulations in our study states cited evidence of abuse of children as grounds for suspension.

- Only the California and Massachusetts licensing regulations specified explicit procedures for reporting, investigating and acting on citizen complaints about violations of standards in particular facilities.

- Licensing provisions in all study states except New Jersey provided for exemptions. Some, like California, were given at the discretion of the agency director—others categorically. South Carolina, for example, exempts all religious institutions in existence since 1959.[74] A state official estimated that currently 10-15 percent of the residential child care facilities in the state are unlicensed.

- Arizona, California, Massachusetts and South Dakota included nondiscrimination clauses in their licensing regulations. Ohio, South Carolina and New Jersey stipulated that the facility must comply with the federal Civil Rights Act or ensure the admission of children and provision of services on a nondiscriminatory basis.

In addition to weaknesses in the licensing authority that limit the scope of public accountability for licensing procedures, we also learned of serious operational problems within the licensing units.

- Licensing units were uniformly understaffed. Massachusetts had *one* staff person in each of nine regions with responsibility for over 300 foster care and day care facilities. In Ohio, the licensing staff reported it was lucky to visit each facility once every two or three years, although the licensing statute required annual visits.

- Even if facilities met licensing requirements at the time of a scheduled visit, the mechanisms for ensuring continuing compliance were inadequate.[75]

- Licensing staffs in California, Ohio and New Jersey reported that even if they identified facilities that should be closed, it was very difficult to carry out a closing.[76] New Jersey alone reported a policy of trying to force substandard facilities out of business by not placing any children in them.

- Licensing was, in general, isolated from other placement processes. Licensing evaluations were not even routinely shared with, or made available to those who must make decisions about where to place children, including the courts.[77]

- Only one state, Massachusetts, required that foster care and adoption programs administered by the Department of Welfare be approved by the licensing office and evaluated for compliance with the state's licensing regulations.[78] All the other study states required only that facilities in which children were placed meet state standards.

Program Reviews

In recognition of the general weakness of licensing as an effective regulatory tool, and particularly as a response to the need to evaluate program content more thoroughly, New Jersey and Massachusetts have been experimenting with the use of program reviews. In Massachusetts, the Department of Youth Services, which is responsible for delinquent youths, had established a special program evaluation unit. In New Jersey, program evaluations were conducted by the Bureau of Residential Facilities, a special unit within the state child welfare agency.

---

[74]The exemption of religious institutions from state licensing requirements reflects a longstanding pattern that results in the exclusion of large numbers of children from any protection from the state. There is little rationale for assuming that religious institutions are more likely to provide appropriate care to children than facilities established under other auspices. Therefore excluding them from the purview of the state is unjustified, particularly when the state itself places children in such facilities. However, often religious groups providing services (as well as other providers) are effective lobbyists for continuing exemptions or maintaining standards at a minimal level.

[75]Only Arizona and California reported making unscheduled visits.

[76]We were told that a major reason why so few facilities were actually closed related to the alleged political influence of the owners. We were not able to investigate these allegations adequately but evidence from licensing enforcement failures uncovered in investigations of nursing homes suggests this is not unlikely. See, M. Mendelsohn, *Tender Loving Greed* (New York: Alfred A. Knopf, 1974). We note, that while the CHAMPUS staff at the time of our visit was routinely sending reports of the facilities it inspected to state licensing agencies, including specific information on violations of the CHAMPUS standards, few states were reported to be interested in following up on violations. Arizona was identified as an exception.

[77]In Chapter 3, for instance, we reported that several state administrators were concerned about the refusal of other states to share licensing information about facilities to which out-of-state children were sent. At the local level, those with direct responsibility for placing children must rely on informational brochures, or the grapevine. In Los Angeles County, for example, the child welfare staff had developed its own internal "do not refer list," although they did not share this list with other counties. Yet, California, on paper, had the strongest licensing regulations of our study states.

[78]See Massachusetts Office for Children, "Approval Study Report of Foster Care Services" and "Approval Study Report, Adoption Placement Services."

RIGHTS OF CHILDREN SPECIFIED IN GROUP CARE LICENSING STANDARDS IN THE STUDY STATES

Arizona
Prohibits corporal punishment and one child punishing another as a form of discipline, but specifies no restrictions on the use of seclusion or the administration of drugs. Protections for handicapped children are the strongest, including the requirement that discipline and control policies be posted and available to parents.

California
Guarantees all persons in community care facilities such rights as: the right to be informed of complaint procedures; to have family informed of progress; and to be given (or have parents given) copies of rights upon admission. Provisions for children further require that rules of discipline be in writing and available to staff working with children.

Massachusetts
Prohibits research or experimentation involving children, but does not mention corporal punishment, seclusion, or the use of drugs. Specifies the right of parents to summaries of a child's progress reports.

New Jersey
Prohibits an agency from admitting a child to a facility without evidence in the child's referral material that institutional placement is the most appropriate plan for the child. Prohibits any form of convulsive therapy except in JCAH-accredited facilities and in accordance with JCAH standards. Parents and other individuals important to the child have the right to reasonable visiting privileges at the discretion of the administration. Written disciplinary policies must be explained to staff and children (there is no mention of parents). Prohibits group punishment for individual misbehavior, humiliating or degrading punishment, corporal punishment, withholding of food, denial of visitation, isolation for more than two hours in any 24-hour period, delegation of punishment authority to other children or to persons on duty not known to the children.

Ohio
Licensing standards do not specify rights of children.

South Carolina
Licensing standards do not specify rights of children.

South Dakota
Licensing standards do not specify rights of children.

There are no standard criteria for conducting program reviews, but in general they require on-site visits and include reviews of case records and interviews with individual children at the facilities, as well as some assessment of the quality of services provided, the comprehensiveness of the program and the adequacy of staff qualifications.

Program evaluation is relatively uncharted territory. Yet, as efforts to assess program quality get underway, a number of problems attached to the process are beginning to emerge.

- In Massachusetts, the program evaluations prepared within the Division for Youth were not shared with either those who placed children directly or with those negotiating new contracts for service. Moreover, evaluations were usually conducted only in response to a specific crisis or complaint.

- In New Jersey, CDF staff were told the program evaluations were shared with the unit negotiating rates and contracts with the facilities providing out-of-home care. However, in reviewing explanatory materials sent to facilities prior to the evaluation, we saw no indication that the evaluations would be part of the rate setting process.

Thus, the program review process risks being as isolated from the mainstream of decision making as is the licensing process. At the same time, it has the potential of being a viable mechanism for increasing knowledge about facilities to which children are sent, and increasing the extent to which those facilities are held accountable for the care they provide. For program reviews to be effective however, the results of such reviews must be widely disseminated to and used by those who actually place children and those who negotiate purchase-of-service contracts. They include information critical to the rate setting process and to the procedure for rejecting facilities for state children.

Administrative Structure Not Related to Quality Services

The organization of children's services is varied and complex. Yet we found anti-family policies, public neglect, and failure of state responsibility regardless of the organizational structure.

There are many who argue that reorganization is the key to more effective services for children and families. Indeed, between 1970 and the time of our visits,[79] major reorganizations affecting children's services had occurred in four of our study states—Arizona, California, Massachusetts, and South Dakota. We were particularly interested in the administrative location and structure of children's services because it provides an indication of the official visibility of children's services in the state, and a clue to the extent of cross-system coordination.

We found considerable variety in organizational patterns and in the extent to which children's services were given organizational priority in the study states at the time of our visits.[80]

- In Arizona and California, children's services were buried in large conglomerate agencies.[81] The subdivisions dealing with children had very little influence on policy or practice.

- In New Jersey, Massachusetts and South Dakota, children's services were also lodged in umbrella agencies, but were given greater visibility.[82]

- In Ohio and South Carolina, children's services were divided among traditional agencies.

The Structure of Child Welfare Services

We also examined the organization of child welfare services within the overall state framework for children's services. Four of the study states, Arizona, Massachusetts, New Jersey and South Dakota are state-administered, while the remaining three states are county-administered. In a county-administered system the staff are county employees. In a state-administered system the staff, even in district or local offices, are state employees.[83] Within this scheme, however, tremendous organizational variety and complexity exists.[84] Below we highlight a few of the complexities we found:

- In Massachusetts the child welfare system was decentralized and regionalized, with different functions at different levels of government. For example, a referral of an abused child for long-term foster care required a shift from the regional agency to a local agency. But if the child was an adolescent needing placement in a group home after an unsuccessful stay in a foster home, the placement responsibility moved from the local office to the state group care office. In the meantime, the child's family had to deal with workers from both regional and local levels and the child with staff from regional, local and state levels. This process, coupled with high staff turnover, does not facilitate a sustained relationship between a worker and either a child or a family.

- In California, New Jersey and Massachusetts, the adoption unit was separate from the other child welfare services. In California, adoptions were entirely state-administered, while the other child wel-

---

[79]Since then, we have learned of further changes in almost all the study states.

[80]Appendix M. identifies for each of the study states the state systems responsible for children in out-of-home care in 1976.

[81]In the Arizona Department of Economic Security, for example, children's concerns competed for political and policy attention with veteran and employment concerns. In California, children's services were in the department which also had responsibility for state hospitals, Medical (California's Medicaid program) and community services and licensing. Since our visit, California has passed and implemented legislation to reorganize once again: this time to dismantle the huge umbrella agency and create a Department of Social Services separate from the Department of Health. Arizona is considering a similar strategy.

[82]In New Jersey, the child welfare agency, the Division of Youth and Family Services, had standing equivalent to other major units within the umbrella agency. In Massachusetts, the Office for Children seemed to be a factor in focusing attention on children's services. In South Dakota, the relatively small size of the bureaucracy facilitated communication. Since the time of our visit, South Dakota has also created an Office on Children and Youth.

[83]As of December 1977, 19 states described their welfare systems as county-administered, the remainder as state-administered. (Telephone conversation with personnel at the American Public Welfare Association, January 6, 1978.)

Regardless of whether child welfare is county or state-administered, the state usually provides some financial support, although the extent of support varies by state. In South Carolina, for example, the state provided all non-federal funds. In Ohio, a survey of 71 of the 88 counties found that state funds accounted for only four percent of the child welfare costs, county funds 61 percent and federal funds the remainder. Citizens Committee for Ohio Children's Services, *The Citizen's Survey of Ohio County Children's Services Program, 1977.*

In California, the county share varied depending upon whether a federal program was involved. For federally eligible children, the federal share was 50 percent; the state paid 33.75 percent of the first $120, the county the remainder. For non-federally eligible children, the state paid 67.5 percent of the first $120, the county the remainder. California Department of Benefit Payments, *Public Assistance Facts and Figures, December 1975* (Sacramento: Department of Health, February 9, 1976).

[84]See Appendix N. for a description of the structure of child welfare functions in each of the study states at the time of our visits.

fare services were county-administered. In New Jersey, the Bureau of Resource Development, responsible for adoptions, was a separate unit within DYFS established to free adoption workers from other tasks and allow lower caseloads. In Massachusetts, an adoption referral required a shift from a local office to the state adoption unit. In practice, the referral flow of potential adoptive children from foster care units to adoption units was a problem in all three states.

- In Ohio, South Carolina and Arizona, the licensing unit for children's facilities was located within the basic family and children's service unit. In California, licensing of children's facilities was carried out by a central state licensing unit responsible for all facilities, including hospitals and nursing homes for the elderly.

Organizational complexity does not necessarily mean that services to children must be fragmented or that decisions must be drawn out and inconsistent with a child's sense of time. We therefore looked at the organization of the state's child welfare system in conjunction with state efforts to see that the system worked effectively.

What we found was very disturbing. Regardless of whether the system was administered by states or counties, the state child welfare agency failed to exercise adequate oversight over the local offices (regional, district or county), or to provide meaningful technical assistance or training to them. As one Ohio child welfare worker commented: "State oversight is absolute except when it is important."

- In California, the Family and Children's Service Unit had official responsibility for child protective services, family planning services, 24-hour out-of-home services, information and referral, and health care services for children. Responsibility for preventive services had just been eliminated. The Unit was charged with providing technical assistance to the counties, drafting and supervising implementation of regulations and taking corrective action when necessary. But it is not surprising that, with a total staff of six to cover 58 counties, no one we talked to within the counties knew the name of the one foster care

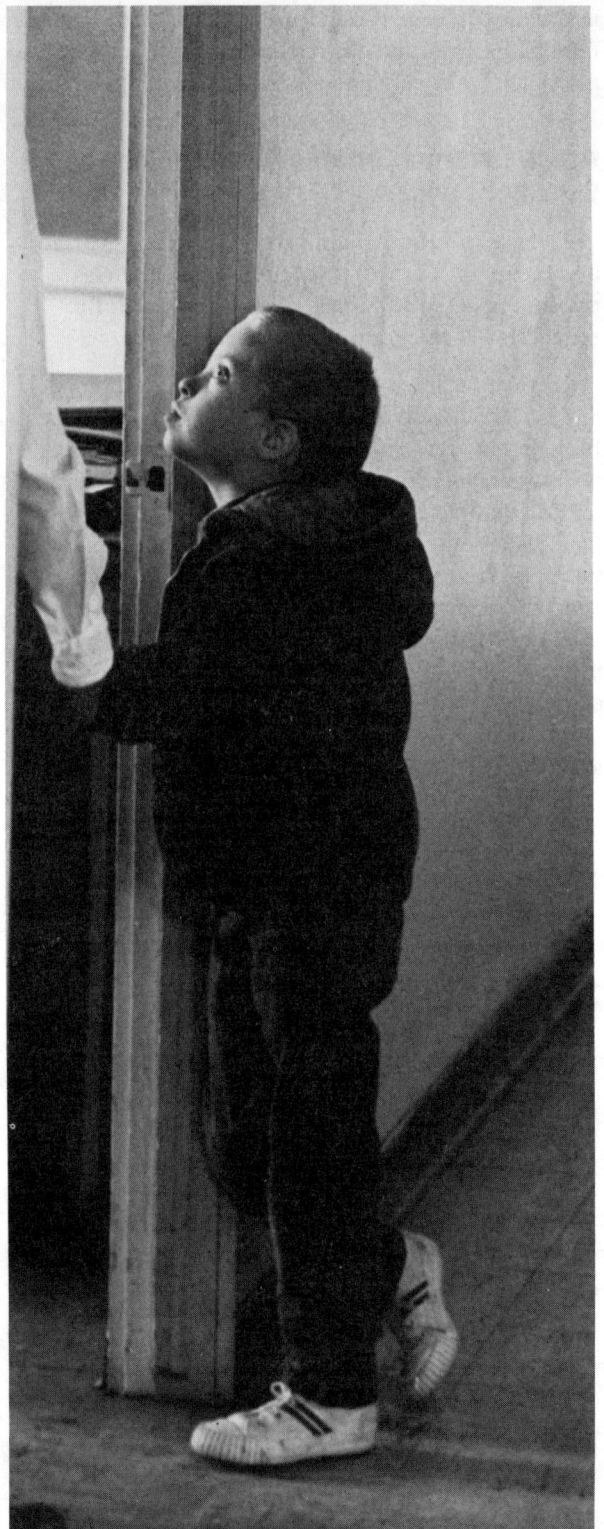

consultant at the state level.[85]

In reality, the state staff told us they spent most of their time working with federal and state officials and legislators and drafting regulations. When questioned about their oversight function, the staff said that in the past they had at least tried to review some case records; now all they could do was review county statistics. The only formal training conducted by the state in the counties for the two years preceding our visit was on how to complete federal forms accurately.

- In Ohio, the state staff concerned with child welfare was demoralized. According to the Director of Social Services in a letter to CDF: " . . .continuous efforts are made to update materials which affect the administration of child welfare services."[86] In fact, at the time of our visit, the child welfare manual had not been revised since 1961, and the licensing regulations since 1959. We heard of a staff member who had developed a handbook on adoption under one administration, but was refused funds to distribute it to the counties after a new administration took office. Further, the state had taken the position that it could offer technical assistance to a county only if the county requested it.

- In South Carolina we learned that although at least one county reported receiving substantial help from the state in relation to adoption, two years after a new statute on termination of parental rights was enacted, the state had done little to ensure that caseworkers knew about its provisions.

Theoretically, a state office should have more control over its own employees in local offices than over county employees in a county-administered child welfare system. However, in practice, there appeared to be no differences in the oversight role of the state, regardless of the administrative structure.

- In Arizona, the complex state structure mitigated against any real accountability. The director of Family and Children's Services, the unit responsible for child welfare services, had relatively low status in the organizational chart of the Department of Economic Security. She had no direct responsibility for the child welfare staff in the local field offices who were accountable to the Assistant Director of the Field Services Division.

- In New Jersey, the central staff recognized the problem of inadequate oversight, but had been unable to solve it. In that state, part of the problem stemmed from demoralization within the district offices in the face of caseload pressures and inadequate basic support from the central office. In one district office, for example, even as the state was asking its citizens to report child abuse, the office phones were so overused that the caseworkers were giving clients phone numbers of two public phone booths outside the office.

- In Massachusetts, the state's deliberate efforts to regionalize responsibility without any effective overall coordination strategy, coupled with the absence of any effective staff training, appeared to be a significant factor in the failure of state oversight.[87]

- Only in South Dakota did the problem of oversight seem manageable, in part because of the relatively small numbers of children and staff involved, and in part because of the general energy and commitment of the state staff.

- No study state had established any specific procedures for monitoring discriminatory treatment of minority children in out-of-home care on a statewide level. We did find that several counties, on their own initiative, were making special efforts to improve services delivered to minority children and their families.

There are many reasons for the lack of oversight. In California, the state had failed to staff the Family and Children's Services unit adequately. In Ohio, the political climate and lack of leadership conveyed to the state employees a message to do nothing. In New Jersey, a conscious effort to strengthen the organization

---

[85] In 1974, the California Auditor General's report found staff in the Family and Children's Service Unit inadequate for exercising its oversight responsibility for children in foster care. It recommended the staff be increased to twelve. Office of the Auditor General, *The State's Role in Foster Care in California* (Sacramento, California: January 1974, p. 17). At that time, there were three full-time foster care consultants. At the time of our visit two years later one consultant was responsible for both oversight and working with foster parent associations in all the counties.

[86] Letter to CDF staff from the Director, Division of Social Services, Ohio Department of Public Welfare, February 12, 1976.

[87] A Massachusetts study of all state systems serving children reported, "Staff training consists of. . .crash courses in basic survival techniques, the indoctrination of procedures and the completion of forms. Virtually no professional staff development exists. True professional development is discouraged and often denied a worker. No agency offers a comprehensive training program to their staffs and there are none that are planned. Training, inservice or otherwise, is given lip service, and only that. Most training is on-the-job, a technique that insures that mistakes will be made with children's lives." D. M. Sheehan, *The Children's Puzzle: A Study of Services to Children in Massachusetts* (Boston: Institute for Governmental Services, University of Massachusetts, February 1977), p. 39. (Recall the comment to CDF staff in one local Massachusetts office that administrative case reviews were conducted not for the children, but to train new workers.)

and staffing in the central office had occurred at the expense of the district offices. In Arizona, the structure of the umbrella agency, and in Massachusetts, the decision to regionalize were important. But, regardless of the reason, the outcome was the same. The states had no first-hand knowledge or control over what was happening to the children who were their responsibility. Neither, as we have shown, did the local offices.

The Structure of Other Child-Placing Systems

Juvenile Justice

Responsibility for children brought before the courts as juvenile delinquents or status offenders is often shared by the courts, probation officers, and correctional agencies. Most typically, probation offices are locally administered,[88] either by the court or the county. There is also often a state juvenile correctional authority to which a court may commit a juvenile. Sometimes this state authority is part of the adult correctional system, sometimes it is independent. In three of our study states—Arizona, South Dakota and New Jersey—the state juvenile correctional program was part of the adult system; in the remaining four it was independent. Yet, as in the child welfare system, responsibilities and obligations varied widely regardless of organization.

- In Arizona, within the adult correctional agency, no one person had designated responsibility for juvenile corrections.

- In South Dakota, an Office of Juvenile Corrections within the Adult Corrections Division had responsibility for developing alternatives to commitment to state training schools.[89] The training schools themselves were run by the South Dakota State Board of Corrections and Charities.

- In Massachusetts, the Department of Youth Services was responsible for the placement of adjudicated delinquents in community-based and other facilities.

The Department purchased services in these facilities. Massachusetts training schools were eliminated several years ago,[90] but the Department had secure detention facilities for limited commitments.

Mental Health and Mental Retardation

Few mental health or mental retardation systems in our study states had designated specific administrative units responsible for meeting the needs of children.

- Massachusetts had an Assistant Commissioner for Children's Services at the state level and regional assistant directors for children's services. These positions were created in response to a highly critical report by the Massachusetts Advocacy Center.[91]

- The Office for Children in the Ohio Division for Mental Health was a token unit with a part-time director and an assistant. At the time of our visit, the director of that office had not ever met the Commissioner of Mental Health and Mental Retardation.

- In two other study states, South Carolina and California,[92] individuals within the mental health structure had some designated responsibility for children, but lacked a clearly defined organizational base.

None of the seven states had specific organizational units for retarded children. This at least partly reflects, as one official explained, the distasteful but traditional view that "*all* retarded citizens are children"—a view

---

[88]Thirty-two states had state-administered welfare systems, but only 11 had totally state-administered probation systems for juveniles. In some states, county probation offices had the option of contracting for state administration. National Council on Crime and Delinquency, *Probation and Parole Directory* (Hackensack, N.J.: NCCD, 1976).

[89]Since our visit, the Youth Services Program, initiated in 1974 to provide diagnoses and placements for children referred by local courts, has been abolished. Placement is now the responsibility of a new Unified Court Services Program.

[90]See Chapter 2, footnote 41 for further discussion of deinstitutionalization efforts in Massachusetts.

[91]Task Force on Children Out of School, *Suffer the Children: The Politics of Mental Health in Massachusetts* (Boston: Task Force on Children Out of School, 1972).

[92]While California had only one state staff person working full time on children's mental health issues, there had been some effort at state leadership. In 1975, local mental health directors adopted minimum standards for children and youth mental health that included general principles, management, planning and coordination and treatment service standards. The standards required that at least one mental health professional in each county be identified as responsible for planning, implementing and administering mental health services for children and youth. They also required the identification of a budget for children and youth mental health services and that special services be available to dependent/neglected children and juveniles in the juvenile justice system. Resolution of the Conference of Local Mental Health Directors, "Minimum Standards for Children and Youth Mental Health Services," October 1975.

In at least two California counties we visited, mental health services were perceived as a helpful resource to the child welfare agencies. While this may or may not be related to the state effort, California was the only state in which such a comment was spontaneously made. At the same time, the state oversight role in children's mental health services was clearly limited. So, for example, although the state conducted program reviews of county mental health services for children, and shared the reports with the counties, it had no leverage for requiring the counties to make any changes.

In South Carolina, the Commissioner had created an Office of Youth Services to serve as a resource to the Commissioner of Mental Health. It had no planning or standard setting function.

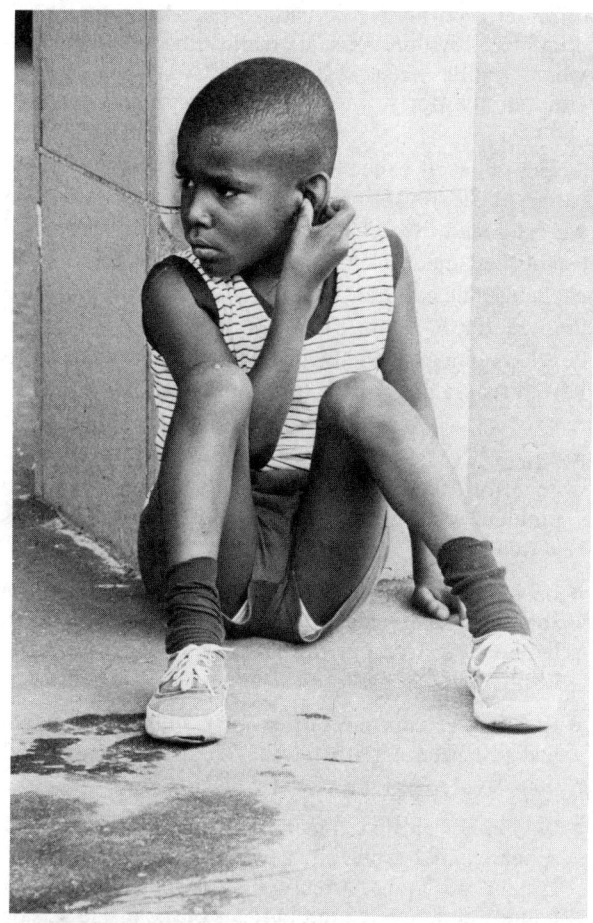

were we able to examine the adequacy of the study states' efforts to educate institutionalized children.[94]

Weak Links Across Child-Placing Systems

Children who are the responsibility of different child-placing systems often have similar needs, but efforts to reduce fragmentation and ensure the children high quality care across systems are virtually nonexistent.

In theory, each of the public child care systems responds to children with different needs.[95] The mental health system, for example, is responsible for severely emotionally or behaviorally disturbed children or children with psychotic disorders.[96] The juvenile corrections system is responsible for delinquent children and children who commit status offenses. The child welfare system has historically cared for children without handicaps whose parents could not care for them.

But in reality, the boundaries between systems are much more vague and frequently overlap. Increasingly, for instance, as a result of broader reform efforts to decriminalize and deinstitutionalize status offenders, services to and placement of status offenders fall to child welfare systems. In the CDF survey of probation offices, for example, 19 percent of the children for whom placement was ordered were referred to child welfare agencies.[97] Countless others may be referred without any court proceeding, as part of diversion efforts. Massachusetts, by statute, has transferred most

coming repeatedly under challenge. The South Carolina Department of Mental Retardation did purchase foster care for retarded children and could provide supplemental medical funds to assist a family in maintaining a child at home. California had created 20 nonprofit referral centers under contract to the state Department of Health to serve California's handicapped, including the retarded. Yet, the director of the program could not tell us how many of the 39,000 people served were children, either in or out of their homes.[93]

As only two of our study states placed substantial numbers of children out of home through special education, we did not explore this system in detail. Nor

---

[93]She also admitted that often the children and their workers got separated from one another and that monitoring by the state was inadequate. Counties reported great frustration with the regional centers, some saying it took up to four months just to get a diagnostic assessment of a child. An independent commission also found evidence of discrimination against minority groups in the provision of mandated services.

[94]We note here, however, that two of the study states did have special bureaus for this purpose. New Jersey had established the Garden State School District with responsibility for the education of all institutionalized persons. However, at the time of our study, the district was concentrating on the educational needs of prisoners, not children. Massachusetts had created the Bureau of Institutional Schools Program to maintain a school department for school-age children in public institutions maintained by the departments of mental health, public health and youth services. The Bureau was responsible for approximately 2500 school-aged children in 13 state institutions and hospital schools. The Bureau of Institutional Schools Program, "What We Are; Where We're Going." (Undated mimeo.) The Bureau has been plagued by budgetary and staff difficulties, and has only been responsive to a small group of children within its jurisdiction. In fact, the Massachusetts Association for Retarded Citizens filed suit in 1975 to force the agency to provide services for all children under its mandate, and has continued to put pressure on the agency. *Mass. Assn. for Retarded Citizens, Inc. et al v. Michael S. Dukakis et al.* C.A. No. 75-5024-C (D. Mass.). In Ohio we were told that when the Division of Special Education requested permission to budget for the education of children in institutions, permission was refused.

[95]The court, as discussed earlier, may be involved with all of these children. (See footnote 1, supra.)

[96]Community mental health centers are, in fact, serving a broader range of children, but typically they are run by counties and loosely linked to the state system, which often has a strong institutional bias.

[97]These include delinquents, status offenders and dependent and neglected children. See Appendix C. for a full discussion of the findings.

of the authority for status offenders from the juvenile justice system to the child welfare system.

All public child care systems deal with adolescent children exhibiting mild to moderate behavioral difficulties. Moreover, often the child welfare system also deals with severely retarded or mentally ill children who have been refused care or discharged by the other child care systems. Sometimes, in jurisdictional debates about which system should have responsibility, the children get completely lost and no one accepts responsibility until there is an explosive crisis.

Harry, a 14-year-old, was declared a child in need of supervision and referred by the court to a child welfare office. While waiting for placement, he set fire to a building, causing extensive damage. No private treatment facility or secure setting would accept Harry. The Community Mental Health Center said he was too disturbed for them to treat as an outpatient. He was placed, in desperation, in a regular foster home, which he systematically destroyed. No one could get him help until he set fire to himself. Then he was accepted for inpatient care in a psychiatric hospital. Throughout this period Harry kept asking for help, saying he was frightened and knew something bad would happen.

The fact that there are "exchangeable children"—children with similar needs who become the responsibility of different systems—leads to a number of consequences. Often several public agencies may provide the same services. Competition is fostered in purchasing services from private providers, with each public system negotiating different rates for the same service from the same provider.[98] It often means different reporting and visiting procedures for children placed within the same facility, depending upon which public agency is paying. And it leads to children like Harry being rejected by one system after another.

The plight of exchangeable children was mentioned to varying degrees in each of our study states. Therefore we examined the extent to which the study states had established mechanisms to: monitor what happens to exchangeable children; equalize protections for all children in out-of-home placement across systems; and develop comparable data available across systems. We have discouragingly little to report.

- Arizona, California and Ohio appeared to have made no effort at all even to identify the extent of the problem within the state or compare policies across systems.

- In New Jersey, the Director of the Division for Youth and Family Services had assigned some of his staff to be liaison personnel with juvenile justice and mental health staff.

- In South Dakota, an Office for Children and Youth had just been administratively created, but its functions were as yet undefined.

- In South Carolina, the Office of Child Advocacy appeared to be making an effort to address cross-system problems affecting children out of their homes, although the initial focus of the office was on the child welfare system.

- The most formal coordinating mechanism existed in the Office for Children (OFC) in Massachusetts. By statute,[99] the OFC has a mandate to: act as the standard-setting and licensing agency for children's facilities; provide information and referral services; organize and provide technical assistance to a network of regional councils for children; and provide for interdepartmental program coordination, evaluation and monitoring. Significantly, it is also responsible for preparing a children's budget showing state expenditures for children across systems.

---

[98] The California Association of Children's Residential Centers reports that in its 61 member facilities, 46 percent of the children were referred by child welfare agencies, 33 percent by probation, three percent by mental health agencies, and seven percent by other agencies. Seven percent of the referrals were private.

In Massachusetts, at the request of the Chairman of the Massachusetts House Ways and Means Committee, a study was conducted of publicly supported children's services, including children out of their homes. It cited figures showing that in 1975-76, the Department of Public Welfare and the Department of Youth Services each spent over three million dollars to purchase care in the same facilities. The same report also related the problem of exchangeable children to the heavy use in Massachusetts of purchase of services, noting: "There is a discernible pattern emerging. The state agencies and the local schools are responding to an escalating demand for services by a population of children with similar needs, and they are contracting with identical agencies in the private sector to serve those children. The major differences between all of the contracting agencies are most often not determined by type of client, methods of service, or type of private provider; the differences are dollars, numbers of clients, bargaining strength, and the organizational maze a child must travel in order to get the service." Sheehan, *The Children's Puzzle*, pp. 29 and 36.

[99] *Mass. Gen. Laws Ann.* Ch. 785.

Massive Information Gaps on Children and Programs

Adequate systems[100] for gathering data on children at risk of or in placement within and across child-placing systems seldom exist.[101]

- Only two study states, California and New Jersey, had, at the time of our visit, developed statewide, comprehensive information systems enabling the routine gathering of aggregate data.[102]

- No study state could provide information on: the types and extent of in-home services received by children; the number of children entering into foster care after receiving in-home services; the numbers of children moving from one system to another (e.g., child welfare to mental health) or repeatedly entering and exiting from the child welfare system.

- Study states varied considerably in the amount of information available on efforts to ensure children permanent homes. In Massachusetts, for example, we were told data would have to be compiled manually to provide information on adoptions. Only two study states, California and South Carolina, could tell us how many foster parents had adopted foster children in the past year; only three, California, New Jersey and Ohio, how many subsidized adoptions had been approved.[103]

Because the California and New Jersey data systems showed some signs of promise in this otherwise bleak picture, they are described briefly below.

The California data collection system[104] incorporated information on children in foster care who were the responsibility of not only the child welfare system, but other systems as well.[105] A foster care registry was filled out for each child at the point of placement, annually and at discharge. The registry included information on age, race, sex, type of facility, number of moves, monthly payment rate, date of last evaluation, legal status, type of service provider, child's problem, reason for initial placement, and what happens to the child at the point of discharge: i.e., transfer to another system, return home, adoption. Data were fed into a

WHAT A GOOD DATA COLLECTION SYSTEM SHOULD TELL ABOUT ALL CHILDREN IN CARE

A good data collection system should enable a state to compile periodically aggregate statistical reports describing *all* children in out-of-home care including:

▶ The number of children by age, race and sex in various types of placements and the length of time they have been in care

▶ The number of children by age, race and sex for whom parental rights have been terminated but who have not been placed in adoptive homes

▶ The number of children by age, race, sex and type of placement who entered care during the preceding year

▶ The number of children by age, race, sex and type of placement entering care during the preceding year who first received services to prevent the need for placement; and a description of the services

▶ The number of children by age, race and sex for whom dispositional reviews were conducted during the preceding year and the outcomes of these reviews

▶ The number of children by age, race and sex for whom parental rights were terminated during the preceding year; and the number of those who have been placed in adoptive homes

▶ The number of children by age, race and sex who moved out of care during the preceding year and the disposition of these cases

▶ The number of children by age, race and sex adopted with subsidies by foster parents, relatives or others during the preceding year

---

[100]The boxes detail the types of information which we believe good data collection systems should provide.

[101]For a discussion of data gaps from a national perspective, see Chapter 5.

[102]South Dakota was willing to gather special information for us, but did not do so routinely. Ohio collected only data on numbers of children in care and the cost, as required by the federal government. (We were told county reports to the state were often inaccurate.) The new Ohio review legislation requires information on reviews be made public and thus more comprehensive data should be available in the future. South Carolina published basic data in an annual report on child welfare. Neither Massachusetts nor Arizona had any systematic procedures for routinely gathering data on children within or across systems. However, since our visit, Arizona has developed, but not put into full operation, a computer system.

[103]See Appendix O. for an analysis of the available adoption related data in the study states.

[104]See the series of publications on children in foster care, California Department of Health, Center for Health Statistics, *Data Matters Topical Reports*.

[105]The usefulness of this approach is further dependent upon the availability of adequate within-system data. In this context, recall that the Director of the Regional Developmental Centers in California could not tell us how many children the centers served or how many of the children were out of their homes.

WHAT A GOOD DATA COLLECTION SYSTEM SHOULD TELL ABOUT EACH CHILD IN CARE

A good data collection system should enable a state to know at least the following about *each* child in its care:

▶ Date of birth, sex, age, race and religion
▶ Family structure, including nuclear and extended family members
▶ Any handicapping conditions. If so, whether the child has been evaluated and provided free special educational services
▶ How the child entered care (court order or voluntary placement) and the nature of the custody agreement
▶ Geographic location upon entry into care
▶ How placement is funded
▶ Reason for placement
▶ Date and type of initial placement
▶ Services provided to child and family prior to placement
▶ Placement status of siblings
▶ Dispositional goal for the child and time by which the goal should be attained
▶ Other agencies providing services to or having responsibility for the child and the family
▶ A record of case transactions including:
    — dates of and changes in legal status
    — dates, type and location of subsequent placements
    — dates of case reviews
    — dates and description of outcomes of dispositional reviews
    — dates and description of services provided to the child and family by the responsible agency and other agencies with which the child or family has contact
    — dates of visits between agency and child, agency and natural parents, agency and foster parents, and child and natural parents
    — date of termination of parental rights
    — barriers to adoption when parental rights are terminated
    — date of discharge and discharge status (e.g., with natural parents or relatives; adoptive placement; transferred to other state agency; reached majority; marriage; death; other)
    — whether child was adopted with the assistance of a subsidy and by whom (i.e., foster parents, relatives, other)
    — dates child reenters placement through this or another agency

computer system and the aggregate information made public.

The California system did have weaknesses. For example, it did not provide data on the types of previous placements, or on changes in legal status during the course of placement.[106] And at the time of our visit, there were no plans to link the system in any way with periodic reviews of the progress of children in out-of-home care. Moreover, all non-child welfare reports were lumped together and not reported by system.

The development of the New Jersey data collection system was tied to the administrative review system described earlier.[107] It gathered information similar to the California system, but only on children placed by the Division of Youth and Family Services. Reports of child-caseworker and parent-caseworker contacts were also included. However, unlike the California system, there was no provision for periodically making aggregate data public.

As we argued in discussing periodic reviews for

---

[106] A 1974 auditor general's report recommended additional inclusions such as the number of children moved from the foster care program in the county welfare departments to county probation departments, the California Youth Authority or other public assistance or probation programs; the number of times a child had been returned to his parents and subsequently re-entered foster care programs; and the types of services provided. Office of the Auditor General, *The State's Role in Foster Care in California*. These suggestions were not adopted.

[107] It is not yet known what data will be collected under the new New Jersey Review System, to become operational October 1, 1978.

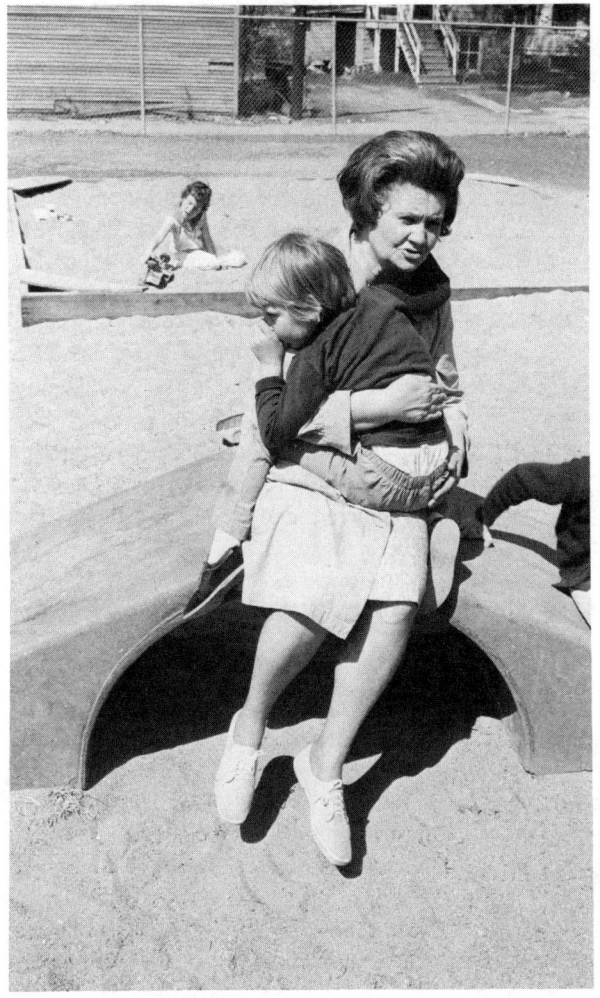

individual children, an efficient data system is no guarantee that care for children will be improved. It is merely an enabling device essential for planning, program evaluation[108] and monitoring.[109] But the absence of a data system makes protecting children against banishment that much more difficult.

Minimal State Efforts to Give Families a Voice

Children and families are provided with few avenues for information or action on their complaints.

Complex human service bureaucracies are a fact of life. Too frequently individual parents and children are at a loss when trying to work their way through these bureaucracies to secure appropriate services. Further, when they have complaints they have nowhere to turn. Yet only two of our study states, Massachusetts and New Jersey, had created any special mechanisms within the state structure to provide a voice, either individually or collectively, for the children and families at risk of or in out-of-home placement or for foster parents and others who care for the children.

- The Massachusetts Office for Children, mandated to provide information and referral services, has created Help for Children (HELP), a telephone "hot line." Staff provide service information and, if necessary, also intervene with other agencies to try to act as case advocates for the children.[110] HELP also controls a small amount of discretionary purchase-of-service funds.

- In 1974 the New Jersey Department of the Public Advocate was created by statute to provide a voice for New Jersey citizens with complaints or problems.[111] The Department represents individual children in abuse and neglect cases, and has established a small child advocacy project to deal with more general problems affecting New Jersey's children.[112]

Neither of these strategies has been evaluated, yet they both represent at least an acknowledgement by the state that consumers of children's services are entitled to some assistance in coping with bureaucracies and in ensuring that they receive the services to which they are entitled.

---

[108]It is, for instance, difficult to set goals for adoption if there is no information on how many children have had no contact with natural parents for a defined period. If there are no data on the types of placements available in each area, it is difficult to determine why a particular county is sending too many children out of state. If there are no adequate data on placements by race, it is difficult for the state to identify discriminatory practices.

[109]An overview of child welfare in 25 states reported, "Few states were observed to have developed operative links between monitoring systems and needs assessment and corrective actions." Department of Health, Education and Welfare, Office of Human Development, Children's Bureau, *Child Welfare in 25 States—An Overview* (Washington, D. C.: HEW, 1976), p. 87.

[110]The Fiscal Year 1975 OFC Annual Report noted that Help for Children received over 50,000 phone calls, 17,172 of which required more than information. Of these latter calls, 5,759 could not be resolved because services did not exist.

[111]*N.J. Stat. Ann.* §52:27E-1-47. The Office includes the Division of Citizen Complaints, the Division of Rate Counsel, involved in setting utility rates, the Division of Public Interest Advocacy, which is empowered to bring class action suits, the Division of Mental Health Advocacy, with a dual mandate to protect persons at risk of institutionalization or institutionalized (both as individuals and as a class), and the Office of the Public Defender, which is comparable to a legal services program.

[112]For example, the office has been challenging the inappropriate out-of-state placement of New Jersey children and the continuing illegal placement of status offenders in secure detention facilities.

What Can Be Done?

The problems of children out of their homes have not been taken seriously enough by states. Their callous and costly inaction must be challenged until corrected by the development of a strong protective framework that holds state systems accountable for the outcomes to children and for public moneys expended in their behalf. Below are detailed recommendations about what can be done for children *now* out of their homes, and for children who in the *future* may be at risk of out-of-home placement.

Reviewing Children Now In Care.

1. **Each state should review promptly the plans for every child currently in out-of-home care to ensure the child permanence. Priority should be given to children out of their homes for more than 18 months.**

   a. Each state should immediately identify those children in out-of-home care who can be returned to parents or relatives, those children who should be placed for adoption, and those who cannot be returned home or adopted, but who should be placed in less restrictive settings such as permanent group care or foster family homes.

   b. Each state should ensure that an appropriate plan for permanence for each child is developed and implemented within a reasonable period of time.

   c. Each state should monitor at periodic intervals the speed with which such plans are implemented.

   d. Each state should report publicly and regularly about the outcomes for all children reviewed.

Ending Inappropriate Out-of-State Placements

2. **Each state should analyze the extent to which its children are banished to other states. Children inappropriately placed out-of-state must be returned to their own families or provided appropriate in-state placements. New procedures to prevent inappropriate future out-of-state placements should be devised and new in-state services created as necessary.**

   a. There should be written documentation for every out-of-state placement showing that appropriate care cannot be received in state. The treatment and care children receive should be monitored periodically to ensure its continuing appropriateness.[113]

   b. Each child in an out-of-state facility should be visited periodically by a caseworker. Standards for caseworker-child contact should be no less stringent than for children in in-state facilities. Funds for at least annual parent-child visits should be provided by the state.

   c. Each out-of-state facility should be periodically inspected by officials of the sending state.

   d. Analyses of new in-state services necessary to prevent the overuse of out-of-state placements must be conducted and necessary funds and support generated to ensure adequate in-state resources.

Preventing Unnecessary Placements

3. **Each state should take concrete steps to ensure that no child is removed from his natural family unnecessarily.**

   a. State child welfare statutes should define the state's responsibility to provide specific services to prevent out-of-home care prior to removal unless a parent refuses service or an emergency removal is required for a child in danger of substantial and immediate physical or emotional harm.

   b. State statutes pertaining to the commitment of children to mental health or retardation facilities should ensure due process protections to the children and mandate that less restrictive alternatives first be considered except in emergency admissions.

   c. Local legal and community groups should review placement practices to determine whether out-of-home placement is being used appropriately. Any abuses should be challenged.

   d. Budgetary processes, including the distribution of federal funds, must be carefully monitored. Advocates should challenge the disproportionate

---

[113]States for example might establish interagency review teams when children from several state agencies are placed out of state.

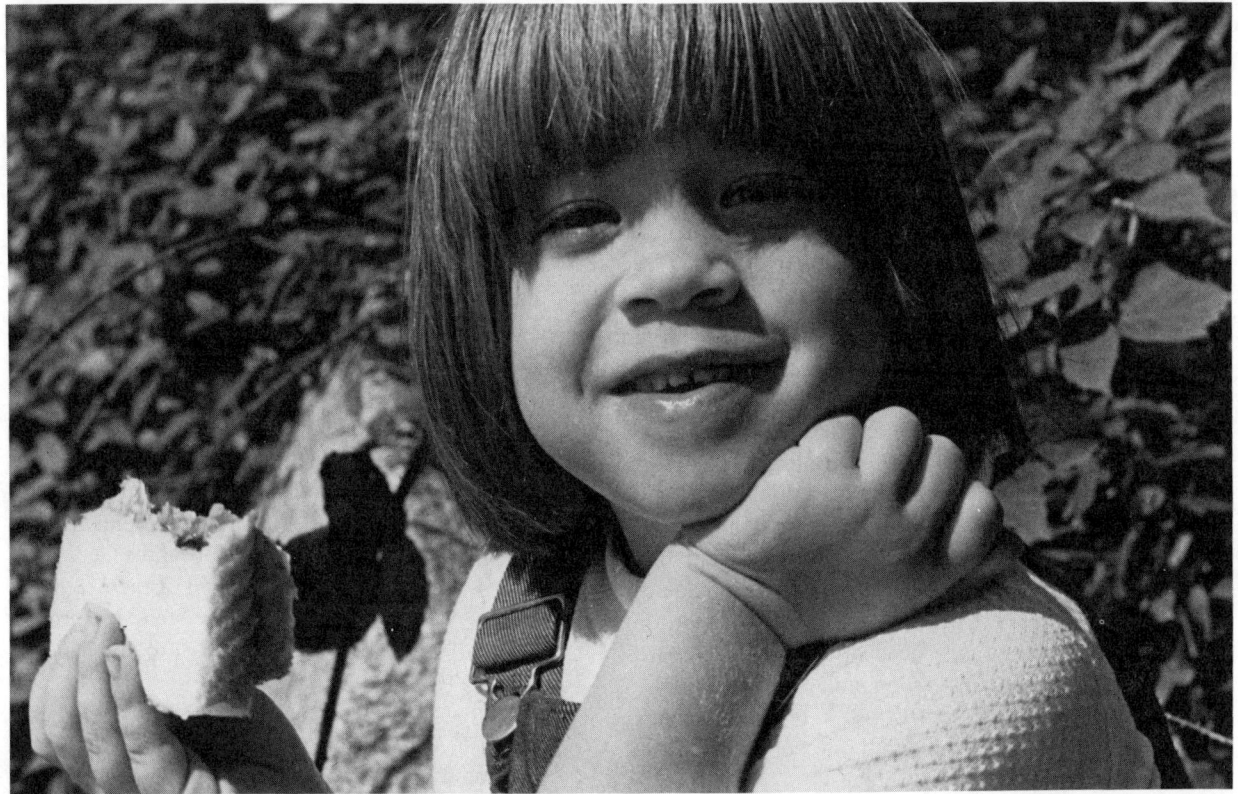

allocation of resources for out-of-home care in comparison to services to the family and/or child in his or her own home.

e. Each state should develop and then evaluate clearly defined preventive service projects. A percentage of foster care funds should be reallocated or new state resources allocated for this purpose.

Guaranteeing Children Families

4. Each state should take concrete steps to reverse anti-family practices and policies affecting children who are removed from their homes.

a. Parents who enter into voluntary placement agreements must be informed in writing of their responsibilities and rights, including their right to have the child returned upon request unless dependency or neglect proceedings are instituted or parental rights terminated. Parents must also be informed of the procedures by which to request the return of their child.

b. The possibility of placement with caring relatives should be explored prior to a child's placement with strangers.

c. Funds should be made available for reunification services, including transportation for parent-child visits, trial home visits, transition and follow-up services.

d. Each child care system should separately or together provide an ombudsman whose functions include responding to complaints from parents, foster parents, children who are in out-of-home care, and advocates on their behalf.

e. Public officials should have a statutory obligation to maintain and encourage parent-child ties wherever possible and to document the extent of parent-child contacts in order to facilitate timely decisions about reunification or termination of parental rights.

f. Specific guidelines directing caseworkers when to consider termination should be promulgated.

g. When adoption is appropriate, interested foster parents should be granted priority for consideration as adoptive parents for children in their care.

Ensuring Quality Care

5. **Every state should take concrete steps to end the abandonment by public systems of children in placement and to ensure quality care to them.**
   a. States should establish maximum caseload standards and provide the necessary resources to reduce the caseload burdens on those who work directly with children and their families.
   b. Written policies specifying caseworker-child contact should be reviewed. While flexible rather than specific standards are desirable as long as minimal levels of contact are defined, no state or locality should permit *uniformly* less contact for children in group homes, residential treatment facilities, and institutions than for children in foster family homes. Regardless of where the child is living, the amount of contact should reflect the child's needs.
   c. No child should be placed in a residential treatment setting or institution unless there is clear documentation about why a less restrictive alternative, such as a group home or specialized foster home, is not possible.
   d. Each state should develop and publicize specific mechanisms for reporting institutional abuse. Licensing statutes should specify reporting procedures and state sanctions for such abuse. Child care staff should be trained in identification and reporting procedures. All confirmed reports of institutional abuse should be reported to the purchase-of-service units.
   e. Training should be provided at the direct service level to enable workers to work effectively with and plan adequately for children in their care, review their cases periodically, and implement permanent plans within the shortest time possible.

Increasing Protections

6. **Each state should take concrete steps to increase and equalize the statutory and administrative protections afforded to children by public systems having major responsibility for them.**
   a. Every child entering the child welfare system should have his case reviewed administratively at least once every six months. Parents should be notified of this review and have the right to be present and to be accompanied, if they wish, by an advocate.
   b. Statutes should mandate that no later than 18 months after a child's entry into care through the child welfare system, a dispositional review take place. At that review, a determination should be made as to whether the child should be returned to his family, freed for adoption, placed in another permanent setting, or permitted to remain in a foster care setting for a specific time period. The review should be open to interested parties and be conducted either by a court or by a specially constituted review board. The decision of such a board should be appealable to a court, with full due process protections. Parents, foster parents and the child should be provided with written notice of the review and of their right to counsel. There should also be statutory provisions for follow-up action to ensure the disposition is implemented.
   c. Parents and children should have the right to counsel at all legal proceedings related to out-of-home care for a child. They should receive notice of this right. Counsel should be appointed if parents are indigent. Parents and children should have mandatory separate counsel at termination proceedings. Counsel for the child should always be independent of the public agency charged with the child's responsibility.
   d. Other public child care systems charged with responsibility for the out-of-home care of children should develop periodic review mechanisms to guard against children becoming lost in the system. These review mechanisms should include both internal administrative reviews and reviews independent of the agencies administering and/or providing services. Various due process protections—the right to notice, to participate in and to be represented by advocates or counsel at review proceedings—should be afforded to parents and children.

Improving Data Systems

7. **Each state should develop data collection systems that provide up-to-date information on**

the status of individual and groups of children at risk of removal and in placement, the amount of funds expended on their behalf, and the effectiveness of these expenditures.

  a. Each state should develop a data collection system to track a child while in the system and to provide basic aggregate information on all children in publicly funded out-of-home care.
  b. Each state should, at periodic intervals, make public aggregate data on children out of their homes on a system-by-system and county-by-county basis.

Enforcing Compliance

8. **Each state should eliminate patterns of discriminatory treatment of children at risk of or in out-of-home care by virtue of race, ethnic background or handicapping conditions.**

   a. In states with large percentages of minority children, the state human rights commission or its equivalent should investigate discrimination in: placement practices; care provided to minority children out of their homes; efforts to ensure the adoption of minority children; and patterns of in-state institutionalization and out-of-state placement. The findings should be made public. Advocates should take action as required, including legal action.
   b. The state human rights commission, a state office for civil rights, or its equivalent, should be charged with ongoing responsibility for monitoring discrimination toward children out of their homes.
   c. States should assume responsibility for monitoring agencies' compliance with Section 504 of the Rehabilitation Act of 1973, which prohibits discrimination on the basis of handicap.

9. **Each state should review the adequacy of its licensing statutes, program evaluations and purchase-of-service contracts, as well as its enforcement capacity.**

   a. Licensing statutes should address the quality of care provided and the rights of children in residential treatment centers and institutions.
   b. Statutes and administrative regulations governing program evaluations and licensing reports should require their distribution to agencies responsible for placing children and their public availability.
   c. Purchase-of-service contracts should specify performance standards. Contracts should require facilities to reach out to parents, to report to parents about their child's progress, and to provide the agreed-upon level of care, remediation and education to each child in care. Noncompliance should result in loss of service contracts.

10. **Each state should monitor local compliance with existing state policies more vigorously.**

    a. Special audits of local programs should be conducted periodically.
    b. States should ensure funds or provide directly for ongoing substantive in-service training to local staff.

Eliminating Fragmentation

11. **Each state should develop specific strategies to eliminate fragmentation both within and across systems in the administration and delivery of services to children.**

    a. State offices for children or their equivalents should be mandated to act as advocates on behalf of children out of their homes, and given specific responsibility for monitoring the state's budgetary commitments for preventive and restorative services.
    b. States should establish a special review team to examine problems within and across systems affecting children at risk of removal or in out-of-home care. Such a team should recommend specific statutory, regulatory, and organizational changes to ensure equal treatment across systems and to minimize fragmentation in the decision-making process.
    c. Every state department of mental health or its equivalent should be required to assign specific high-level responsibility for planning and oversight of children's mental health services, including linkages between institutional and community-based services. Greater organizational and programmatic efforts should be made to ensure an appropriate education to children in institutional care.

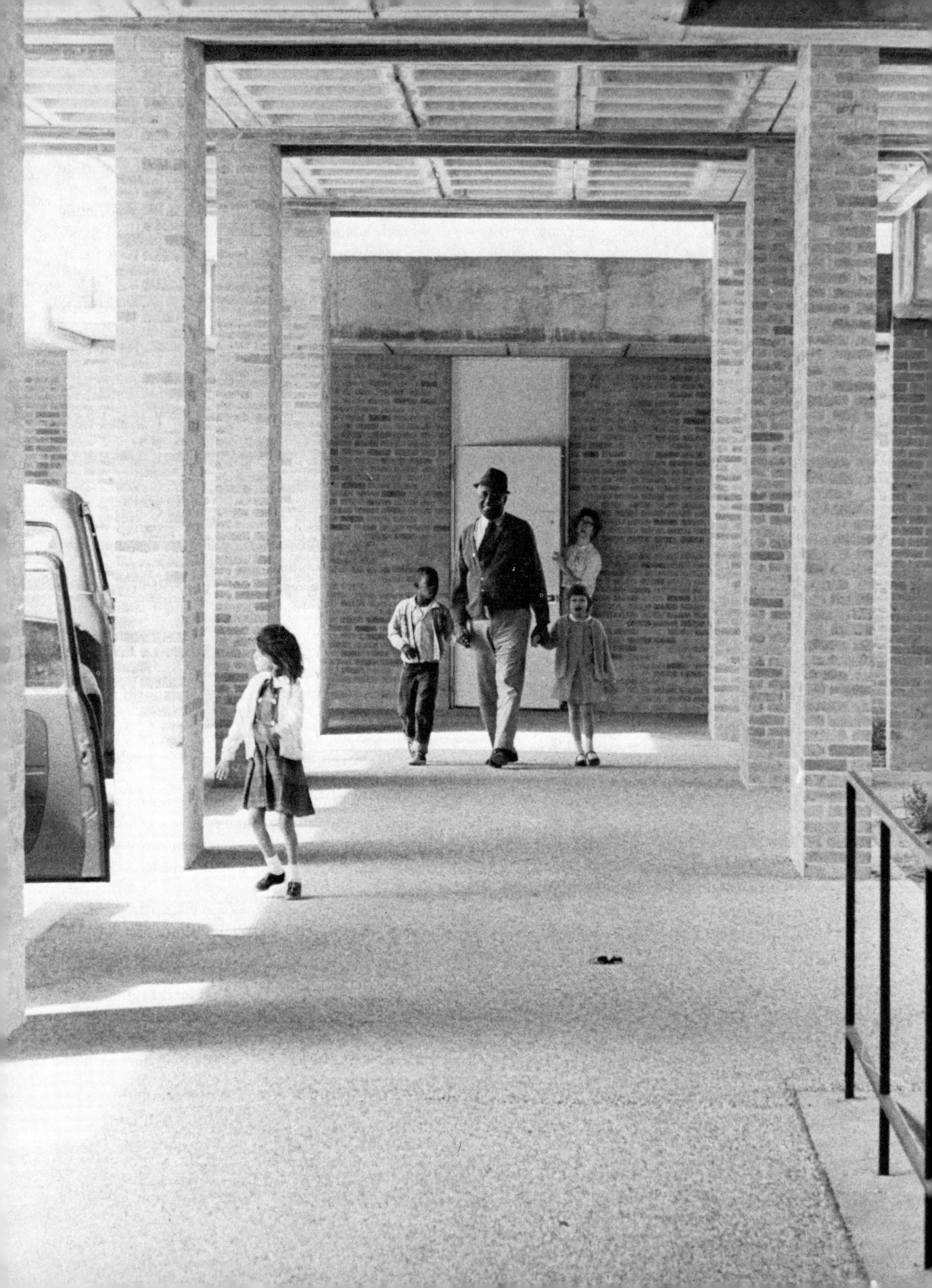

5 The Federal Role

In Search of a Viable Federal Policy

In the United States, services for children have historically been considered the sole responsibility of states and local communities. But with the first White House Conference on Children in 1909[1] and the subsequent establishment of the Children's Bureau, the federal government took its first active steps toward making the welfare of children a legitimate national concern. Before 1935, child labor and maternal and child health were the federal government's primary emphases.[2] The passage of the Social Security Act in 1935, however, created a program designed specifically to stimulate child welfare services as well as programs addressing other needs of children, such as a public assistance program to help needy families deprived of parental support stay together.[3]

Since 1935, the federal government has gradually expanded its role in children's services. Today, interest in national family policy is high, and whatever action the federal government takes or does not take has a major impact on the quality of life for children and families.

Our findings substantiate the extent of federal influence on children at risk of placement and in out-of-home care. They also show that despite the significance of the federal role, there has been little detailed analysis of the impact of federal dollars, programs and administration on this vulnerable group of children. Without such analysis and subsequent reform of national strategies and programs, it is unlikely that the destructive patterns identified in the report will end.

An effective national effort on behalf of these children and families is necessary for two very specific reasons. First, the problems we and others have identified are national in scope. They are not confined to one geographic area, or one group of children and families. Indeed, one of our most startling overall findings is the universality of system-wide problems. These problems demand national attention.

Second, the availability of federal dollars often determines what a state does and does not do. States typically seek federal funds to offset their expenditures. Fiscal incentives and disincentives implicit in federal programs therefore become extremely significant in

---

[1] Subsequent White House Conferences on Children have been held every decade. For an analysis of the outcomes of these conferences, see R. Beck, "White House Conferences on Children: An Historical Perspective," *Harvard Educational Review* 43 (November 1973): 653-668.

[2] The Sheppard-Towner Act passed in 1921 was the first federal grants program for children. Essentially a maternal and child health program, it was administered by the Children's Bureau until the legislation expired in 1929. The program was subsequently re-enacted as part of the Social Security Act. For a detailed description of the early history of the Children's Bureau, as well as a discussion of its later development, see G. Steiner, *The Children's Cause* (Washington, D. C.: The Brookings Institution, 1976).

[3] In addition to the child welfare services and aid to dependent children programs, the Social Security Act established the crippled children's services program and the maternal and child health services program.

shaping the services available on the state and local levels, as do specific protections, regulations and monitoring procedures required by federal programs. Crucial too is the extent to which the federal government monitors and enforces compliance with its regulations.

Major Federal Programs: An Overview

At least 34 federal programs have either a direct or indirect impact on the families and children described in this report.[4] Taken together, they comprise an unwieldy, haphazard, often contradictory set of policies that are confusing to public officials, to recipients, and to outside advocates.

The 34 programs are administered from 17 offices in 6 federal agencies producing a maze that is difficult to chart. They vary significantly according to:

- Purpose
  - service programs
  - financial assistance payments
  - reimbursement for maintenance costs
  - special project grants
  - research and evaluation projects
  - demonstration projects
  - training grants
  - planning and coordination
  - technical assistance

- Eligibility Requirements
  - income
  - age
  - residence
  - handicapping conditions
  - need for services
  - educational needs
  - state performance standards

- Funding Patterns
  - formula grants to states
  - discretionary grants
  - direct payments
  - grants to local communities
  - grants or contracts to public or private agencies, organizations or institutions
  - allocation formulas
  - set-asides for particular groups or purposes
  - state-federal match
  - authorizations and appropriations

- Administration
  - statutory authority
  - regulations and guidelines
  - administering agencies and offices
  - responsible Congressional committees

- Other Provisions
  - state plan requirements
  - due process protections
  - parental involvement provisions
  - public participation requirements
  - monitoring and enforcement mechanisms
  - reporting requirements

These variations result in a patchwork of programs which are theoretically available to children at risk of placement and in care. However, their conflicting and confusing requirements and provisions often work to undermine the very purposes the programs were intended to serve. In the following pages, we discuss each of the major programs most relevant for childen without homes and critique its impact.[5]

---

[4]Appendix P. sets forth for each of these programs the administering agency and appropriate citations to legislative authority and regulations. More detailed descriptions of each program appear in the following pages of this chapter.

[5]Others have compiled inventories of federal programs affecting broader categories of families and children. See, for example, Family Impact Seminar, *Toward an Inventory of Federal Programs With Direct Impact on Families* (Washington, D. C.: Family Impact Seminar—Staff Report, December 1977), and Office of Juvenile Justice and Delinquency Prevention, Law Enforcement Assistance Administration, Department of Justice, *Federal Juvenile Delinquency Programs–First Analysis and Evaluation, Volume 2* (Washington, D. C.: LEAA, DOJ, December 1976). Our scope is more limited. We have addressed primarily those programs which focus on children in particularly vulnerable situations. We have not, for example, included the numerous federal education, employment, housing, health care and nutrition programs which, by attempting to improve the general quality of life, can eliminate family stress and possibly reduce the risk of needless or lengthy separations of children and families. Nor have we discussed youth employment programs, although all of these obviously affect the well-being of the children described in this report.

Promoting the Welfare of Children

First there are programs specifically designed to promote the welfare of children.

AID TO FAMILIES WITH DEPENDENT CHILDREN PROGRAM

The AFDC Program, authorized under Title IV-A of the Social Security Act, provides federal funds to states for cash assistance payments to needy children and their families.[1] Although the stated purpose of the program is "to encourage the care of dependent children in their own homes or the homes of relatives," the low level of aid and manner in which it is administered in many states make the program insufficient to enable families to care for their children adequately.

The rate of federal reimbursement varies inversely with state per capita income. Matching rates range from 50 percent in the wealthiest states to 78 percent in Mississippi. In September 1977, almost two-thirds of the 10.9 million AFDC recipients were children.[2] Coverage and eligibility requirements vary widely and benefits are generally inadequate. Average monthly payments for an adult and two children ranged from $47.23 in Mississippi to $370.47 for a family of comparable size in New York.[3] AFDC payments in Fiscal Year 1977 amounted to $5.6 billion.[4]

---

[1]As of September 1977, in 24 states payments were limited to families in which at least one parent was deceased, disabled or absent from the home. The remaining states and the District of Columbia also extended benefits to families with unemployed fathers.
[2]Committee on Finance, United States Senate, *Staff Data and Materials on Public Welfare Programs* (Washington, D. C.: U. S. Government Printing Office, 1978), Table 7.
[3]Ibid, Table 7.
[4]Ibid, Table 17.

AFDC FOSTER CARE PROGRAM

All states are required to provide foster care as a regular part of their AFDC Program. Under the AFDC Foster Care Program (AFDC-FC), authorized in Section 408 of the Social Security Act, federal reimbursement is provided *only* for out-of-home care for children otherwise eligible for AFDC who are placed, as a result of a judicial determination, by the local welfare agency or another public agency, in licensed or approved foster family homes or private nonprofit child care institutions. Semi-annual periodic reviews and case plans are required for each AFDC-FC child,[1] but there is no limit to the length of time children are eligible for federal reimbursement under the program.

In Fiscal Year 1976, states received approximately $176 million in federal funds[2] for approximately 100,000 children in care under this open-ended entitlement program.[3] States vary significantly in the extent to which they participate in the program.[4]

---

[1]42 U.S.C. §608(f); 45 C.F.R. §233.110(a)(2).
[2]Department of Health, Education and Welfare, Social and Rehabilitation Service, Division of Finance, Office of Financial Management, *State Expenditures for Public Assistance Programs Approved Under Titles I, IV-A, X, XIV, XVI, XIX, XX of the Social Security Act, Fiscal Year 1976* (Washington, D. C.: HEW, 1977), p. 11, as adjusted for Illinois. Illinois figure compiled from monthly estimate of expenditures.
[3]An "entitlement program" is one in which the legislative authority requires the payment of benefits to any person meeting the requirements established by law. General Accounting Office, *Budgetary Definitions* (Washington, D. C.: GAO, November 1975), p. 11. Under the current AFDC-FC Program federal matching must be provided for all children who are legitimately claimed by the states as participating in the program, with no fiscal ceiling imposed.
[4]Appendix Q. shows, by state, Fiscal Year 1976 federal expenditures for this program and children participating in the program in June 1976. The variation is in part due to the extent to which children enter foster care through the courts. Several states have revised their intake procedures to require a judicial determination prior to placement for all children coming into care in order to increase the number of children for whom federal reimbursement can be claimed.

CHILD WELFARE SERVICES PROGRAM

The stated purpose of the Child Welfare Services Program, authorized under Title IV-B of the Social Security Act, is to enable the federal government to assist the states in establishing, extending, and strengthening a system for public social services which supplements or substitutes for parental care and supervision. Under the program, funds are provided for a broad range of services which are available to families regardless of income. Although preventive and reunification services are among those authorized, program funds are primarily used for maintaining children in out-of-home care. Regulations for the program require states to develop a case plan, which is to be reviewed periodically, for each service recipient,[1] but the requirement is generally ignored.

Federal participation in this program is limited, representing less than ten percent of total local, state

---

[1]45 C.F.R. §220.40(b)(3).

and federal expenditures for child welfare services.² In Fiscal Year 1977, only $56.5 million in federal funds were available under the program—over $200 million less than the legislative authorization.

---

²The ten percent figure is a percentage of expenditures nationwide. The proportion of child welfare services expenditures which is federal varies from state to state, but is generally small. In a survey of child welfare services in 25 states, all but three of the 21 states for which data were available reported that federal expenditures under Title IV-B comprised five percent or less of the total child welfare expenditures in the states. Department of Health, Education and Welfare, Children's Bureau, *Child Welfare In 25 States–An Overview* (Washington, D. C.: HEW, 1976), pp. II 53-54.

EMERGENCY ASSISTANCE PROGRAM

Under the Emergency Assistance Program, funded under Title IV-A of the Social Security Act, states may provide cash payments and selected services, including shelter care, to needy families with children to avoid destitution of the children or to provide other living arrangements for them. States may establish their own conditions for eligibility; describe which emergency needs will be met; and establish the services that will be provided.¹ Federal matching is available only for emergency assistance furnished for no more than 30 days in any 12-month period.

Only 20 states were participating in the federal Emergency Assistance Program as of August 1, 1977.² Fiscal Year 1977 federal expenditures for the program were $30.9 million.³ Figures are not available to indicate the extent to which such assistance was used to prevent the need for extended out-of-home care of children.

---

¹For example, in the District of Columbia, emergency assistance funds are used for such things as cash payments to help reunite families whose children have been in foster care and to provide temporary shelter and services to dependents under 21 years of age who are neglected or abandoned.
²Department of Health, Education and Welfare, Social Security Administration, Office of Family Assistance, State Programs and Characteristics Branch, Branch Report—August 1, 1977.
³Executive Office of the President, *The Budget of the United States Government, 1979-Appendix* (Washington, D. C.: U. S. Government Printing Office, 1978), p. 448.

INDIAN CHILD WELFARE ASSISTANCE PROGRAM

The Indian Child Welfare Assistance Program provides financial assistance for the maintenance of Indian children in foster homes or non-medical care facilities, if such care is not otherwise available from state or local child welfare agencies.¹ Services to the children are provided under the Indian Social Services Counseling Program.² Payment levels are supposed to be limited to the AFDC Foster Care levels. In Fiscal Year 1976, $8 million was expended to provide out-of-home care to approximately 3,000 Indian children.³ Fiscal Year 1977 expenditures are estimated to be approximately $12 million.

---

¹Federal regulations for the Child Welfare Assistance Program and other Indian social services programs were promulgated for the first time in February 1977. See 25 C.F.R. §§20.1-20.30.
²See description of program at p. III, infra.
³Department of Interior, Bureau of Indian Affairs, Office of Indian Services, "Child Welfare—1976."

CHILD ABUSE AND NEGLECT PREVENTION AND TREATMENT PROGRAM

The Child Abuse and Neglect Prevention and Treatment Program is authorized under the Child Abuse Prevention and Treatment Act of 1974, which was recently extended for a four-year period.¹ The program assists states, localities and other organizations to develop preventive programs and services for abused and neglected children and their families. To be eligible for grants states must meet a number of requirements relating to the reporting and care of abused and neglected children.² A major portion of the funds available under the Act must be used for research, demonstration and training grants or contracts to public and private nonprofit agencies. The National Center on Child Abuse and Neglect, established by the 1974 Act, has directly supported 16 regional resource projects to provide training and technical assistance on the state and local level. A total of $18.2 million in federal funds was expended for this program in Fiscal Year 1977.³

---

¹P.L. 95-266, approved April 24, 1978.
²42 U.S.C. § 5103(b)(2). These include, among others, requirements that a guardian ad litem be appointed to represent a child in any judicial proceeding in an abuse or neglect case, and that a procedure for protecting the confidentiality of records be developed. Thirty-seven states plus the District of Columbia qualified for grants under the Act in Fiscal Year 1977. The Act also specifies that states may operate child abuse and neglect programs under Title IV-B of the Social Security Act only if they have a child abuse reporting law; procedures for investigating reports of abuse and neglect; and provisions for immediate protection of a child, confidentiality of records, and cooperation among various state agencies having responsibility in abuse and neglect cases. 42 U.S.C. § 5103(b)(3).
³Executive Office of the President, *Budget of the U.S., 1979–Appendix*, p. 461. In addition to programs funded by the National Center on Child Abuse and Neglect, child abuse projects are also funded by the Administration for Public Services in the Office of Human Development Services, Office of Education, the Public Health Service, and the National Institute of Education within HEW, as well as by the Departments of Agriculture, Defense, Housing and Urban Development, Interior, Justice and Labor.

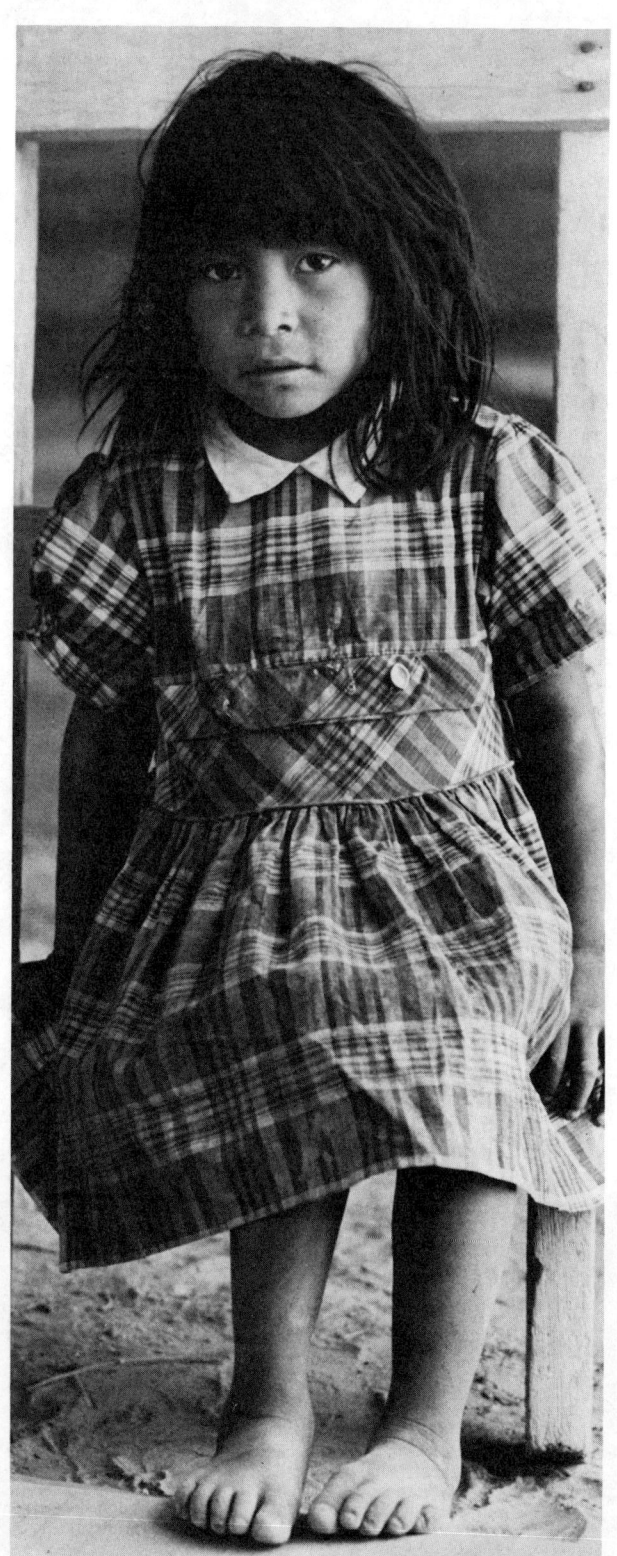

Strengthening the Juvenile Justice System

The juvenile justice programs have historically been directed primarily toward juvenile delinquents. However, as a result of recent attention given to diverting youths from the juvenile justice system and providing alternatives to institutionalization for those within it, there is increasing overlap with the population addressed by programs just described.

JUVENILE JUSTICE AND DELINQUENCY PREVENTION PROGRAM

The Juvenile Justice and Delinquency Prevention Act of 1974, as recently amended,[1] authorizes funds[2] to improve the quality of juvenile justice, to divert juveniles from the traditional juvenile justice system and to provide critically needed alternatives to institutionalization. To be eligible for funding under the Act, a state must make a number of assurances in its state plan that it will try to improve its juvenile justice system. States must provide among other things, that:

— status offenders and dependent or neglected children will not be placed in juvenile detention or correctional facilities;[3] and

— juveniles alleged or found to be delinquent, status offenders and dependent or neglected children will not be detained or confined in any facility in which they have regular contact with adult prisoners.[4]

States are also required to establish systems to monitor compliance with these and other plan requirements.

---

[1] P.L. 95-115, approved October 3, 1977.

[2] The Act authorized funds for formula grants to the states, discretionary funds for special emphasis programs, and funds for the research, information and training functions of the National Institute for Juvenile Justice and Delinquency Prevention. In addition to appropriations under the Juvenile Justice and Delinquency Prevention Act LEAA is required to allocate 19.15 percent of its non-Juvenile Justice and Delinquency Prevention Act funds for juvenile justice and delinquency prevention programs. In Fiscal Year 1978, this additional amount was expected to be about $330 million.

[3] 42 U.S.C. §5633(a)(12)(A). By October 1978, states must have achieved, "substantial compliance" with this requirement (at least 75 percent of the juveniles deinstitutionalized) and may then have an additional two years to achieve full compliance. 42 U.S.C. §5633(c). A state is further required to submit annual reports to the Office of Juvenile Justice and Delinquency Prevention in LEAA. These reports must assess the state's progress relative to deinstitutionalization and, pursuant to the 1977 Amendments, its progress in providing that the juveniles are placed in facilities which are the least restrictive alternatives appropriate to their needs and the needs of the community, are in reasonable proximity to their family and home community, and are provided appropriate services. 42 U.S.C. §5633(a)(12)(B).

[4] 42 U.S.C. §5633(a)(13).

Funding for the juvenile justice programs has been slow and limited. The Fiscal Year 1977 appropriation was $75 million; the authorization $150 million. Over half of the amount appropriated ($47.6 million) was for grants to the states;[5] the remainder for special emphasis grants ($18.9 million);[6] research, training and information functions of the National Institute for Juvenile Justice and Delinquency Prevention ($7.5 million)[7] and a special report on the concentration of federal effort regarding juvenile delinquency.[8] The Fiscal Year 1978 appropriation is $100 million.

---

[5]Forty-six of the 56 states and territories eligible to receive funds participated in the program in Fiscal Year 1977. In large part, non-participation was due to the states' inability to accept the deinstitutionalization and separation mandates. Non-participating states included Kansas, Mississippi, Nebraska, Nevada, North Carolina, North Dakota, Oklahoma, Utah, West Virginia, and Wyoming. U.S. Congress, Senate Committee on the Judiciary, *Juvenile Justice Amendments of 1977*, S. Rept. 95-165 on S.1021, 95th Cong., 1st Sess., 1977, p. 130.

[6]Under the special emphasis program, direct grants are available to public and private agencies and organizations to develop innovative projects in the area of juvenile delinquency. At least 30 percent of the funds must go to private nonprofit agencies, organizations or institutions that have had experience dealing with youth. 42 U.S.C. §5634(c). Initial priorities in awarding special emphasis grants were deinstitutionalization and diversion.

[7]By statute, the National Institute for Juvenile Justice and Delinquency Prevention was established to serve as a national clearinghouse and information center regarding juvenile delinquency, to provide multi-disciplinary training and to conduct research and demonstration projects, evaluations and studies. 42 U.S.C. §5651. Its progress in performing all its mandated functions has been slow.

[8]Senate Committee on the Judiciary, *Juvenile Justice Amendments of 1977*, p. 125.

RUNAWAY YOUTH PROGRAM

The Runaway Youth Program is authorized under Title III of the Juvenile Justice and Delinquency Prevention Act of 1974 (the Runaway Youth Act), as recently amended.[1] Grants under the program, which are administered within HEW rather than in LEAA,[2] are made available for the purpose of developing temporary care programs for runaway youth and other homeless youth outside of the law enforcement structure and the juvenile justice system.

Grant applications must specify arrangements that will be made for reuniting children with their families or providing alternative living arrangements, aftercare counseling, and services for the youth and their

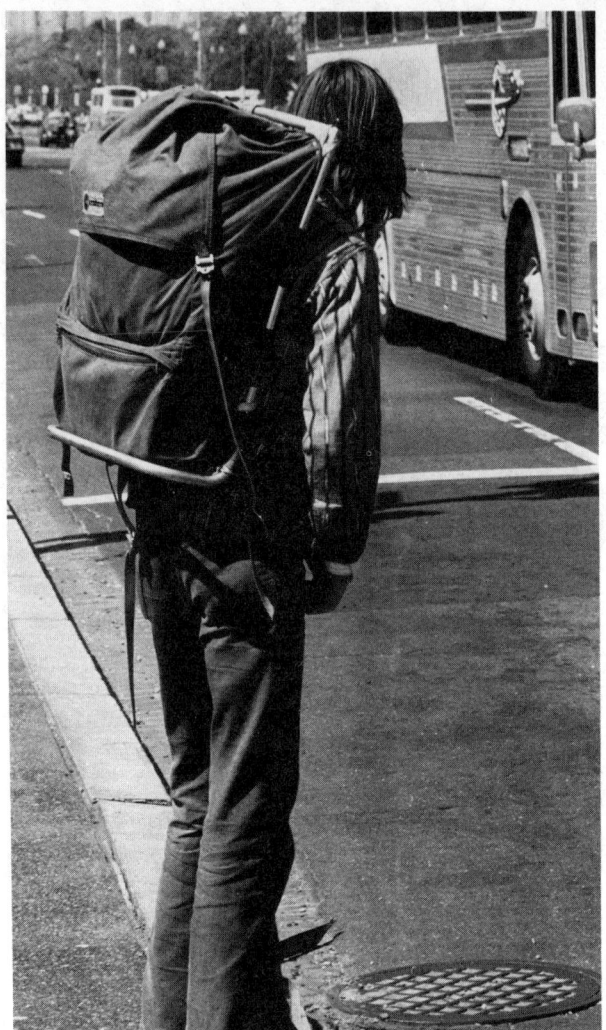

families. Grants are awarded on the basis of the number of runaway or otherwise homeless youth in the community and the availability of shelter facilities. Programs with experience in dealing with such youth have priority.[3] In Fiscal Year 1977, expenditures under the program were $7.7 million for 128 service projects and a national toll-free runaway switchboard. Approximately 33,000 youth received services from the runaway facilities.[4] The Fiscal Year 1978 appropriation is $11 million.

---

[1]P.L. 95-115, approved October 3, 1977.

[2]Although the program is currently administered by the Administration for Children, Youth and Families in the Office of Human Development Services at HEW, the 1977 Juvenile Justice Amendments provide for authorization of Presidential transfer of the program to ACTION or the Office of Juvenile Justice and Delinquency Prevention in LEAA after April 30, 1978.

[3]42 U.S.C. §5711.

[4]Statement of G. J. Ahart, Director, Human Resources Division, General Accounting Office, before the House Subcommittee on Economic Opportunity, Committee on Education and Labor, on the Management and Operation of the Runaway Youth Program, March 7, 1978, pp. 3-4. An evaluation of the program by a private contractor is underway and due to be completed in December 1978.

Providing Social Services to Children and Youth

Children at risk of placement or in out-of-home care also benefit from federal social services programs which address the needs of adults as well as children.

TITLE XX PROGRAM

The social services program authorized under Title XX of the Social Security Act is a type of "special revenue sharing" program.[1] It provides $2.5 billion to the states for a broad range of social services programs.[2] States receive funds and are generally free to decide what services they will provide and who will receive them.[3] Although eligibility for most services is income-related, it is not limited to traditional public assistance categories.[4] Furthermore, eligibility and fee levels for services may vary by geographic area within a state.

States are required to provide at least one service directed toward each of five goals, three of which relate specifically to children at risk of placement or in out-of-home care. The goals are:

— Achieving or maintaining self-support

— Achieving or maintaining self-sufficiency

— Preventing or remedying neglect, abuse or exploitation of children and vulnerable adults, or preserving, rehabilitating or reuniting families

— Preventing or reducing inappropriate institutional care

— Securing institutional care when appropriate or providing services to individuals in institutions.

Title XX funds cannot be used for room and board costs in foster care, except for temporary emergency shelter for a limited period (up to 30 days in any six month period) when a child is endangered by abuse or neglect, or for group home or residential care for up to six months if the costs of room and board are subordinate to the costs of the social services being provided.[5] Funds are available too for certain services to children with special needs in foster family homes.[6] Although funds potentially can also be used for a continuum of other child welfare services, including preventive, reunification and adoption services,[7] the poor data available make it difficult to determine to what extent Title XX funds are actually used for such purposes.

Title XX requires that states involve the public in the planning process for the use of Title XX funds. Each state must develop a Comprehensive Annual Services Plan, which is available for public review, and an administrative state plan.[8] Both of these must be submitted annually to the regional office of the Administration for Public Services in HEW for certification and approval.

---

[1]Title XX, enacted in 1975, is the successor to the open-ended social services programs which were part of the Title IV-A and Title VI Programs authorized by the Social Security Act.

[2]P.L. 95-600, approved November 7, 1978, increased the Title XX funding level to $2.9 billion for a one-year period.

[3]The federal match for family planning services is 90 percent; 75 percent for all other services.

[4]There are three main types of Title XX eligibility. Certain persons are eligible because they are recipients of certain categorical programs, AFDC and SSI. Others may be determined eligible because their family income is within the limits set by the state. A third group is persons who are in need of services which the state has the option of making available without regard to income: family planning, information or referral, or protective services for children and adults. 45 C.F.R. §228.60(b).

[5]45 C.F.R. §§228.41, 228.46. Reimbursement is not possible under Title XX for room and board in a facility which provides only care or supervision. However, room and board in a residential treatment center would be reimbursable if inpatient care was necessary to the treatment being received.

[6]45 C.F.R. §228.45.

[7]Title XX funds can be used to cover certain costs associated with adoption including costs incurred in locating an adoptive placement and in freeing a child for adoption. They may not be used for adoption subsidy payments because they are considered to be cash assistance payments and thus ineligible costs under Title XX. It is estimated that only about 1.2 percent of the Title XX funds were used for adoption services in Fiscal Year 1976.

[8]For an indication of the types of services provided under Title XX, see E. Wolff, Office of the Assistant Secretary for Planning and Evaluation, Department of Health, Education and Welfare, *Technical Notes–Summaries and Characteristics of States' Title XX Social Services Plans for FY1978*, May 1, 1978, Appendix.

INDIAN SOCIAL SERVICES COUNSELING PROGRAM

The Indian Social Services Counseling Program provides counseling services to recipients of general assistance, to children in the Indian child welfare assistance program, and to other Indians, both children and adults, in need of social services. Regulations specify that foster care services to Indian children in out-of-home care who are recipients of child welfare assistance payments must include an assurance that a placement is suitable, that services to the child and the caretaker are provided, and a plan for each child is developed and reviewed periodically.[1] Only limited funds are avail-

---

[1]25 C.F.R. §20.24(b)(4).

Addressing the Special Needs of Children

A number of federal programs address the special needs of children at risk of placement and in out-of-home care. These include health, mental health, nutrition and education programs.

MEDICAID PROGRAM

The Medicaid Program, authorized under Title XIX of the Social Security Act, provides federal reimbursement to the states for medical assistance payments to certain low income individuals, including children.[1] In Fiscal Year 1977, an estimated ten million children under 21 received services under Medicaid (42 percent of the total recipients).[2] Approximately $2.3 billion (15 percent of the total Medicaid expenditures) was expended for services for these children.[3]

In addition to providing Medicaid coverage to children in the categorical assistance programs and certain other medically needy children, 17 states, as of December 1977, extended eligibility to all financially needy children under 21, and 30 other states extended coverage to financially eligible children in publicly supported foster care.[4]

States have considerable latitude in administering the Medicaid Program, in determining what services will be provided, and determining who will be eligible for those services. Thus Medicaid programs differ significantly among states and within states. All states, however, are required to provide certain services under Medicaid,[5] including preventive and curative health care services for children under 21. Many states also extended Medicaid coverage for services to children in

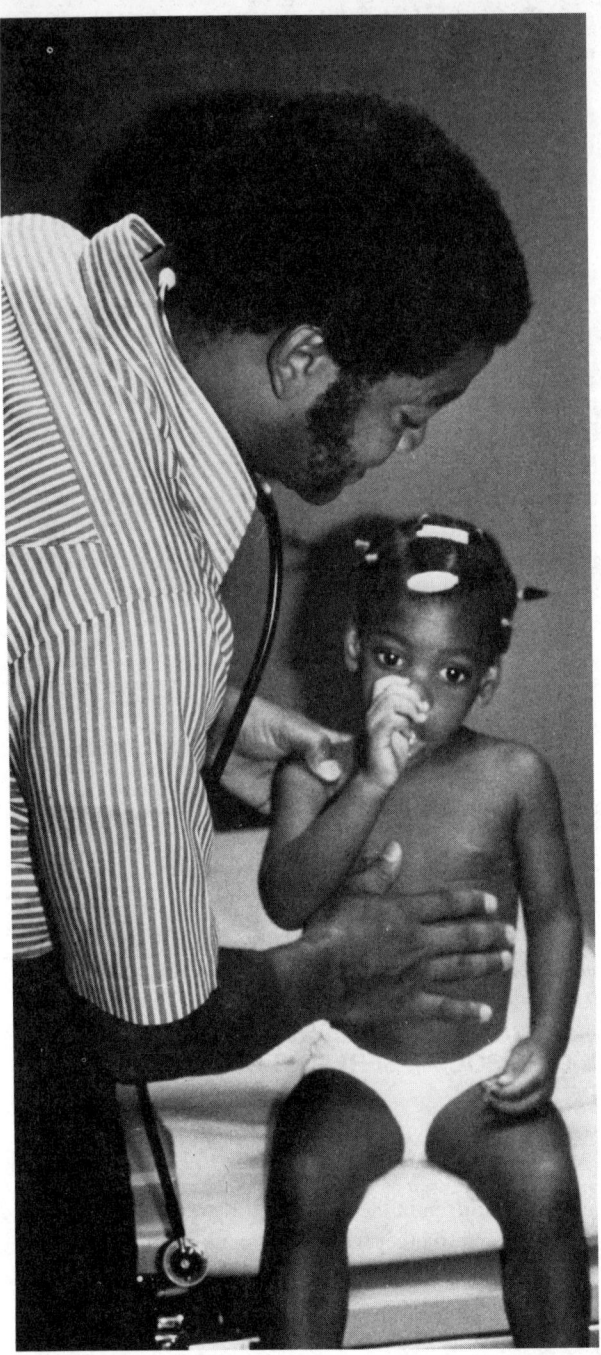

able for the program. Fiscal Year 1977 expenditures were $9.8 million. From the data available it is not possible to determine what percentage of the expenditures were for services to children, or for specific services to prevent placement or reunite children with their families.

---

[1]Medicaid is an entitlement program. Federal reimbursement percentages range from 50 to 78 percent, depending on the population and income of the state. Arizona is the only state that has not initiated a program under Title XIX.

[2]Department of Health, Education and Welfare, Health Care Financing Administration, Office of Policy Planning and Research, *Medicaid Statistics, Fiscal Year 1977* (Washington, D. C.: HEW, April 1978), pp. 4, 16.

[3]Ibid, pp. 20-22.

[4]For a list of these states, and states extending coverage to financially needy children in intermediate care facilities, inpatient psychiatric facilities and subsidized adoptions, see Appendix R.

[5]The Medicaid statute requires states to provide at a minimum: certain inpatient and outpatient hospital services; other laboratory and X-ray services; early and periodic screening, diagnosis and treatment of children under 21; skilled nursing facility services for some persons 21 or older and some health services for persons in nursing homes; physicians' services, whether furnished in the office, patient's homes, a hospital, a skilled nursing home or elsewhere; and family planning services. 42 U.S.C. §1396 d (a)(1)-(5).

various out-of-home settings, including hospitals, intermediate care facilities and inpatient psychiatric facilities.[6]

---

[6]As of June 1977, 43 states extended Medicaid coverage to include services in intermediate care facilities for the mentally retarded; 42 states covered services to at least some patients under 21 in skilled nursing facilities; and 31 states extended Medicaid coverage for services for children under 21 in psychiatric hospitals. Department of Health, Education and Welfare, Health Care Financing Administration, Medicaid Bureau, Division of State Management, "Medicaid Services State by State, June 1, 1977."

EARLY AND PERIODIC SCREENING, DIAGNOSIS, AND TREATMENT PROGRAM

The Early and Periodic Screening, Diagnosis and Treatment Program (EPSDT) was enacted in 1967. Every state operating a Medicaid program is required to provide EPSDT services to all children eligible for Medicaid, including children in out-of-home care. EPSDT requires that states not only reimburse for services but also insure the provision of periodic medical screening, diagnosis and treatment to all eligible children.

Broadly construed, treatment under EPSDT includes the prevention, correction or limitation of the effect of a disease or abnormality detected through screening and diagnosis. States are required to pay for treatment covered by their Medicaid plans, as well as eyeglasses, hearing aids, other kinds of treatment for visual and hearing defects, and some dental care, regardless of coverage under the state plan. States are given wide latitude in the implementation of EPSDT. Generally, the program is run by state welfare or health agencies which arrange for health department clinics, individual physicians, community clinics, and a variety of other providers to deliver services.

Estimated costs of the program in Fiscal Year 1977 were $205 million, $115 million of which were federal expenditures.[1] EPSDT has failed to reach many eligible children. Only 25 percent of needed screenings were provided in 1976, and many children did not receive the indicated follow-up care.[2]

---

[1]Department of Health, Education and Welfare, Health Care Financing Administration, "Medicaid and EPSDT Cost Estimates, Fiscal Years 1976 to 1979," May 9, 1978.

[2]For a further discussion of the EPSDT Program, see Children's Defense Fund, *EPSDT: Does It Spell Health Care for Poor Children?* (Washington, D.C.: Children's Defense Fund, 1977).

SUPPLEMENTAL SECURITY INCOME PROGRAM

The Supplemental Security Income Program (SSI),[1] authorized under Title XVI of the Social Security Act, provides direct federally financed supplemental income payments (currently $189.40 a month for an eligible individual and $284.10 a month for an eligible couple) to financially needy aged adults and to adults and children who are blind or disabled.[2] The SSI Program affects disabled children in their own homes and in institutional settings, as well as children in transition from institutions to less restrictive settings. The approximately 175,000 children receiving SSI in December 1977 represented 4.1 percent of the total SSI recipients[3] and only about half, if that many, of the potentially eligible children. A total of $4.7 billion was expended for federal benefit payments under this program in Calendar Year 1977.[4]

The 1976 Amendments to the SSI legislation established the SSI Disabled Children's Program.[5] It requires that all SSI children under 16 be referred to the state's crippled children's agency or another appropriate agency to determine their need for services. Children six years of age or under (or other children who have never attended public school) must be *provided services* which will help them benefit from subsequent education or training or otherwise enhance their opportunities for self-sufficiency or self-support as adults. Older children must be *referred for services*. The Amendment authorized funds annually for three

---

[1]This program, which went into effect in January 1974, replaced three former Social Security Act grant-in-aid programs which provided federal matching for programs for the elderly and for blind and permanently and totally disabled adults, but not for children under 18. It is an open-ended entitlement program.

[2]Final regulations defining the medical criteria to be used in determining whether a child is disabled and eligible for SSI were published in March 1977. The primary standard used was the effect an impairment has on a child's development, although the developmental norms used were not specific. Generally, the regulations provide that a child under 18 will be considered disabled if he or she has a medically determined physical or mental impairment of comparable severity to that which qualifies an individual 18 or over. The disability must be such that the child "is not engaged in substantial gainful activity" and must be of extended duration. See 42 *Federal Register* 14705-14713 for a further description of the disability requirements including a listing of the medical impairments which must be present.

[3]Department of Health, Education and Welfare, Social Security Administration, Bureau of Supplemental Security Income, Office of Research and Statistics, *Program and Demographic Characteristics of Supplemental Security Beneficiaries, December 1977.* (Forthcoming.)

[4]Ibid.

[5]P.L. 94-566. 42 U.S.C. §1382(d). Interim regulations for the program were published on December 16, 1977. 42 *Federal Register* 63568-63572.

years for states to provide services to the pre-school children—up to ten percent of which can be used for referral and monitoring of the older children. A maximum of $30 million in federal funds is available annually under this program and is allocated to the states in relation to the number of children under the age of seven in the state.

CHAMPUS PROGRAM

The Civilian Health and Medical Program of the Uniformed Services (CHAMPUS) provides for financial assistance for medical care for dependents of active duty members of the military, retirees and deceased members on a cost-sharing basis with the recipients. CHAMPUS includes the Basic Program and the Program for the Handicapped. Under the Basic Program, general medical services, both inpatient and outpatient, including psychiatric services for children with emotional and behavioral disorders, are provided. The Program for the Handicapped covers remedial and medical services to children and spouses of active duty members who are moderately or severely mentally retarded, or seriously physically handicapped and in need of specialized institutional care, training or rehabilitation. Coverage under the latter program is limited by regulation to situations in which required services are not available from public facilities or agencies. Neither the Basic Program nor the Program for the Handicapped provides services for children that are not medically necessary.

Fiscal Year 1976 expenditures for the two CHAMPUS programs were $503.4 million. This figure includes $4.9 million under the Program for the Handicapped, 60 percent of which was for residential services, primarily for the mentally retarded. The remainder was for expenses under the Basic Program, of which $409.5 million was for inpatient care.[1] A breakdown of expenditures for children's services is not routinely prepared by OCHAMPUS.

Program regulations published in April 1977 detail the scope of benefits under both the Basic Program and Program for the Handicapped, and the procedural and substantive protections that must be afforded beneficiaries of both programs.[2] These include the CHAMPUS Standards for Psychiatric Residential Treatment Centers Serving Children and Adolescents[3] developed in response to severe Congressional criticism of abuses in the program. All CHAMPUS approved residential treatment centers for emotionally disturbed children must comply with these standards.

[3]32 C.F.R. §199, Appendix A.

CRIPPLED CHILDREN'S SERVICES PROGRAM

The Crippled Children's Services Program authorized under Title V of the Social Security Act, awards grants to state health departments to extend and improve medical and related services to crippled children and children suffering from conditions that lead to crippling.[1] Emphasis in distribution of funds under the program is to be given to rural areas and areas suffering from economic distress. Funds are also used for special project grants related to the development of crippled children's services. Other than the existence of the handicapping condition, there are no eligibility requirements in the federal program. Each state's plan stipulates the crippling conditions covered and eligibility requirements.[2]

Funds under the program may be used for locating crippled children and providing a range of preventive, diagnostic and treatment services.[3] These services may include medical care, hospitalization, and other institutional care and aftercare, as well as provision of appliances and the facilitation of services to restore crippled children to maximum physical and mental health.[4] In Fiscal Year 1977, $97.6 million was available for this program.[5]

---

[1]Department of Defense, OCHAMPUS, Statistical Division, "Quarterly Statistical Phaseback Report Based on Claims Processed Through December 1977."
[2]32 C.F.R. §§199.1-199.16.

[1]Although historically the program has focused on the physically handicapped child, the statute defines "crippled child" more broadly to mean a child under 21 "who has an organic disease, defect, or condition which may hinder the achievement of normal growth and development." 42 U.S.C. §714.
[2]The Crippled Children's Services program was combined with the Maternal and Child Health Services program in 1967. State plans address services under both portions of the combined program.
[3]Regulations require that diagnostic services for crippled children must be available to any child without charge. 42 C.F.R. §51a.109. Crippled children's services are also defined more broadly to include the development of standards relating to the provision of services, training and administration.
[4]42 C.F.R. §51a.101(k). Eligible out-of-home care can include convalescent and foster home care for children receiving medical services. See 42 C.F.R. §51a.107.
[5]The funds available for this program comprise only a portion of the total appropriation made pursuant to 42 U.S.C. §701.

COMMUNITY MENTAL HEALTH CENTERS PROGRAM

The Community Mental Health Centers Program, authorized under the Mental Retardation and Community Mental Health Centers Act of 1963, as amended, provides grants to nonprofit private or public organizations or agencies to provide comprehensive mental health services. From 1970 to 1975, a portion of the funds was earmarked for improving underdeveloped services to children in community mental health centers and for creating innovative children's mental health services.[1] However, new legislation in 1975 mandated the phasing out of grants for special child mental health programs and incorporation of services for children and adolescents in the range of services to be provided by community mental health centers.[2]

Community mental health services may include preventive services such as day treatment or respite care, reunification services, alternatives to placement, and alternative placements for children in institutional care.[3] In Fiscal Year 1977, $231.7 million was available for the program, $20.8 million of which was earmarked for children's mental health services.[4]

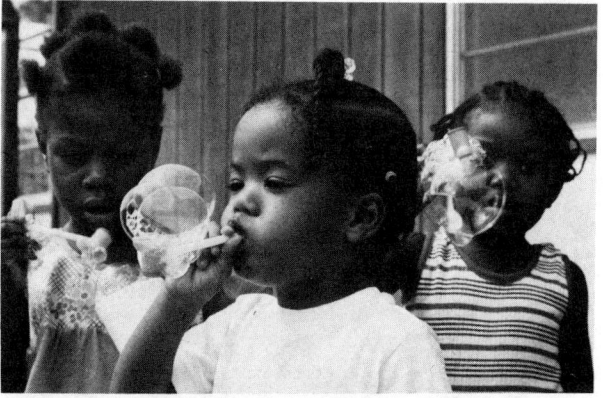

SPECIAL SUPPLEMENTAL FOOD PROGRAM FOR WOMEN, INFANTS AND CHILDREN

Young foster children may be eligible for participation in the Special Supplemental Food Program for Women, Infants and Children (WIC), a special nutrition program for pregnant, post-partum and breastfeeding women, infants and young children under five years of age determined to be at nutritional risk.[1] The program was authorized in 1972 under the Child Nutrition Act of 1966, as amended. Cash grants are given to state health departments or comparable state agencies and recognized Indian tribes or the Indian Health Service (IHS). They are administered locally through public health or welfare agencies, private nonprofit agencies, Indian tribes, or IHS service units.

The program provides supplemental foods or food vouchers and nutrition education to program recipients who reside in an approved project area and qualify under the nutritional risk standard. The supplemental foods may not be issued for use in institutional settings where meals are provided.[2]

Fiscal Year 1977 expenditures for the program were $274.7 million.[3] No figures are available on the extent to which children in foster homes may have been aided by the program.

---

[1]P.L. 91-211 authorized grants for developing specialized service programs, training personnel, and conducting surveys and field trials in services concerned with the mental health of children, as well as grants for the construction and staffing of treatment facilities concerned with the mental health of children.

[2]P.L. 94-63. Specialized services for children is now included as one of a number of services which must be provided through community mental health centers, in order for the centers to be eligible for federal funds. Others include inpatient and outpatient services, day care and other partial hospitalization services, emergency services, specialized services for the elderly, mental health consultation and education services, screening prior to admission for inpatient treatment, follow-up for patients discharged from mental health facilities, half-way house services and, where necessary, services related to alcohol and drug abuse. 42 U.S.C. §2689. The Secretary of HEW is required by P.L. 94-63 to prescribe the full range of diagnostic, treatment, liaison and follow-up services for children which must be provided but as of this writing final regulations for the program had not been published.

[3]Funds available through Comprehensive Health Service grants may also be used for these purposes, although there is no specific targeting for children's services. 42 U.S.C. §246, et seq. To be eligible for grants, states must establish and implement a plan to eliminate the inappropriate institutionalization of persons with mental health problems, ensure the availability of appropriate non-institutional services, and improve the quality of care for persons for whom institutional care is appropriate. Ninety million dollars was available under the program in Fiscal Year 1976 for formula grants to state health and mental health authorities. At least 15 percent of a state's allotment has to be used for mental health services, and 70 percent of that amount for community services. However, because these federal dollars represent such a small portion of the states' total mental health budgets, the impact of these requirements is limited.

[4]Department of Health, Education and Welfare, Public Health Service, National Institute of Mental Health, Mental Health Services Programs, Services Support Branch, "Community Mental Health Centers Community Programs Budget," December 20, 1977. The total includes $112.6 million available under P.L. 94-63, for which a breakdown of children's services was not available, and $119.1 million in continuation grants under P.L. 91-211, which included targeted funds for children's services.

[1]The program regulations define "nutritional risk" to mean special risk by reason of inadequate income and nutritional need. For an infant or child, "nutritional need" means one or more of the following: anemia, abnormal pattern of growth, inadequate nutritional pattern, or status as an infant under six months old whose mother was a WIC recipient during pregnancy. 7 C.F.R. §246.2. There is no federal income standard for the WIC program. A state may establish its own income eligibility standard for the program. However, recipients must meet the income requirements, if any, in use in other health programs operated by the local agency administering WIC. 7 C.F.R. §246.7.

[2]7 C.F.R. §246.10(c)(9). For example, women in maternity homes are not eligible for WIC.

[3]Executive Office of the President, Budget of the U.S., 1979—Appendix, p. 198.

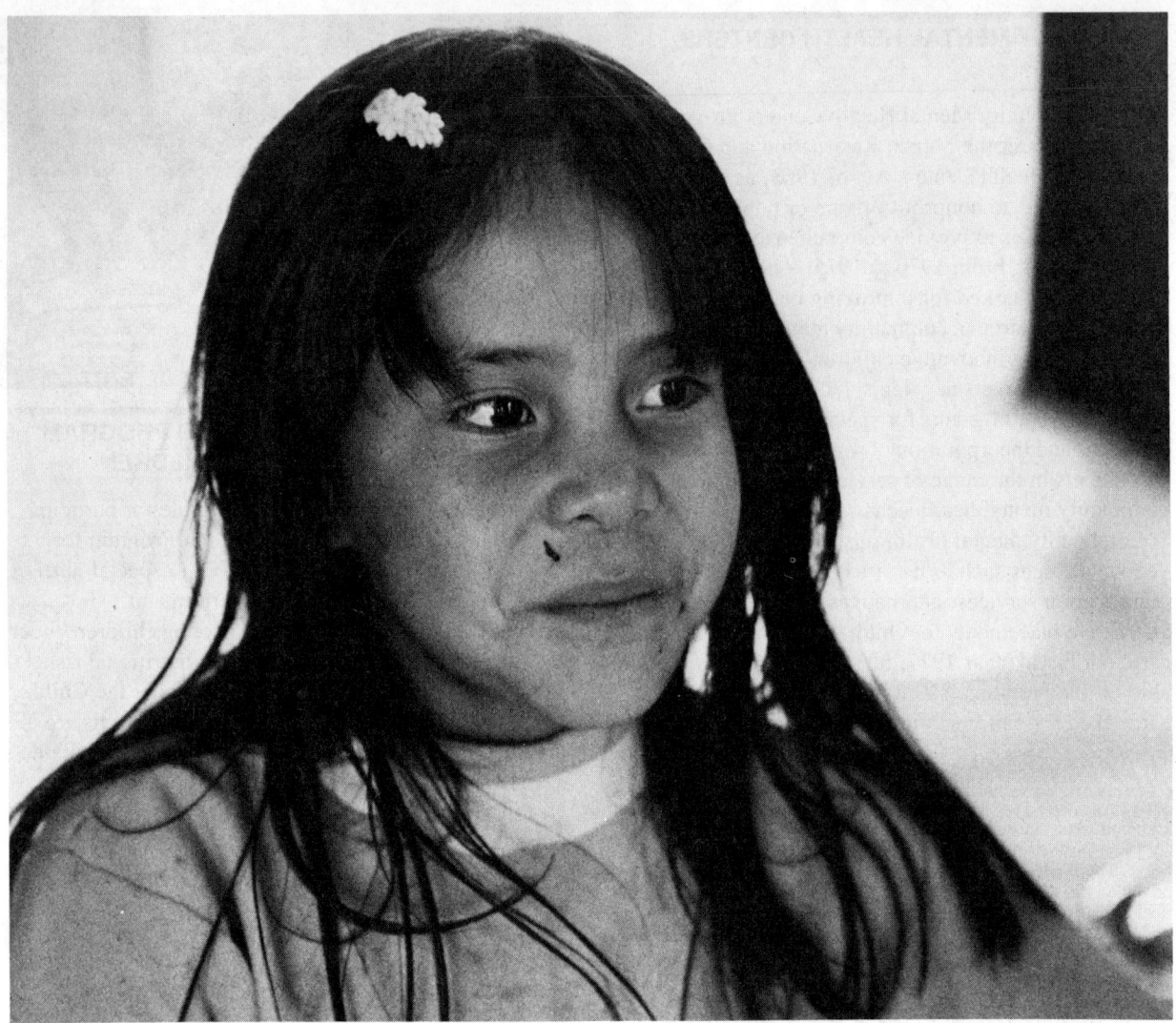

Some of the programs addressing the special needs of children focus specifically on institutionalized children.

TITLE I EDUCATION PROGRAMS FOR INSTITUTIONALIZED CHILDREN

Handicapped Children

The Title I program for handicapped children in state-supported facilities (P.L. 89-313) provides funds to states, based on the attendance of handicapped children (ages 5 to 21) in state-operated and state-supported schools. Funds are distributed to facilities within a state on a grant basis.[1] Eligible schools include state-run residential programs for the handicapped, state-run day programs which have educational components, and schools with which state agencies contract for special education programs for handicapped pupils.[2] Funds under the program are to be used to supplement the basic educational programs provided

---

[1] For a detailed overview of the operation of this program, see M. LaVor, House Committee on Education and Labor, "Public Law 89–313—Past, Present and Future: A Review of the Law and the Program," set forth as Appendix 3 in *Record of Hearings Before the House Subcommittee on Elementary, Secondary and Vocational Education on H.R. 15, Part 14: Title I—State Handicapped Program,* Hearings held October 4, 1977.

[2] These facilities may be run by state educational agencies, or departments of health, mental health, mental retardation or comparable agencies. In Fiscal Year 1978, 144 state agencies received funding under P.L. 89–313. M. LaVor, "Public Law 89–313," p. 156.

with state funds. P.L. 89-313 also allows for funds to follow a child who leaves a state-operated or state-supported program in order to attend a program operated by a local education agency.³

Program funds have increased significantly since the handicapped program was started in 1965. The Fiscal Year 1966 appropriation was approximately $16 million to serve 65,440 children, 98 percent of whom were in residential programs. The Fiscal Year 1977 appropriation was $111 million to serve 201,428 children, 44 percent of whom were in residential programs.⁴ The Fiscal Year 1978 appropriation is still higher—$121.6 million. Approximately 60 percent of the P.L.89-313 funds are expended on behalf of mentally retarded children.

Neglected and Delinquent Children

Title I also makes funds available to states and local education agencies to provide programs designed to meet the special educational needs of children in institutions for neglected or delinquent children or in adult correctional institutions. In Fiscal Year 1977, almost $44 million in Title I funds was allocated to state and local education agencies for this purpose, based on a count of over 118,000 children in 2,186 institutions.⁵ About half of these were institutions for neglected children. The other half were facilities for delinquent children and children adjudicated in need of supervision. Twenty percent were adult correctional facilities.⁶ The majority of the funds are spent for remedial programs in reading, math and language arts.

The funds for services to children in local institutions are given to the local education agencies, which are responsible for providing the services. Funds are allocated, in part, on the basis of the number of children, ages 5-17 residing in local institutions for 30 or more consecutive days.⁷ Funds for services to state educational agencies are allocated on the basis of the attendance of children in educational programs in state-operated institutions.⁸ The state agencies then make grants to individual institutions (not necessarily to all of those originally counted) for special education projects.

Fiscal Year 1977 expenditures were $14.5 million for the local institutions and $28.8 million for the state institutions.⁹

---

⁸Funds for the Title I state agency programs for neglected and delinquent children and for handicapped children are guaranteed to be at least equal to the preceding year's appropriation. The local educational agency programs are funded at a lower rate with remaining funds.

⁹The GAO has recently completed an examination of this program and has concluded that program resources "should be directed at the target population on a more selective basis, with priority consideration given to institutions that provide services over a longer term and serve younger children." (p. 22) See GAO, *Reevaluation Needed of Educational Assistance for Institutionalized Neglected or Delinquent Children* (Washington, D.C.: GAO, December 1977). The U. S. Office of Education has also completed the first phase of a national evaluation of the program for neglected and delinquent youth in state institutions. See, U. S. Department of Health, Education and Welfare, Office of Education, Office of Planning, Budgeting and Evaluation, *Title I of the Elementary and Secondary Education Act of 1965 in State Institutions for the Neglected and Delinquent: A National Evaluation, Phase I, October 1977.* (Revised.)

BIA BOARDING SCHOOL PROGRAM

In addition to the approximately 3,000 Indian children who received out-of-home care under the Indian Child Welfare Assistance Program in Fiscal Year 1976, approximately 28,000 Indian children were cared for in 72 schools through the Bureau of Indian Affairs' Boarding School Program.¹ Over one-fourth of these children attended elementary and secondary boarding schools off the reservation, often at great distances from their families. In Fiscal Year 1977, $82.4 million was expended for the BIA boarding school program, 34 percent for off-reservation schools.² The boarding schools which house orphans and neglected children as well as children for whom no other educational programs are available, are increasingly attended by children with serious learning problems.³

---

³P.L. 93-380.

⁴Statement by Edwin W. Martin, Jr., Deputy Commissioner, Bureau of Education for the Handicapped, U. S. Office of Education, HEW, before the House Subcommittee on Elementary, Secondary and Vocational Education, October 4, 1977, p. 1a.

⁵Although statutory and regulatory references are to "institutions," our review of the data submitted by these facilities indicate that many of the facilities are not institutions but group homes, youth homes and various youth ranches. Six-hundred and six of them were state-operated facilities, the remainder were locally operated.

⁶Department of Health, Education and Welfare, Office of Education, "Elementary and Secondary Education Act of 1965, as amended, Title I, Assistance for Educationally Deprived Children in Programs for Neglected and Delinquent Children," Fiscal Years 1967-1977.

⁷A count of children ages 5-17 living in foster homes supported by public funds is also included in the Title I allocation formula. The 1977 Title I formula count for children in foster homes was 200,261. OE, 1977 Formula Children Count for Local Educational Agencies.

---

¹Department of Interior, Bureau of Indian Affairs, Office of Indian Education Programs, *Fiscal Year 1977 Statistics Concerning Indian Education* (Lawrence, Kansas: Publications Service, Haskell Indian Jr. College), Table 4.

²Figures obtained from Management Support Staff, Office of Indian Education Programs, Bureau of Indian Affairs.

³For further discussion of the use of boarding school placements for children who require foster care, see Chapter 2, pp. 52-54. See also, "A Special Report of Off Reservation Boarding Schools" in Indian Education Task Force, *Report on Indian Education, Final Report to the American Indian Policy Review Commission* (Washington, D. C.: U. S. Government Printing Office, 1976), pp. 241-256.

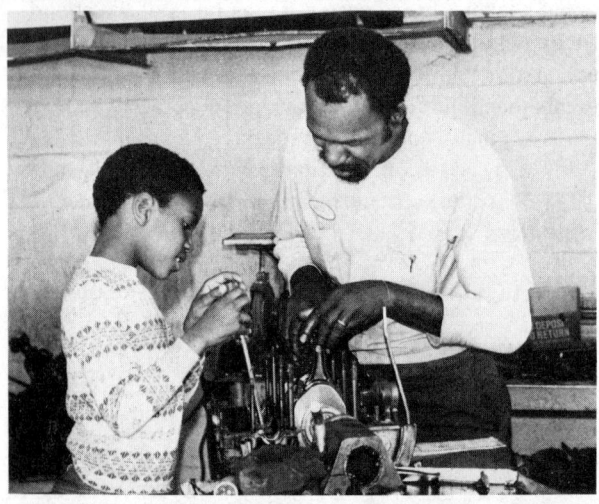

NUTRITION PROGRAMS IN INSTITUTIONS

The federal government, until 1975, paid little attention to the adequacy of food programs in residential facilities.[1] Up until that time, the Food Commodity Distribution to Institutions Program was virtually the only source of federal food assistance to institutions,[2] and residential facilities were specifically excluded from several of the other food programs. In 1975, the National School Lunch Act was amended to make children's residential institutions eligible for federal reimbursement under the school lunch program and the school breakfast program.[3] Foster homes are specifically excluded from the provision, but public and private nonprofit facilities for handicapped children, maternity homes, group homes, halfway houses, shelters for abused and runaway children, long-term care facilities for chronically ill children and juvenile detention centers are eligible facilities.[4] In Fiscal Year 1978, $20 million was budgeted for the Food Commodity Distribution to Institutions Program, but only a small portion of the commodities went to children's facilities.

[1] In 1974 and 1975, the Children's Foundation, a Washington-based child nutrition advocacy organization, did an extensive study of the food service needs of children in residential institutions. The findings addressed the poor quality of the food these children were receiving and pointed out how many of these children were denied the benefits of the various federal child nutrition programs. See, Children's Foundation, *Whose Children? An Assessment of Food Service Needs in Children's Residential Institutions*, (Washington, D. C.: Children's Foundation, April 1975).

[2] Some institutions, which operated school programs, were eligible for the Department of Agriculture supported school food programs. However, these facilities were then denied commodities. BIA boarding schools receive federal food program support through the BIA.

[3] P.L. 94-105.

[4] 7 C.F.R. §210.2.

The Fiscal Year 1977 appropriation for the National School Lunch Act was approximately $586 million, only a very small percentage of which (less than one percent) went to residential facilities.[5]

[5] The Children's Foundation estimates that only about 45 percent of the eligible children's residential facilities have chosen to participate in the program.

VOLUNTEER PROGRAMS

The Foster Grandparent Program is a volunteer program in which indigent elderly persons receive a stipend to provide support and companionship on a one-to-one basis to children with a range of special needs. Foster grandparents work with physically handicapped, delinquent, emotionally disturbed, mentally retarded or dependent and neglected children in hospitals, correctional facilities, other residential institutions, schools, day care facilities, and private residences. In Fiscal Year 1977, the program budget was $34 million, with volunteers in 184 programs serving approximately 30,000 children. Although ACTION has made an effort since 1974 to expand the placement of foster grandparents in non-institutional settings, the progress has been slow.[1] There is no requirement, for example, to ensure that a foster grandparent who has worked with a child in an institution will maintain contact with the child when he or she moves to a community-based setting.

The Retired Senior Volunteers Program (RSVP) is also a potential resource for assisting in efforts to alleviate the numerous problems facing the vulnerable families and children discussed in this report. Participation in RSVP is limited to retired persons aged 65 or over, but no economic guidelines are imposed, nor is a stipend paid. Volunteers may serve in a variety of settings such as schools, courts, day care centers, hospitals, welfare agencies, nursing homes and institutions. The Fiscal Year 1977 appropriation for RSVP was $19 million, with 233,000 volunteers participating in the program.

[1] The Pittsburgh Foster Grandparent Program has worked with the Allegheny County Welfare Department to develop a home visitors program in which foster grandparents are assigned to work with troubled families in their homes in order to prevent or delay institutionalization of the children. The role of the home visitors is to "parent" the parents, model appropriate parenting behavior, and to provide stimulation for the child and siblings. See, S.D. Arch, "Older Adults as Home-Visitors; Modeling Parenting for Troubled Families," *Child Welfare* (In Press).

Protecting Children With Handicapping Conditions

Several federal initiatives targeted at handicapped persons offer significant procedural protections for children and families, including children without homes.

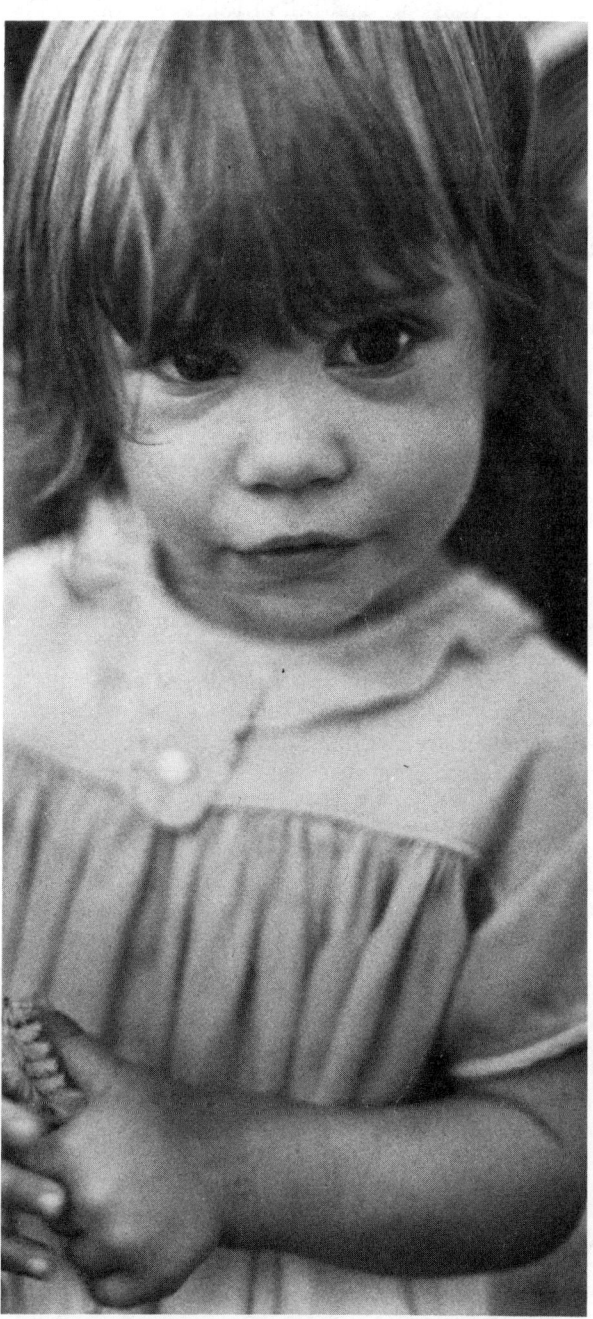

THE EDUCATION FOR ALL HANDICAPPED CHILDREN ACT OF 1975 (P.L. 94-142)

To be eligible for federal funds under the Education for All Handicapped Children Program, states must provide, pursuant to P.L. 94-142, a "free appropriate public education" to all handicapped children[1] ages 3-18 (including children in public and private institutions) by September 1, 1978.[2] The children must be educated in the least restrictive environment, as much as possible with children who are not handicapped. The Act and its regulations include additional substantive and procedural safeguards for such children and their parents, including children who are wards of the state or whose parents are unknown or unavailable.[3] The protections include a child's right to an individual evaluation and education plan, periodic reviews of progress, and the parents' right to participate in all decisions concerning a child's evaluation and placement, including notice of any anticipated change in the child's program. The Act also gives a parent the right to challenge a placement and contains extensive procedural safeguards to be used in this process.[4]

The Education for All Handicapped Children Act authorizes a formula grant program which makes federal funds available to local school districts, through the state education agencies, to pay a portion of the cost of providing educational and related services to handicapped children at the pre-school, elementary and secondary levels.[5] Federal funds are available only

---

[1] Handicapped children are defined to include children who are mentally retarded, hard of hearing, deaf, speech impaired, visually handicapped, seriously emotionally disturbed, orthopedically impaired, deaf-blind, multi-handicapped, or have specific learning disabilites, and other health-impaired children who require special education and related services. Precise definitions of each of the handicapping conditions are set forth at 45 C.F.R. §121a.5.

[2] All children ages 3-21 will be eligible by September 1, 1980, unless state law or practice does not allow serving 3-5 or 18-21 year olds. The same exception applies to 3-5 year olds who will be eligible in September 1978.

[3] The Act provides for designation of a "surrogate parent" to advocate on behalf of these children. Regulations require that surrogate parents have no interests which conflict with the interests of the child, and have the knowledge and skills to ensure adequate representation of the child. A surrogate parent may not be an employee of a public agency involved in education or care of the child. 45 C.F.R. §121a.514.

[4] For a guide for parents and advocates to educational services and the processes for getting them under P.L. 94-142, see Children's Defense Fund, *94-142 and 504: Numbers that Add Up to Educational Rights for Handicapped Children* (Washington, D. C.: CDF, 1978).

[5] P.L. 94-142, like the Title XX Program referred to earlier, requires public participation in the development of the state's annual program plan. Regulations specifically provide that there must be public hearings, adequate notice of such hearings, and an opportunity for comment from the general public prior to the adoption of policies, programs and procedures. 45 C.F.R. §§121a.280-121a.284.

for amounts in excess of the regular per pupil costs. The Fiscal Year 1977 appropriation for the program was $300 million, and is approximately $550 million in Fiscal Year 1978.

SECTION 504 OF THE REHABILITATION ACT OF 1973

Section 504 of the Rehabilitation Act of 1973 prohibits any recipient of federal funds from operating a program in a manner that discriminates against persons who are handicapped or have a record of handicaps.[1] Recipients of federal funds may include social services departments, child-placing agencies, special schools and other facilities for the handicapped, prisons and jails, as well as state education agencies, public school systems and hospitals.

Regulations implementing Section 504 address the right of a child to a free appropriate public education, as does P.L. 94-142, and include many of the same substantive and procedural protections for children and their families.[2] These protections apply to all handicapped children—children in foster homes, group homes and institutions, as well as children living with their own families.

Section 504 also applies to handicapped children who are served by health, welfare and other social service programs and activities that receive or benefit from federal financial assistance.[3] In these areas, providers must integrate their programs and services and make reasonable accommodations to facilitate participation of handicapped individuals. For example, a handicapped child in a foster home has a right to the same social services as a non-handicapped child. Section 504 further requires modification of these services to make them suitable to a foster child's particular handicapping condition. So, if training for foster parents and after-school day care are made available for non-handicapped children, they must also be made available for handicapped children. Similarly, if a child-placing agency recruits foster homes for non-handicapped children, special efforts must also be taken to locate foster homes for handicapped children.

[1]Section 504 is a Civil Rights Act, and does not include an authorization for funds to assist providers in their efforts to comply with the non-discrimination requirements.
[2]See, 45 C.F.R.§§84.31-84.39.
[3]See, 45 C.F.R.§§84.51-84.54.

DEVELOPMENTAL DISABILITIES PROGRAM

The Developmental Disabilities Program, designed to improve and coordinate services to individuals with developmental disabilities,[1] was significantly strengthened by the passage of the Developmentally Disabled Assistance and Bill of Rights Act of 1975. The 1975 Amendments require each state to establish a protection and advocacy system to protect the rights of developmentally disabled persons.[2] The system should address children, although children were not singled out in the legislation.

The Program provides formula grants to the states for the purpose of filling in gaps in existing services or expanding services and developing a plan for a coordinated and integrated service delivery system. It also provides special project grants, and grants to university-affiliated facilities to assist them in operating demonstration facilities and interdisciplinary training programs for personnel serving developmentally disabled persons. Overall, the Developmental Disabilities Program provides only approximately one percent of all funds available from federal, state and local sources for services to the developmentally disabled.[3] Thus, the thrust of the program is to improve the effectiveness of the rest of the funds. In Fiscal Year 1977, program expenditures were $57.6 million.[4]

The 1975 Act established a number of protections, procedures and important principles which apply to developmentally disabled children. It also specified the obligation of the state and federal governments to enforce these protections, which include:

— The right of developmentally disabled persons to appropriate treatment, services and habilitation designed to maximize their developmental potential, and provided in the least restrictive setting.[5]

[1]A developmental disability for purposes of this program includes mental retardation (or related conditions), cerebral palsy, epilepsy, autism, or dyslexia, resulting from one of the above disabilities. The disability must have originated before age 18, be expected to continue indefinitely and constitute a substantial handicap to the person's ability to function normally in society. 42 U.S.C. §6001.
[2]The establishment of such systems, which had to be independent of any state agency providing developmental disabilities services, was a requirement for funding in Fiscal Year 1978. 42 U.S.C. §6012.
[3]U. S. Congress, House, Interstate and Foreign Commerce Committee, *Developmentally Disabled Assistance and Bill of Rights Act*, H. Rept. No. 94-58 on H.R. 4005, 94th Cong., 1975, p. 6.
[4]Executive Office of the President, *Budget of the U.S., 1979–Appendix*, p. 461.
[5]42 U.S.C. §6010(1)(2).

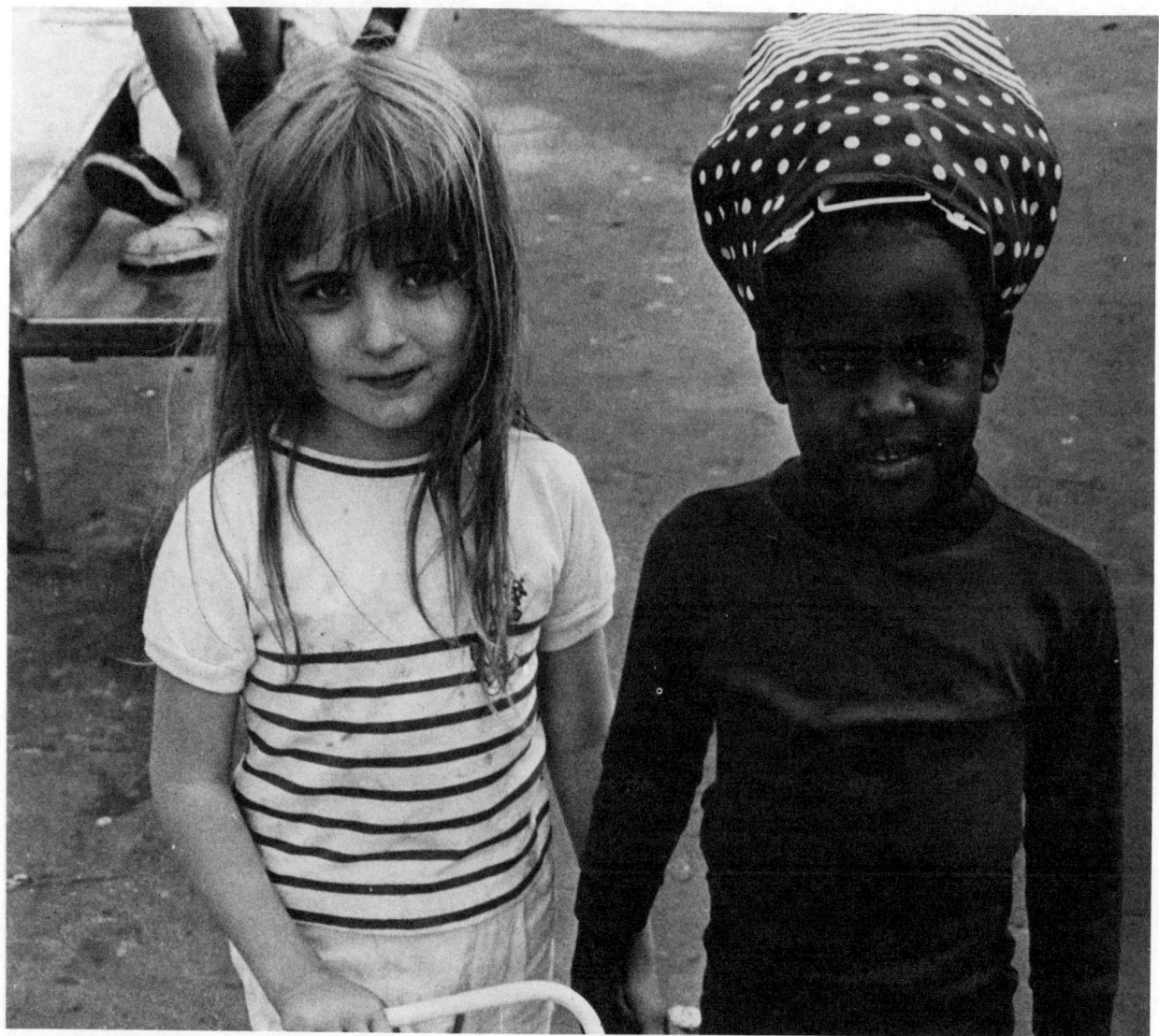

— The right of developmentally disabled persons to habilitation plans and periodic reviews.[6]

— The requirement that public funds not be used for residential programs which do not provide appropriate treatment and habilitation, nourishing meals, sufficient medical and dental services, freedom from physical and chemical restraints, and visits from relatives at reasonable hours without prior notice.[7]

— The requirement that 30 percent of the state's allotment be targeted toward the elimination of inappropriate institutionalization, and that states present a plan for deinstitutionalization and for improving the quality of necessary institutional care.[8]

— The requirement, as a condition for continued funding, that states establish an advocacy system for developmentally disabled persons, independent of any state agency providing treatment or services to such persons.[9]

[6] 42 U.S.C. §6011.
[7] 42 U.S.C. §6010(3).
[8] 42 U.S.C. §6063.
[9] 42 U.S.C. §6012.

Offering Technical Assistance

A major focus of the federal role with respect to children out of their homes has been to support research, demonstration and training efforts, with the delivery of ongoing service programs left to the states. Provisions for research, demonstration and training are scattered throughout a number of the programs previously discussed.

RESEARCH AND DEMONSTRATION PROGRAMS

Research and demonstration efforts have been funded under both Title IV-A and Title IV-B of the Social Security Act, as well as under the Child Abuse Prevention and Treatment Act, the Juvenile Justice and Delinquency Prevention Act, and several of the programs for handicapped persons: the Education for All Handicapped Children Program, the Developmental Disabilities Program and the Crippled Children's Services Program.

Section 426 of Title IV-B of the Social Security Act specifically authorizes funds for special research or demonstration projects to improve the quality of child welfare programs and demonstrate new service approaches. In the past, administration of these funds was split within HEW among the Office of Child Development, the Office of Youth Development and the Social and Rehabilitation Service (SRS).[1] The funds are now administered by the Administration for Children, Youth and Families within HEW.

In Fiscal Year 1977, the Office of Child Development administered $14.7 million in grants and contracts under Section 426. Approximately 40 percent of that amount ($6.3 million) went for projects related to children at risk of placement or in out-of-home care (including child abuse prevention programs).[2] The Office of Youth Development expended approximately $1 million in Section 426 funds in Fiscal Year 1977, used for the most part for projects addressing the problems of runaway youth. The remainder of the Section 426 funds were administered by SRS, which expended $3.9 million for research and demonstration projects in Fiscal Year 1977.[3]

The focus of research and demonstration efforts under the other programs is broader, but encompasses the development of appropriate services for children with special needs, including abused children, juvenile offenders, and children with handicapping conditions. There have also been efforts under various programs to develop alternatives to institutionalization.

---

[1] The Office of Child Development and Office of Youth Development are now part of the Administration for Children, Youth and Families, and many of the functions of SRS have been transferred to the new Administration for Public Services.

[2] The remainder was used for projects related to the delivery of day care services and other projects related to child and family development issues.

[3] This figure included 426 funds as well as monies authorized under Sections 1110 and 1115 of the Social Security Act. Sections 1110 and 1115 provide funds for research and demonstration projects to promote the general purpose of the Social Security Act. The funds were used for research and development efforts in the areas of income maintenance, health and social services. In the social services area, efforts were concentrated in four areas: (1) improving the delivery of services to Indians; (2) preventive services; (3) improving program administration; and (4) understanding the economic, political and legal dimensions of social services.

TRAINING PROGRAMS

Training grants, as well as research and demonstration grants, are also authorized under the child welfare, juvenile justice and handicapped programs described previously, as well as under Title XX of the Social Security Act.

Just over $8 million was expended for child welfare related training under Section 426 of Title IV-B of the Social Security Act in Fiscal Year 1977. The majority of 426 training funds are used for teaching grants and traineeship grants to institutions of higher learning, but funds may also be used for short-term, in-service training grants to be administered through universities and colleges.[1] This latter category may be used for training foster parents and homemakers, as well as child welfare personnel, lawyers, law enforcement and court personnel. Approximately $1 million of the Fiscal Year 1977 appropriation was awarded for projects "of national significance," directed to specific areas such as program administration and delivery of preventive services. Over 80 percent of the remaining funds were used for long-term training grants rather than short term, in-service training. We were not able to determine the extent to which any grants were used to train foster parents.

Training monies under Title XX of the Social Security Act, available at a 75 percent federal match, may also be used for training foster parents and staff who work with children with special needs.[2] Figures on expenditures for this purpose, however, are not available. Title XX training funds are open-ended and do not have to be claimed under the $2.5 billion ceiling in the Title XX services program. In Fiscal Year 1977, $45.7 million was expended under the program, but figures on expenditures for child welfare related training are not available.

Training funds available under the other programs may be used for a range of training efforts related to the development of preventive services, alternatives to institutionalization, and the care of children with special needs.

---

[1] Funds other than those awarded for projects "of national significance" are allocated to the various HEW regions for training projects in direct proportion to the amount of federal funds expended in each region in Fiscal Year 1976 for social services programs under the Social Security Act.

[2] The training of foster care providers covers foster parents preparing to take a child with special needs as well as those who already have children in their care who require such services. It may also be used for more general foster parent training, if the home is a resource for the Title XX agency's foster care services program. 45 C.F.R. §228.81.

The CDF Findings

Taken together, these federal programs define a national policy toward children at risk of removal or in out-of-home care, as well as toward state and local child-caring agencies involved with them. It is a policy that, with only few exceptions, reflects an anti-family bias. It is a policy that affords few statutory protections to children and families, and provides for little federal monitoring of state and local performance. It permits the federal government year after year to claim ignorance about the magnitude of the problem of children without homes and to discount the negative impact of a fragmented federal administrative structure. In short, it is a policy that must be redirected.

In this section, we summarize the evidence of federal failures, based on the programs just described. We then set forth a series of specific recommendations for federal reform.

Fiscal Disincentives

Federal funding patterns act as disincentives to the development of strong family support programs.

The major federal foster care program encourages the break-up of families.

- Under the AFDC Foster Care Program (AFDC-FC), open-ended, unlimited federal reimbursement is available only for room and board of children in out-of-home care. The program does not pay for services to prevent placement, services to reunite families,[6] services related to termination of parental rights, or services related to adoption. It does not condition federal reimbursement on the length of time a child is in care without good faith efforts by the state to ensure the child permanence. Audits by the HEW Audit Agency reveal, in fact, that children in the federal foster care program often linger in care

---

[6] The legislation mentions such services, but the lack of funds and stringent enforcement makes the reference virtually meaningless. Although foster care services to AFDC-FC recipients were mandatory under Title IV-A prior to institution of Title XX, current Title XX regulations (when revised in Janaury 1977) deleted the reference to mandatory foster care services and the requirement that such services be available statewide.

indefinitely.[7]

There is no federal child welfare money or legislation specifically targeted to develop alternatives to placement, although states may use resources from several sources, including the Emergency Assistance Program, Title IV-B and Title XX of the Social Security Act, to pay for such services. In fact, only a small proportion of funds are so used.

- The potential of the Emergency Assistance Program to provide special funds to aid a family with a financial crisis that might otherwise result in the removal of children from the home has never been fully tapped. Only half of the states even participate in the program. Moreover, federal aid is limited to one 30-day period each year. Family crises may well not fit this timetable.

- While the Child Welfare Services Program funded under Title IV-B theoretically goes far toward fulfilling the needs of the vulnerable population described in earlier chapters, the actual federal investment in the program has been minimal and the focus of funds misdirected. Consistently there has been a staggering gap between the Congressional authorization for the program and the appropriation. Until Fiscal Year 1979, the Administration had never requested more than $56.5 million for the program, even though the authorization had increased to $266 million. Without strong federal leadership, states have used most of the little money available for out-of-home care. There has been no federal initiative in targeting the funds for preventive, restorative or adoption services. In Fiscal Year 1976, for example, less than ten percent was spent for day care, a smaller amount for protective services, and two percent for adoption services.[8]

- Theoretically, the Title XX Social Services Program could provide funding for a range of family-oriented service programs. The allocation of funds within each state, however, is largely determined by the strength of the constituencies arguing for the funds. Systematic advocacy for a range of services specifically for children at risk of removal or out of their homes and for their families is limited. Therefore, it is not surprising that the few funds actually allocated for this population have been crisis-oriented and directed toward families who abuse or neglect their children.[9]

No federal funds are specifically targeted for adoption-related services or for adoption subsidies. Even more significantly, current policies provide explicit disincentives for the adoption of hard-to-place children.

- If adoption requires the total utilization of state or local funds, it is of fiscal benefit to the states to keep children, particularly those with special needs, in the AFDC Foster Care Program for which the state receives some federal funds to offset state and local expenditures.

- Although Title XX funds may be used for a variety of activities related to adoption, they may not be used for adoption subsidies because such expenditures are considered to be maintenance costs. States are not allowed, however, to claim federal reimbursement for adoption subsidies under the AFDC Foster Care Program even though maintenance costs are reimbursable under that program.

- Children in foster care who are eligible for Supplemental Security Income (SSI) and Medicaid may lose their eligibility if they are adopted by a family whose income is over the eligibility standards for these programs.[10] Yet often these families do not have the financial resources, without federal benefits, to cover necessary medical expenses, particu-

---

[7]Statistics gathered in the Philadelphia County Assistance Office showed that in a one-year period only 6.7 percent of the 2,181 children in the AFDC-FC Program returned home. Almost 40 percent of the participants in the program had been in care seven years or more. A report of the Virginia audit concluded that three out of every four children in the program could be expected to remain there until age 18. See reports by the HEW Audit Agency's Philadelphia Regional Office, *Review of AFDC Foster Care Program Administered by the Department of Public Welfare, Commonwealth of Pennsylvania* (Washington, D. C.: HEW Audit Agency, May 1976), p. 4, (Audit Control No. 03-60254); and *Report on the Aid to Families With Dependent Children Foster Care Program, Commonwealth of Virginia* (Washington, D. C.: HEW Audit Agency, June 1976), p. 3, (Audit Control No. 60253-03). Audits of the AFDC Foster Care Program have been conducted, are underway or are planned for 27 states which receive funds under the program. See Appendix B. for a list of these states.

[8]Budget Division, Public Services Administration, Social and Rehabilitation Service, Department of Health, Education and Welfare, "Child Welfare Services Expenditures by Type of Service, Fiscal Year 1976."

[9]Precise figures are unavailable due to the data collection problems described more fully later in this chapter. However, it is estimated that in Fiscal Year 1978, 17 percent of the total Title XX expenditures will be for protective services and substitute care for children. (The largest percentage of Title XX expenditures for children's services is for day care for children of working mothers, estimated to be 22.3 percent of total expenditures in Fiscal Year 1978). E. Wolff, *Technical Notes–Summaries and Characteristics of States' Title XX Social Services Plans for Fiscal Year 1978*, p. xi.

[10]States do have the option of extending Medicaid eligibility to children in subsidized adoptions. 45 C.F.R. §248.1(c)(4). As of December 1977, 17 states extended Medicaid eligibility to all financially needy children under 21 and seven additional states extended eligibility to children receiving adoption subsidies. Appendix R. includes a list of these states.

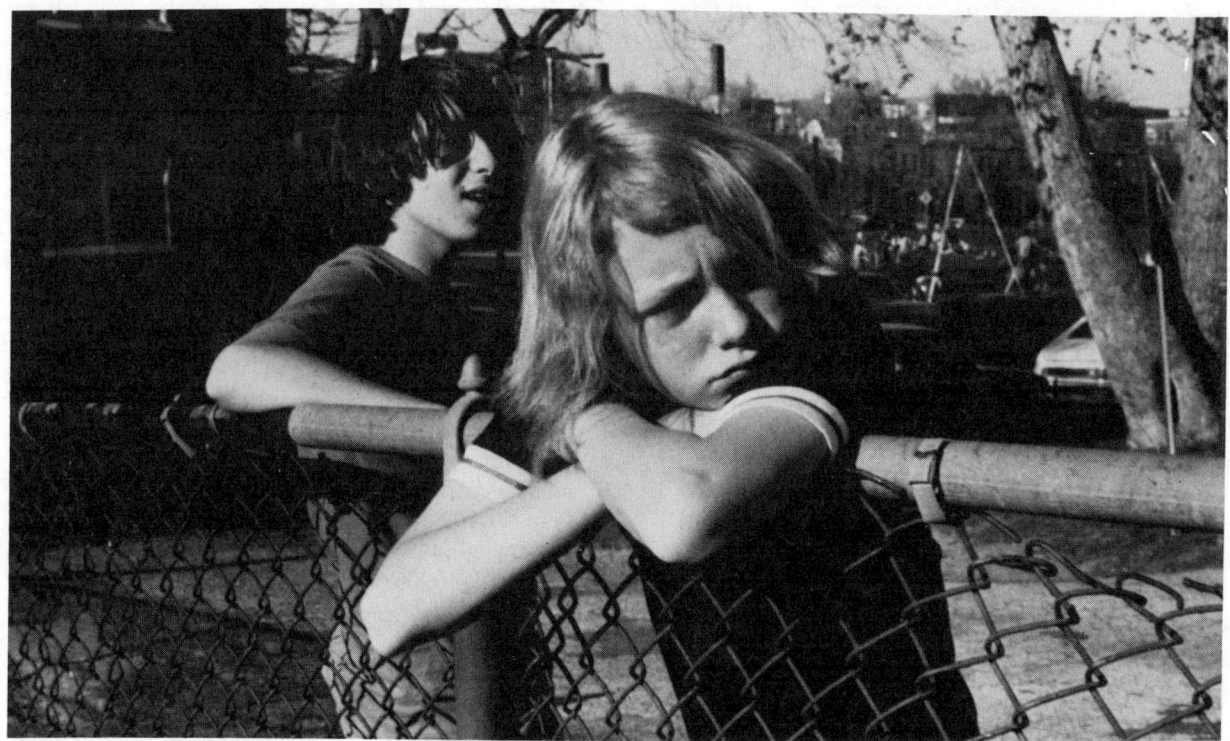

larly since they may not be able to get insurance coverage for children with pre-existing disabilities. This problem creates a particular impediment to permanence for children with handicapping conditions.

Inadequate Protections

Current federal policies fail to ensure adequate procedural and substantive protections to children at risk of removal and in placement, or to their families.

Ensuring adequate protections against the arbitrary, intrusive or inappropriate acts of the child caring systems is a complex task. Statutorily defined protections are a necessary first step. But there must also be sufficient fiscal resources to ensure that states can institute case plans, reviews and required grievance mechanisms. And there must be ongoing efforts by the states and federal government to ensure compliance with mandated protections. Our review of federal programs revealed inadequacies in all three aspects.

The AFDC Foster Care Program, Title IV-B Program, and Indian Child Welfare Assistance Program all lack adequate statutory provisions to protect families and children. The few requirements that do exist are not enforced.

- None of these programs requires that, prior to a child's removal, the family be offered preventive services (except in emergency situations); that the child be placed in the least restrictive setting appropriate to his needs; and that the child be placed within reasonable proximity to his home and community.[11] None requires a dispositional review for children in out-of-home care by an independent body (not involved in the provision of direct services) to ensure children do not linger indefinitely in foster care without permanent homes.

- Eligibility for the AFDC Foster Care Program requires that a child be removed from his home pursuant to a judicial determination that the home condi-

---

[11]The Indian Child Welfare Act, P.L. 95-608, approved November 8, 1978, does establish minimum federal standards and protections affecting the removal of Indian children from their families, and their placement in out-of-home care. It requires, among other things, that efforts must first be made to prevent removal, and that any child accepted for foster care must be placed in "the least restrictive setting which most approximates a family and in which his special needs, if any, may be met" and "within reasonable proximity to his or her own home."

tions are contrary to the child's welfare. This requirement was initially instituted to protect against coercive placements. In some states, however, the judicial determination consists of little more than a rubber stamp process in which all children are funneled through the courts to increase the pool of children eligible for reimbursement under the AFDC Foster Care Program.[12]

- Federal audits have found that even minimal requirements for case plans and periodic reviews in the AFDC Foster Care Program and the Title IV-B Program have been ignored. The most recent GAO review of residential treatment programs receiving funds under the AFDC Foster Care Program found that semi-annual case reviews satisfying federal and state requirements were conducted in less than half of the cases reviewed.[13] In 1975, the GAO conducted a study of children served by both the AFDC Foster Care Program and the Child Welfare Services Program. After reviewing case records of 724 children, selected as protective service cases, GAO concluded: "We found no means being used or proposed for assessing, at specified intervals, the extent of change in and the adequacy of a child's situation."[14] Audits by the HEW Audit Agency revealed similar deficiencies.

- Regulations for the Indian Child Welfare Assistance Program were promulgated for the first time in 1977.[15] These do require that preference be given to placement in Indian foster homes. They refer to case plans and periodic reviews, but give little emphasis to reuniting families or otherwise ensuring a child permanence.

- None of the child welfare legislation defines adequate explicit grievance procedures for parents, children, foster parents and caregivers who feel deprived of a service or benefit to which they are entitled. Although the fair hearing mechanism applicable to public assistance recipients applies to AFDC Foster Care children,[16] fair hearings are not provided to IV-B recipients.

The Title XX Program and Child Abuse Prevention and Treatment Program also provide few protections for children in care who are receiving federally reimbursed services.

- The Title XX Program does pay lip service to concern for quality care by requiring states providing Title XX services to children and others in foster homes and various residential facilities to designate a state authority responsible for establishing and maintaining standards for such facilities. However, the emphasis of such standards is on safety, sanitation, and protection of civil rights, not the quality of the programs.[17] Furthermore, a 1977 report of a GAO analysis of the impact of federal programs on deinstitutionalization noted that Title XX did not require individual service plans or periodic reviews to ensure that placements were appropriate, persons received proper care, or placements continued to be necessary.[18]

- The Child Abuse Prevention and Treatment Act represents an effort to produce widespread systematic reform in the state response to child abuse and neglect. Under the Act, states must meet stringent requirements concerning reporting procedures, definitions of child abuse and neglect, and the provision of representation for children in legal proceedings, to be eligible for funds.[19] However, the Act does not require case plans, periodic reviews, or placement in the least restrictive setting appropriate and within reasonable proximity to family or home community for children in out-of-home care, and participating in projects funded under the Act.

---

[12]For example, at one point, New York was allegedly contemplating returning children who had been in foster care but were held to be ineligible for the AFDC-FC Program to their homes for a brief period and then replacing them in foster care pursuant to court orders so they could claim federal reimbursement for them. Department of Health, Education and Welfare, General Counsel's Opinion on Questions Regarding AFDC-Foster Care, September 23, 1976, pp. 13-16.

[13]General Accounting Office, *Children in Foster Care Institutions: Steps Government Can Take to Improve Their Care* (Washington, D. C.: GAO, February 1977), pp. 9-10.

[14]General Accounting Office, *More Can Be Learned and Done About The Well-Being of Children* (Washington, D. C.: GAO, April 1976), pp. 6-7.

[15] 45 C.F.R.§§20.1-20.30.

[16]In California, the fair hearing procedures were conducted by those administering the larger AFDC program. The child welfare staff did not participate in any way and had no way of knowing what, if any, issues were being raised in AFDC Foster Care related hearings. A national figure on the number of fair hearings held in AFDC-FC cases is not available.

[17]45 C.F.R.§228.12.

[18]General Accounting Office, *Returning the Mentally Disabled to the Community: Government Needs To Do More* (Washington, D. C.: GAO, January 1977), pp. 137-40.

[19]42 C.F.R.§5103(b). Other requirements cover: immunity from prosecution for those who make reports; provisions for investigating reports and appropriate procedures for dealing with child abuse and neglect cases; methods to protect confidentiality; provisions to ensure cooperation of all systems involved in abuse and neglect cases; assurances that federal funds will supplement existing child abuse prevention and treatment efforts; provisions for public dissemination of information regarding abuse and neglect; and assurances that parental organizations combatting abuse and neglect receive preferential treatment.

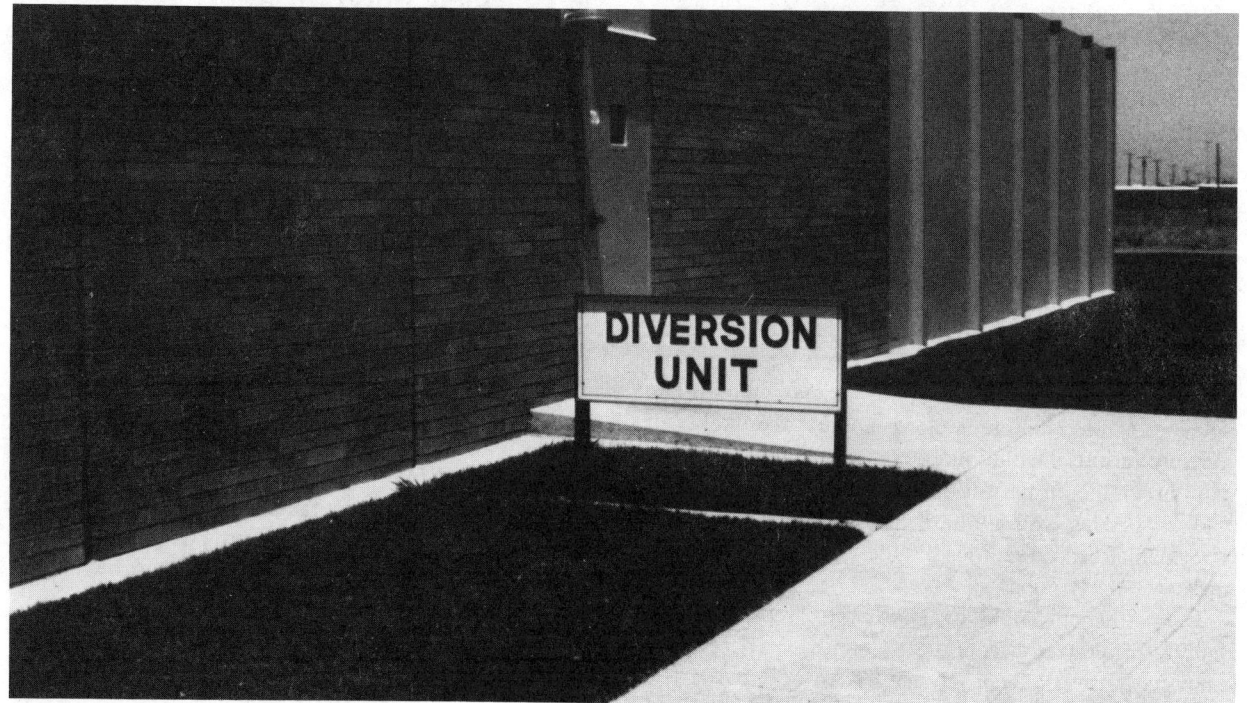

- In the implementation of the Child Abuse Prevention and Treatment Act, little emphasis has been placed on protecting children from institutional abuse and neglect. Child abuse and neglect are defined in the regulations to include harm and threatened harm to a child's health or welfare by a person responsible for their health or welfare, but the focus in programs funded under the Act has clearly been on parental abuse.[20]

There are several pieces of federal legislation which do include adequate, enforceable protections: the Education for All Handicapped Children Act (P.L. 94-142), Section 504 of the Rehabilitation Act of 1973, and the Developmentally Disabled Assistance and Bill of Rights Act of 1975. But there has been little follow-through to ensure the protections are actually afforded to children.

- The Developmentally Disabled Assistance and Bill of Rights Act of 1975 provides strong and important protections to disabled persons, but only limited resources to ensure their implementation. The Developmental Disabilities Program supplies only a very small percentage of the total funds available for services to the developmentally disabled population, and instead attempts to improve the use made of other funds. Yet compliance with the protections in the Developmentally Disabled Assistance Act is not a requirement for receipt of the other federal program dollars which benefit the developmentally disabled.

- Notwithstanding the requirements in P.L. 94-142, the Education for All Handicapped Children Act, educational funds under the two Title I education programs for children in various residential settings are distributed without ensuring that these facilities are in compliance with P.L. 94-142. Attempts to coordinate implementation of P.L. 94-142 and P.L. 89-313 are just beginning.

---

[20]A draft of the proposed Federal Standards for Child Abuse and Neglect Prevention and Treatment Programs and Projects, prepared for the National Center on Child Abuse and Neglect (dated March 1978), does reflect a recognition of the problems of institutional abuse. The Standards for the Prevention and Correction of Institutional Child Abuse and Neglect state that each institution should develop and implement child abuse and neglect reporting procedures; comply with state law in reporting abuse and neglect; and develop a plan for corrective action if a report is founded. The draft standards further suggest the designation of an independent state agency to oversee institutions and assess reports of institutional abuse and neglect; conduct regular audits of all institutions; and establish regional interdisciplinary review boards to conduct pre-placement reviews. This agency should assess reports of suspected institutional abuse or neglect, and establish a conciliation team to assist in negotiations for corrective action. They further recommend that state child abuse and neglect laws should require that all residential child care institutions be licensed, monitored and evaluated on an annual basis in terms of their treatment programs. (Section K, pp. 219-250.) In Chapter 2, we make similar recommendations.

- The Crippled Children's Services Program is a potential source of funds for services to children with special needs, including aftercare, convalescent or foster care. Yet, there is little assurance that children served in the program have treatment plans, or that their need for continuing care and the appropriateness of their treatment plans are reviewed periodically; nor are there requirements for parental participation.

Some of the programs with broad social service mandates are also beginning to take their responsibility to protect children more seriously. Belatedly, there has been an effort to ensure that children receiving financial benefits under the SSI Program receive appropriate services.[21] Medicaid regulations address the quality of care in various institutional settings. Regulations pertaining to the in-patient psychiatric care of children under 21,[22] as well as those pertaining to children in intermediate care facilities for the mentally retarded,[23] are particularly good.

In another example of appropriate redirection of federal effort (four years after Congress exposed horrendous abuses in the program), CHAMPUS has issued strong regulations concerning children in residential treatment facilities, including a clear articulation of the rights of the children and their parents.[24]

These various protections, however, apply only to selected children at risk of or in out-of-home placement and their families. Without strong, uniform protections attached to *all* programs, individual children, families, citizen advocacy groups and public officials are left with few means to enforce their rights and to ensure that program benefits are forthcoming.

---

[21]Initially, the program required that all SSI recipients be referred to the Vocational Rehabilitation Agency, which historically had served only adults and had no experience dealing with children. Now, all children must be referred to the crippled children's agency or another appropriate agency for counseling and referral for services, and children six and under must actually be provided with services. 42 U.S.C. §1382d.

[22]The regulations 45 C.F.R. §249.10(b)(16), state that services can only be made available after certification that "available alternative local community resources for ambulatory care do not meet the treatment needs" of the child; that proper treatment of the child requires inpatient services; and that such services can reasonably be expected to improve the child's condition or prevent further regression. 45 C.F.R. §249.10(b)(16)(iii)). Services to the child in care must also involve active treatment. That is, there must be an individual plan of care for each child "designed to achieve the individual's discharge from inpatient status at the earliest possible time," which must be reviewed every 30 days by an interdisciplinary team of medical professionals. 45 C.F.R. §249.10(b)(16)(iv). The child and the child's parents must be involved in the development of the plan. In addition, the facility must be accredited by the Joint Commission on the Accreditation of Hospitals.

[23]45 C.F.R. §249.12.

[24]32 C.F.R. §199, Appendix A. These protections co-exist with the fiscal disincentive to in-home care described.

Inconsistent Efforts Toward Deinstitutionalization

The federal government has taken an explicit stance in favor of deinstitutionalization. Yet, there has been no concerted effort to ensure that deinstitutionalization efforts are, in fact, working for children. Legislative, regulatory and fiscal provisions are often inconsistent—on the one hand encouraging, and on the other discouraging deinstitutionalization.

A haphazard federal commitment to deinstitutionalization for children is reflected in a variety of ways. There is no one agency or office required to monitor deinstitutionalization efforts in relation to children across agencies and programs. Nor has there been any federally funded research to trace the impact of deinstitutionalization efforts across systems on the children involved.[25]

Federal funds are often not used to ensure care in the least restrictive setting.

- In Fiscal Year 1976, approximately 70 percent of the expenditures under the Indian Child Welfare Assistance Program were for institutional care, with most of the remainder for foster home care.[26] There was no requirement that a child be placed in the least restrictive setting appropriate to his special needs.

- The basic CHAMPUS program calls for families to contribute more of their own funds for the care of a child treated on an out-patient basis in the community than for care of a child in a residential facility.

- Under the Medicaid program, both maintenance and necessary services are reimbursed for children in institutions.[27] For children in less restrictive settings, only medical care is reimbursable. This has promoted the creation of "boarder babies" and the transfer of children from hospitals to equally restrictive but fully reimbursed nursing homes. Home health care, a required service under Medicaid for certain adults, is

---

[25]While the General Accounting Office has done a careful review of the impact of federal programs on deinstitutionalization, children were not singled out for special attention, nor were any of the recommendations directed specifically toward children. See, GAO, *Returning the Mentally Disabled to the Community.*

[26]Department of Interior, Bureau of Indian Affairs, Office of Indian Services, "Child Welfare 1976."

[27]In Fiscal Year 1977, an estimated 70 percent of the *total* Medicaid expenditures were for inpatient services. Department of Health, Education and Welfare, *Medicaid Statistics, Fiscal Year 1977,* pp. 5-6.

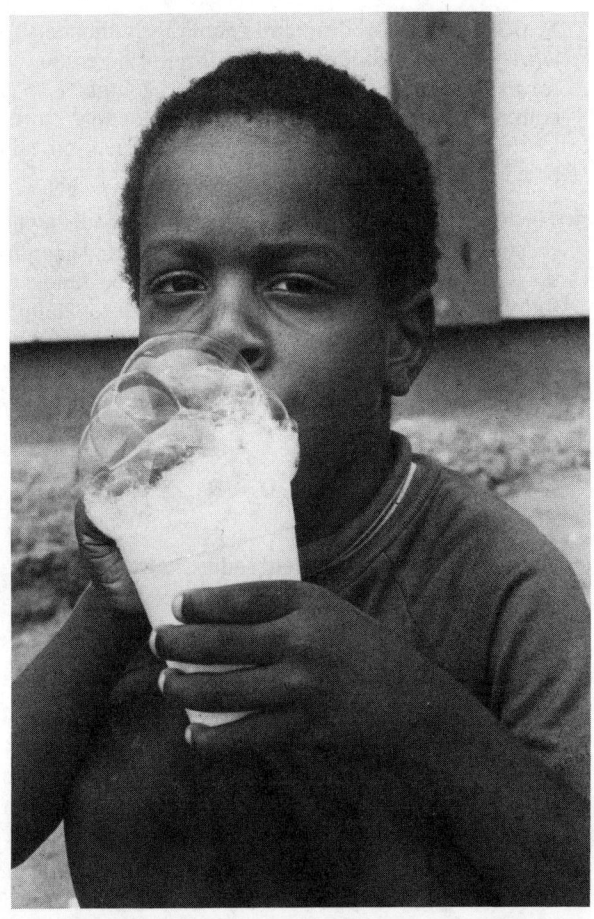

not a required service for persons under 21.²⁸

- States may receive federal reimbursement under Title XX for emergency shelter as a protective service for children, including runaways, as long as it is for not more than 30 days in any six-month period.²⁹ There is no requirement that such shelter must be provided in the least restrictive setting appropriate. The regulations allow placements in institutions, and include no restriction against placements in secure facilities. Similarly, such protections are lacking for more lengthy placements which are reimbursable under Title XX if room and board are an integral but subordinate part of a child's treatment.

- SSI, which has the potential to provide the financial assistance necessary to help keep children in their own homes, has been consistently underutilized for children.³⁰ The failure to mandate, until recently, that services be made available to SSI children has been a disincentive to deinstitutionalize those children already in institutions. It may also have led to the unnecessary institutionalization of some children for whom financial aid alone was not enough. The fact that the SSI program does allow funds to be used for care in public institutions serving 16 or fewer persons should create an incentive for the use of community-based residences.

There are also non-fiscal federal disincentives to deinstitutionalization and the use of less restrictive alternative settings and treatment. In addition, when requirements to encourage deinstitutionalization exist, there is no follow-through to ensure compliance with them.

- The AFDC Foster Care Program does not currently provide federal reimbursement for the care of children in public facilities. It only provides for care in foster family homes and private nonprofit child care institutions. While such a provision acts as a disincentive to the use of large congregate public child care institutions, it also discourages the development of small public group homes for children, despite the critical need for them.

- Although Medicaid regulations include numerous protections for the delivery of services to children in various institutional settings,³¹ inadequate monitor-

---

²⁸The General Accounting Office has recently recommended development of a national policy for home health care with a focus on elderly persons. See GAO, *Home Health–The Need for a National Policy to Better Provide for the Elderly* (Washington, D. C.: GAO, December 1977). While there is a clear need for the development of alternatives to institutionalization for the elderly, the need is as great for children and any comprehensive national home health services policy should recognize the needs of both populations.
²⁹45 C.F.R. §228.46.

³⁰Underutilization of the program for children has been attributed to inadequate outreach efforts, inappropriate disability criteria and the inadequacy of intake procedures and disability determination procedures for child applicants for SSI. N. Solarz and A, Hirschhorn, *A National Study of the Implementation and Implications of the SSI Program for Disabled Children* (Washington, D.C.: National Council of Organizations for Children and Youth, November 1976), Chapter III.
³¹For example, the regulations include numerous protections for the delivery of inpatient psychiatric services to children to try to ensure that children are not placed inappropriately in institutions and left to linger there unnecessarily. See discussion in footnote 22, supra.
Federal statutory and regulatory requirements for the Medicaid Program also require establishment of a utilization review procedure which provides for periodic review of all patients in various inpatient facilities (acute care hospitals, skilled nursing facilities, intermediate care facilities and inpatient mental hospitals) to determine the medical necessity and appropriateness of services. 42 U.S.C. §§1296a(a)(9), (30), (33); 42 U.S.C. §§1396B(g)(1) and (i)(4); 45 C.F.R. §§250.18, et seq. Although the bodies responsible for conducting the review, the standards and frequency vary according to the facility, the utilization reviews are basically cost control mechanisms. However, they have the potential for ensuring that patients are not maintained indefinitely in overly restrictive settings. For a detailed discussion of the various utilization review mechanisms, see S. J. Price, J. Katz, and M. Provence, "An Advocate's Guide to Utilization Review," *Clearinghouse Review* (August 1977): 307-331.

ing and insufficient alternative resources frequently prevent the intent of the regulations from being realized. For example, the failure of states to provide outpatient mental health services under Medicaid reduces the likelihood that children will be discharged from institutions.

- The Juvenile Justice and Delinquency Prevention Act calls for the provision of alternatives to institutionalization and state assurances that status offenders, as well as dependent and neglected children, are not placed in detention or correctional facilities.[32] The federal government, however, has failed to monitor the states' progress, and can provide little information on the impact of the program.[33] The Act also requires that youths placed in adult correctional facilities have no regular contact with adult prisoners. Yet the Title I Education Program for children in institutions for neglected and delinquent children includes no similar requirement, and over 14,000 children were counted as being in adult correctional facilities under that program for Fiscal Year 1977.

In addition to these specific disincentives, there is the more general problem that emphasis on upgrading the quality of institutional care under Medicaid and other programs has in some instances diverted attention and resources away from the development of community-based alternatives.[34] Further, there has been inadequate effort to ensure that federal dollars, services and protections affecting institutionalized children follow them when they are moved to community-based facilities.

- Although two federally supported volunteer programs, the Foster Grandparents' Program and Retired Senior Volunteers' Program, encourage volunteers to work with institutionalized children, there are no formal provisions to ensure that a volunteer may continue to work with a child when he or she returns to the community—assisting in the transition and providing aftercare services.

- The Title I program for the education of handicapped children in state-operated or state-supported institutions was amended in 1974 to allow for funds to follow a child who leaves a state program to attend a locally operated school program.[35] States have found the provision difficult to administer, and the extent to which it is in fact encouraging deinstitutionalization is not clear.[36]

Inadequate Attention to the Quality of Care

There has been insufficient federal attention to the quality and comprehensiveness of care for children in facilities that receive federal funds.

Children, whether in or out of institutions, require adequate health care, food and education. Children who must be removed from their homes frequently require specialized services and treatment. Federal funds are available for these purposes. Yet, there has been no federal effort to examine how all these programs actually affect individual children in particular settings; or whether, in some instances, they are working at cross-purposes. Nor has there been a coordinated attempt to relate the total federal dollars going into institutions to the needs of children in those facilities.

The requirement in federal law that facilities receiving federal funds be licensed in and of itself is not a sufficient safeguard for the children in those facilities. Further, federal and state monitoring to ensure compliance with licensing requirements is inadequate to ensure quality care.

- The regulations for the AFDC Foster Care Program

---

[32]The Act, when passed in 1974, required deinstitutionalization within three years. The 1977 amendments modified this to require that states must have achieved at least 75 percent deinstitutionalization by October 1978, and then gave them an additional two years to achieve full compliance with the deinstitutionalization requirement. 42 U.S.C. §5633(c).

[33]In December 1976, only nine of the 42 participating states submitted complete reports to the Office of Juvenile Justice and Delinquency Prevention. Further, preliminary findings from a GAO study of the state efforts to deinstitutionalize status offenders revealed many problems with the states' own monitoring efforts in the five states it studied. For example, local jails and correctional facilities were often not monitored, state legislation permitted placement of status offenders in detention facilities and funds for alternative facilities were lacking. Testimony of John Rector, Associate Administrator, Office of Juvenile Justice and Delinquency Prevention, LEAA, and William J. Anderson, Deputy Director, General Government Division, General Accounting Office, before the Senate Subcommittee on Juvenile Delinquency, September 27, 1977.

[34]On the other hand, it is encouraging that recognition of the problem of inadequate community-based facilities is growing. Recent legislative efforts recognize that Indian children and others are frequently required to leave their homes and attend distant institutions because other more appropriate facilities are unavailable. See legislative history accompanying the Indian Child Welfare Act, P.L. 95-608.

[35]P.L. 93-380. Such a provision was considered essential to eliminate a potential fiscal incentive to institutionalize children. In 1976, the average per pupil expenditure for handicapped children in the Title I program ranged from $415 to $623 per child, while programs serving handicapped children in local schools under P.L. 94-142 received about $70 per child. M. LaVor, "Public Law 89-313," p. 162.

[36]A review of the program by Martin LaVor reported that 13 of the 40 states responding indicated that the pass-through works, 14 indicated it did not, and 13 said it was difficult to administer. Only half of the states were able to report a specific number of children who had been deinstitutionalized and in nine states that number was zero. M. LaVor, "Public Law 89-313," Part III, p. 235.

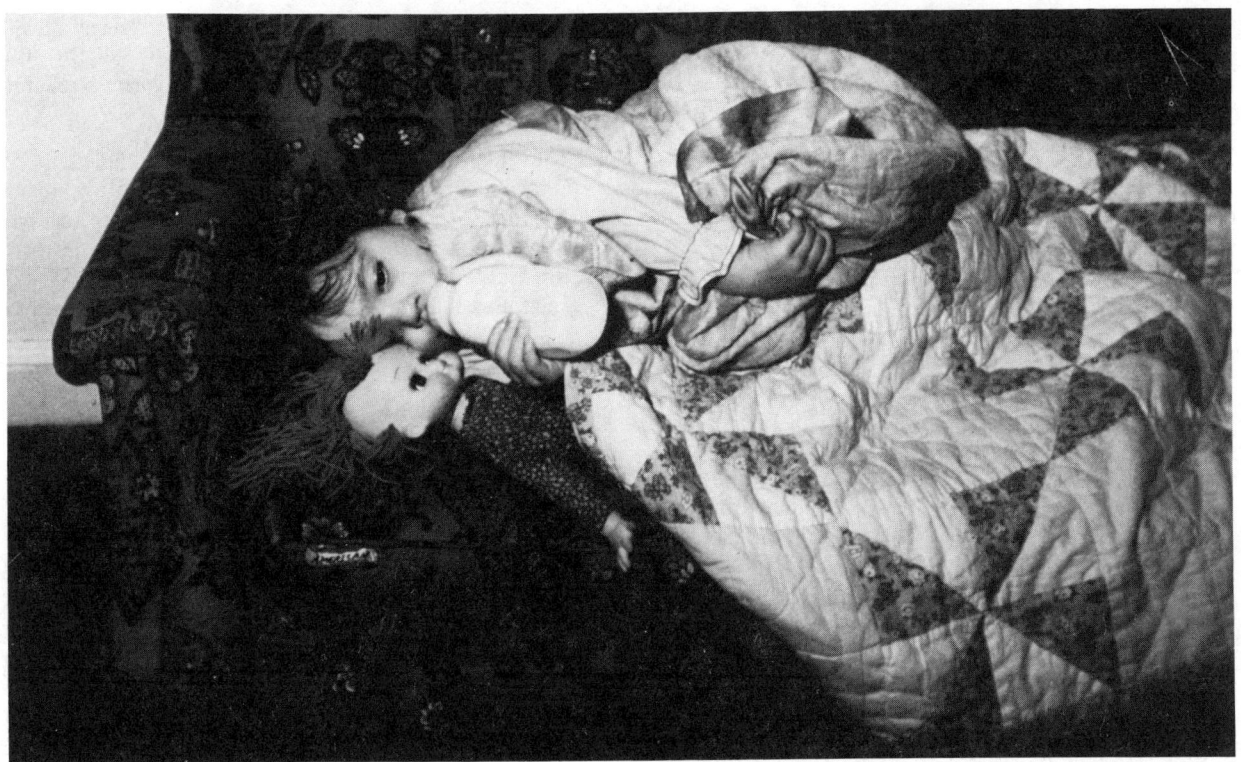

require that children be placed only in licensed or approved facilities.[37] However, a GAO study of 18 institutions in four states that received funds under the AFDC Foster Care Program in 1976 revealed that almost half of the facilities were either unlicensed or had serious physical deficiencies in health and safety conditions.[38]

- Audits of the AFDC Foster Care Program by the HEW Audit Agency also revealed licensing deficiencies. State placing agencies were found to use unlicensed facilities. And frequently, children were placed in facilities and left to remain there for years, without any reevaluation of the adequacy of the facility, although such reappraisals are required by law.[39]

Federal reimbursement for licensing activities is uneven.

- Under the Medicaid program 100 percent federal reimbursement is available to states for costs related to the compensation or training of personnel involved in inspecting long-term care facilities for compliance with Medicaid standards.[40] But there is no comparable federal incentive to help states maintain adequate licensing staff to oversee group care facilities for neglected and dependent children.

Federal funds do not always result in increased or improved services at the state and local level.

- States in some instances use federal dollars simply to replace state and local expenditures. There are too

---

[37] In July 1977, 22.8 percent of the children in AFDC Foster Care in the 46 states reporting data were in child care institutions, and 47 percent of the federal expenditures were used to care for these children. Office of Research and Statistics, Social Security Administration, Department of Health, Education and Welfare, *Public Assistance Statistics, July 1977* (Washington, D. C.: HEW December 1977), p. 12.

[38] The deficiencies included: children sleeping on mattresses on the floor in cramped and dingy rooms; children's beds pushed up against gas heaters that were operating at full power, even though it was a hot summer day; dirty and unsanitary sleeping, living and kitchen areas; and inadequate control over prescription drugs, which in two institutions were left in shoe boxes on desk tops. General Accounting Office, *Children in Foster Care Institutions—Steps Government Can Take to Improve Their Care*, pp. 23-26. In the *Gary W.* suit discussed in Chapter 3, many of the inadequate Texas facilities were receiving AFDC-FC funds.

[39] See, for example, reports by the HEW Audit Agency of reviews of the AFDC Foster Care Programs in Kansas (Kansas City Regional Office, Audit Control No. 07-60251, June 16, 1976), Maryland (Philadelphia Regional Office, Audit Control No. 03-70256, February 11, 1977), and North Carolina (Atlanta Regional Office, Audit Control No. 04-60255, December 17, 1976).

[40] 42 U.S.C. §1396b(a)(4).

few maintenance of effort[41] provisions incorporated in federal programs. For example, there is no maintenance of effort provision in the Child Welfare Services Program.

- When school lunch and breakfast programs were extended to children's residential institutions in 1975, states were not required to maintain their current level of contribution for food programs in these facilities. Thus, there is a need to examine whether the quality of nutrition for children in these facilities has, in fact, improved.

Requirements for monitoring the quality of care provided under federally reimbursable purchase-of-service agreements are vague and poorly monitored.

- Federal statutes and regulations for some child welfare-related programs grant states the authority to purchase services from other public agencies or private sources.[42] Although federal regulations address allowable and unallowable costs and activities in relation to such contracts,[43] ultimate responsibility for monitoring the quality of services or the contracts themselves is not specified. Yet during a single quarter in Fiscal Year 1976 (April-June), almost 50 percent of the expenditures under Titles XX, IV-B and IV-C of the Social Security Act were used to purchase services from public and private vendors.[44] Under Title IV-B alone, 74 percent of the total (federal, state and local) child welfare service expenditures in Fiscal Year 1976 were for purchased services.[45]

There is little attention to ensuring that children in care receive all the services to which they are entitled. Generally, agencies receiving federal funds are not required to notify children's caretakers—when other than their families—of the availability of health, education and nutrition services under various federal programs.

- Current Medicaid regulations do not include procedures for ensuring that children in foster care who are eligible for Medicaid have an opportunity to receive services under the EPSDT program. Outreach efforts are seldom directed to foster family homes and institutions.

- There is no specific requirement that foster parents who care for young children be notified of the child's potential eligibility for supplemental foods under the WIC Program.

- Although P.L. 94-142 provides for the designation of a "surrogate parent" for handicapped children with special educational needs who are wards of the state and whose parents are unknown or unavailable,[46] there is no assurance that agencies in contact with these children will be advised of the provision. Nor are parents of children currently in institutions systematically advised of their rights under P.L. 94-142, even though its provisions for an evaluation, individualized education plan and periodic review might substantially improve the quality of care the child is receiving or allow the parent to return the child to the community.

Training funds have had only minimal impact on the quality of services for children.

- Staff training is an essential component of quality services. Yet only limited federal funds have been aimed at training people who have daily contact with children at risk of placement or in care and their families. In Fiscal Year 1975, approximately 80 percent of the training funds available under Section 426 of Title IV-B of the Social Security Act were used for long-term training relevant to child welfare, such as stipends and institutional support, rather than for short-term, in-service training.

- Training funds available under Title XX can be used for training staff and potential staff of Title XX agencies and individual providers. Training for foster parents is an eligible service, but only for foster parents who contract directly with the Title XX agency for care of Title XX children. States are not currently able to claim reimbursement under Title XX for foster parent contracts with private nonprofit

---

[41] In this context a maintenance of effort provision refers to a requirement that states continue their funding for a particular purpose at the level it was at at a specified time so as not to substitute increased federal funds for state funds. For example, the maintenance of effort requirement for the Title XX Program reads: "Each State which participates in the program shall assure that the aggregate expenditures from appropriated funds from the State and political subdivisions for the provision of services during each services program year with respect to which payment is made under this Part is not less than the aggregate expenditures from such appropriated funds for the provision of services during the fiscal year ending June 30, 1973, or the fiscal year ending June 30, 1974, with respect to which payment was made under the plan of the State. . . ." 45 C.F.R.§228.18.

[42] For further discussion of the purchase of service concept, see Chapter 2.

[43] 45 C.F.R. 74, Appendix F. See also 45 C.F.R. §§228.70, 228.71.

[44] Administration for Public Services, Office of Human Development Services, Department of Health, Education and Welfare, *Social Services U.S.A. (April-June 1976)* (Washington, D. C.: HEW, December 1977), pp. 70-78. The reference to Title IV-C is to the Work Incentive Program (WIN) authorized by the Social Security Amendments of 1967 and 1971.

[45] Social and Rehabilitation Service, Department of Health, Education and Welfare, "Total Expenditures by Purpose, Fiscal Year 1976."

[46] 45 C.F.R. §121a.514.

agencies not providing other Title XX services. National figures on the extent to which states use Title XX funds for foster parent training are not available.

- Training projects have frequently been isolated from the needs of ongoing service programs. Yet without such training, significant legislation, good regulations, and targeted service dollars are insufficient. There has been too little joint funding of interdisciplinary training efforts. And the important role of the social worker as case manager in the child welfare system has been neglected in training.

Enforcement Failures

There has been a striking absence of federal compliance efforts with regard to children at risk of removal or in out-of-home placement. Federal agencies have done little to ensure that existing program requirements are met. They have also failed to monitor and take action against discriminatory treatment of minority children.

For most programs, the only rigorous evaluations of the extent of state compliance with federal laws and regulations have been studies by the General Accounting Office (GAO), initiated at Congressional request. Follow-up of GAO findings by federal agencies has been weak or nonexistent.[47]

- In its reviews of both the AFDC Foster Care and Title IV-B Programs, the GAO reported widespread abuses. HEW, however, has made no effort to impose sanctions on the states or to clarify existing program regulations and reporting requirements.[48]

- The HEW Audit Agency has undertaken an extensive study of the AFDC Foster Care Program in 27 states.[49] Reviews in over half of these states have been completed and have uncovered many program violations, but there appears to be no structured response for follow-up. To date, HEW has conducted no audit of the Title IV-B Child Welfare Services Program.

Federal agencies have not devoted adequate resources or attention to monitoring responsibilities.

- A July 1975 analysis of HEW programs affecting children[50] estimated that .1 percent of HEW's Fiscal Year 1975 budget impacting on children was spent on monitoring and evaluation activities. The Social and Rehabilitation Service, which spent $13 billion for children in Fiscal Year 1975, applied only .006 percent of this money for evaluation and monitoring.

In some instances, responsibility for enforcement has not been adequately defined by statute.

- The litigation experience of the Civil Rights Division of the Department of Justice has shown that basic constitutional and federal statutory rights of institutionalized persons, including children, are being violated on a systematic and widespread basis. Yet there is currently no legislation specifically authorizing the United States to initiate litigation when these rights are violated.[51] Although the Justice Department has argued that it has the authority to initiate such suits, recent court decisions have held otherwise.[52]

- Existing statutes and program regulations provide very few mechanisms for monitoring by parents, child advocates, or other interested parties. Sometimes, too, the obligations upon states are not stated clearly, and self-enforcement at the state level is inhibited.[53]

Insufficient staff has also limited the ability of the federal government to monitor its child welfare programs adequately.

- The Children's Bureau in HEW currently employs one adoption specialist and one foster care specialist, neither of whom has full-time counterparts at the regional level. There are currently two Children's

---

[47]One of the most frequently imposed sanctions resulting from audits is the disallowance of expenditures, frequently several years after the abuses occurred. The use of sanctions to ensure compliance with federal program requirements is a complex issue. Sanctions vary according to when they are applied, their nature and their effect. Financial sanctions may range from positive fiscal incentives to penalties, the most extreme and infrequently used being a total cut-off of funds. Non-financial sanctions may include imposed technical assistance or various administrative or judicial remedies. In fact, however, our review of federal programs indicated that few meaningful sanctions are imposed.

[48]In July 1977, S. 1928 was introduced for the Administration which would have improved both the AFDC Foster Care Program and the IV-B Child Welfare Services Program.

[49]See Appendix B. for a list of the states and the status of the audits.

[50]*DHEW Programs Affecting Children: A Summary Report for FY 1975,* prepared by the HEW Committee On Children, July 1975. No similar report was published for Fiscal Year 1976.

[51]Legislation which would have given the Justice Department standing in such matters was introduced in the 95th Congress. See H.R. 9400 and S. 1393.

[52] See, for example, *United States v. Solomon,* 563 F.2d 1121 (4th Cir. 1977), and *United States v. Mattson,* appeal pending, No. 76-3568 (9th Cir.).

[53]See, for example, General Accounting Office, *Children In Foster Care Institutions–Steps Government Can Take to Improve Their Care,* pp. 14-22.

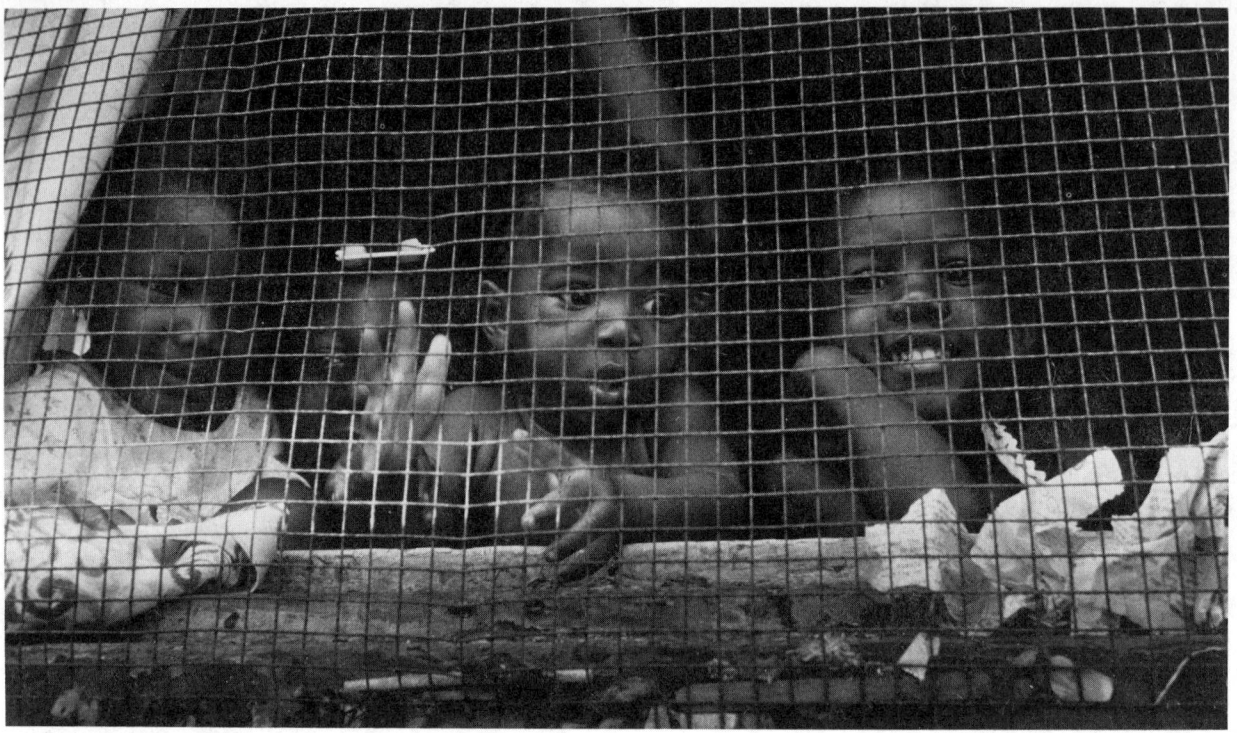

Bureau employees in each of eight of the HEW regional offices and three each in the other two regions, who are responsible for overseeing activities funded by the National Center on Child Abuse and Neglect as well as services, research and training funded under Title IV-B of the Social Security Act.

- At the regional level, the AFDC Foster Care Program is usually the responsibility of the individual who monitors other public assistance programs, and it is thus given relatively low priority. In both dollars expended and number of recipients, the AFDC-FC program ranks far behind the AFDC program.

There have been virtually no federal compliance efforts on behalf of minority children at risk of placement or in out-of-home care and their families.

- Title VI of the Civil Rights Act of 1964 prohibits discrimination on the basis of race, color, or national origin in federally assisted programs. The Office for Civil Rights (OCR), which is responsible for enforcing Title VI in HEW funded programs, has not published policy guidelines for the states to use in monitoring Title VI compliance in the administration of their social services and child welfare programs. OCR conducts periodic surveys of nursing homes and hospitals in order to assess their compliance with Title VI but has not conducted comparable surveys of child-placing and child-caring agencies.[54]

- Longstanding abuses against Indian children have been well documented in Congressional hearings and studies conducted for the American Indian Policy Review Commission and the Children's Bureau at HEW. Great concern was expressed about the fact that Indian children were frequently unnecessarily removed from their homes; placed in non-Indian foster care homes and institutions;[55] and often

---

[54] The inadequacy and ineffectiveness of the Title VI compliance efforts by OCR in the area of social services, particularly child care, have been well documented. See, for example, M. G. Rose and S. Newman, *The Civil Rights Enforcement Program in the Health, and Social Service Programs of the U. S. Department of Health, Education And Welfare–Policy Paper for a New Direction And Approach* (Washington, D. C., 1977); and U. S. Department of Justice, *Implementation of Title VI by the Department of Health, Education and Welfare in the Areas of Health and Welfare* (Washington, D. C.: Department of Justice, 1972).

[55] In response to evidence that AFDC Foster Care Program licensing requirements were preventing the placement of children in foster homes with relatives or on Indian reservations in some states, the Social and Rehabilitation Service in HEW issued a Program Instruction in 1974 advising states that special standards other than state licensing requirements could be applied in approving homes on reservations. Notwithstanding this instruction, the problem continues. Few states have developed special procedures for approving Indian homes. Children's Bureau, Office of Human Development, Department of Health, Education and Welfare, *Indian Child Welfare: A State-of-the-Field Study* (Washington. D. C.: HEW, 1976), pp. 18-19.

adopted by non-Indian families. Yet it is only recently that any attention has been given to ensuring tribal governments and Indian organizations a role in the delivery of services to Indian children.

Little effort has been taken at the federal level to ensure compliance with Section 504 of the Rehabilitation Act of 1973. This civil rights act for disabled citizens makes it illegal for any agency or organization receiving federal funds to discriminate in any way against disabled persons, including children.

- Although Section 504 was enacted in 1973, final regulations were not issued until May 1977, and thus during that period there were only limited federal enforcement activities.

- HEW is charged with responsibility for coordinating 504 enforcement programs throughout the federal government. Within HEW, OCR is responsible for the 504 enforcement program. Although OCR has initiated a series of technical assistance programs to help federally funded institutions and agencies voluntarily comply with the 504 regulations, it has not yet developed an effective enforcement program.[56]

Fragmented Administrative Authority

Administrative responsibility for federal programs affecting children without homes is fragmented. Adequate policy planning and coordination to ensure administrative linkages among programs and among their service, training and research components are virtually nonexistent.

The disorganized structure of federal responsibility for the vulnerable children at risk of or in out-of-home placement is part of a larger fragmented federal policy toward all children and families. This problem will not be fully resolved until there is a more coherent and responsive federal administrative structure for all programs affecting children and families. In the meantime, however, a much clearer focus on the problems of children without homes should be developed.

There are over 17 administrative units within 6 departments of the federal government—10 within HEW alone—with responsibility for programs affecting displaced children and their families. Yet, often these various units operate in a vacuum—aware neither of the activities of other units nor the extent to which needs are being met. There is little joint funding among agencies, and no comprehensive planning to provide a continuum of services to these children and families. The division of program responsibilities between Washington and the regional offices further complicates and fragments program authority. The situation is reflected on the Congressional level, where these programs are addressed, either for funding or oversight, by numerous committees and subcommittees.[57]

Within the past year, there has been a shift in organizational responsibility at the federal level for a number of the social service and child welfare programs. Whether this will lead to significant substantive change and a refocusing of federal responsibility is not yet clear.[58]

- The reorganization of the Office of Human Development Services within HEW has consolidated the Title IV-B programs which include child welfare services, research and training monies, under one administration, but Title XX services are still administered elsewhere. Further, the AFDC Foster Care Program is now administered by the Social Security Administration as an income maintenance program, without regard to service requirements or linkages with other child welfare and social services programs.

- There is no formal mechanism for coordinating the agencies and offices responsible for these various programs. A recent GAO report recommends that "Congress should examine the extent to which ACYF and the Children's Bureau have, or should have, the mandate to advocate and coordinate Federal programs affecting children."[59] The GAO found that although the Children's Bureau has the legislative authority to assume a leadership role with respect to children's programs, it does not have the legislative mandate to carry out specific coordination activities.[60]

---

[56] Such a program should include a meaningful data collection system, a mechanism for acting upon individual complaints, and a design for compliance reviews which reaches local school districts, colleges and universities, and health and social services agencies and institutions.

[57] The programs are authorized, for instance, by 5 committees and 7 subcommittees in the House; and 6 committees and 10 subcommittees in the Senate. A list of the specific authorizing committees for each of the programs is included in Appendix P.

[58] As reported in Chapter 4, recent administrative changes in our study states have had little apparent effect on services delivered to children and families.

[59] General Accounting Office, *Administration for Children, Youth, and Families—Need to Better Use Its Research and Clarify Its Role* (Washington, D. C.: GAO, March 31, 1977), p. 12.

[60] Ibid, pp. 42-52.

There is little attempt to coordinate different programs funding similar services or to ensure that they are not actually working at cross-purposes.

- Although some of the projects funded under the Runaway Youth Program also receive funding under programs administered by LEAA and the Department of Labor, a recent GAO review of the program indicated that program coordination was very limited.[61]
- No one has been assigned responsibility for coordinating and monitoring efforts to facilitate deinstitutionalization of children across federal agencies. There has been no systematic effort to focus on what is happening to deinstitutionalized children.[62]
- A number of programs are designed to meet special needs of handicapped children, but the different requirements for services and protections in each may result in confused and fragmented health care services for these children. Service plans are required under P.L. 94-142, Section 504, the Disabled Children's Program, SSI and Medicaid, but there has been little attention to ensure that the requirements are consistent or offer equal protections to the children affected. Nor are definitions of disability consistent.

Fragmentation, in some instances, has resulted in duplication and impairment of the quality of services provided.

- Under contracts from two separate offices within HEW, two sets of standards relating to the prevention and treatment of child abuse and neglect were prepared. Similar duplication has been evident in the location of child abuse-related training programs.
- A recent GAO review of the use of educational funds available under P.L. 89-313 for institutionalized children found that there has been limited program guidance, technical assistance, monitoring, and dissemination assistance provided to the states by the federal government. The GAO attributed this in part to the fact that fiscal and programmatic authority for the program is split between two administering agencies within HEW. As a result, neither has sufficient interest in the overall management of the program.[63]
- There has been little systematic effort to disseminate the results of research and demonstration programs, either to the states or to federal agencies funding service programs. In a recently released report, the GAO confirmed that funds utilized by the Administration for Children, Youth and Families (ACYF) within HEW for child welfare research and demonstration projects have generally had only limited impact on providers of social services.[64] Until recently, the administration of service programs and research and demonstation efforts funded under Title IV-B were separated.

Even when coordination is mandated by statute or referred to in regulations, the references are often vague and result only, at a maximum, in a statement of cooperation or agreement.

- The Office of Juvenile Justice and Delinquency Prevention has been under a legislative mandate to coordinate federal juvenile delinquency efforts. However, during its first three years of existence, the Office had little to show for its efforts except the publication of two volumes identifying over 100 programs "related" to juvenile delinquency.[65] The document included only program descriptions, and listed almost all programs affecting children, even Head Start.
- Regulations for the Title XX Program require states to include in their Comprehensive Annual Services Plan (CASP) a description of how the provision of services under Title XX will be coordinated with and utilize programs funded under Titles IV-A, IV-B, XVI and XIX of the Social Security Act, as well as other human services programs in the states.[66] How-

---

[61]Statement of Gregory J. Ahart, Director, Human Resources Division, GAO, before the Subcommittee on Economic Opportunity of the House Committee on Education and Labor, on the Management and Operation of the Runaway Youth Program, March 7, 1978, pp. 16-17.

[62]The 1977 Amendments to the Juvenile Justice and Delinquency Prevention Act, however, authorize the Coordinating Council to review federal programs and practices to determine whether any federal funds are used for purposes inconsistent with the Act's mandate for deinstitutionalization. 42 U.S.C. §5616(c). The Coordinating Council was established by the Juvenile Justice and Delinquency Prevention Act of 1974. It is an independent body in the Executive Branch responsible for coordinating all federal juvenile delinquency programs. Chaired by the Attorney General and composed of high ranking officers of various executive agencies and offices, it has been ineffective to date.

[63]General Accounting Office, *Federal Direction Needed for Educating Handicapped Children in State Schools* (Washington, D.C.: GAO, March 16, 1978), p. 43.

[64]See, General Accounting Office, *Administration for Children, Youth, and Families—Need to Better Use Its Research Results and Clarify Its Role*. ACYF has funded special dissemination programs for a relatively small number of its demonstration projects, and has recently established the Child Welfare Resource Information Exchange to disseminate information on successful projects.

[65]See, Office of Juvenile Justice and Delinquency Prevention, *Federal Juvenile Delinquency Programs–First Analysis and Evaluation, Volume 2.*

[66]45 C.F.R. §228.29.

ever, the descriptions are frequently void of detail.[67]

No National Data

The absence of useful national information about children out of their homes and about the impact of relevant federal programs prevents meaningful planning, monitoring and evaluation efforts.

In spite of the fact that there are at least 20 data collection efforts conducted by or under contract with federal agencies which include some data on children out of their homes, very little *useful* data are available on a national basis.

- Data which do exist are not comparable. Different definitions of handicaps, different age breakdowns, different descriptions of the same settings, and different time spans all prevent the compilation of information from these various surveys.[68]

- The U.S. Census contains data on gross numbers of children out of their homes by state, and will be of even greater value when the mid-decade census becomes mandatory in 1985.[69] However, it is not possible to determine from the Census data how many children are in foster homes of either relatives or non-relatives. Nor is it possible to distinguish among out-of-home care in community-based group homes, small residential treatment settings, or large institutions.[70]

- The Current Population Survey, conducted annually by the Census Bureau, includes national data on institutional inmates and other persons living in households or other group quarters where they have no relatives.[71] It does not, however, distinguish foster children from other such persons. Further, the data obtained on institutionalized persons do not include a breakdown by type of facility.[72]

Although HEW is responsible for the majority of federal programs affecting children in out-of-home care, it does not know how many children are in various foster care settings or who is responsible for them.[73]

- Monthly reports are published by the Social Security Administration which include data on children participating in the AFDC Foster Care Program,[74] but no unduplicated count of annual participation in the program is available. Nor are complete data available on children in foster care not eligible for the federal program.

- The former National Center on Social Statistics[75] conducted an annual survey on the total number of children receiving child welfare services and other

---

[67]For instance, in its proposed Fiscal Year 1979 CASP, Massachusetts comments on coordination with other human services programs only by naming other responsible state agencies administering Title XX services for particular client groups—elderly, children, blind, developmentally disabled, alcohol and drug abusers, as well as programs in mental health, mental retardation and corrections.

[68]For example, the Juvenile Detention and Correctional Facility Census, conducted annually by the Census Bureau for the Law Enforcement Assistance Administration, does not specify the ages of children in the various facilities. Similarly, the Master Facilities Inventory, conducted every three years by the National Center for Health Statistics, includes data on the age ranges served by hospitals, nursing homes and other health and correctional facilities, but no data are compiled on the numbers of children served by type of facility. Deficiencies in some of the other data collection efforts are described in the following pages.

[69]The Census data include figures on the sex, age and race of persons in various types of institutions and of persons residing in other group quarters and also include numbers of individuals living in households where they are not related to the head of the household. See, for example, U.S. Bureau of the Census, Census of Population: 1970, *Persons in Institutions and Other Group Quarters*, Final Report PC(2)-4E and *Persons by Family Characteristics*, Final Report PC(2)-4B (Washington, D.C: U.S. Government Printing Office, 1973).

[70]At ten-year intervals, the institutional population is analyzed by type of facility (e.g., training school, mental hospitals, residential treatment settings), based on a 20 percent sample.

[71]This group of unrelated persons is referred to as "secondary individuals."

[72]The Census Bureau also issued in June 1978 a report on a 1976 survey it conducted for HEW, which focused on a national sample of long-term care institutions. The report describes characteristics of the institutions and residents, including data on children in various types of facilities. See, U. S. Bureau of the Census, Current Population Reports, *1976 Survey of Institutionalized Persons: A Study of Persons Receiving Long-Term Care*, Special Studies Series P-23 (Washington, D.C.: U.S. Government Printing Office, 1978).

[73]The Children's Bureau in HEW has awarded a contract for $439,000 for a national survey of public social services for children and their families. This has the potential for producing some valuable data on children in out-of-home care. The survey sample covered approximately 9,500 children in 39 states served by 315 public social service departments during the first quarter of 1977. Variables examined for the child sample include, among others: age, sex and ethnicity of the child, the length of time in placement, numbers of parent-child, parent-agency and child-agency contacts, number of placements, services provided to the family and to the child, number of caseworkers assigned to the child, and reasons why a child is or is not free for adoption. A full report on the results of this survey is expected to be available by the close of 1978. It will include national projections, but no information from particular local agencies or states. An overview of highlights from the survey was released in March 1978, see A. W. Shyne and A. G. Schroeder, *National Study of Social Services to Children and Their Families–Overview* (Washington, D.C.: Children's Bureau, HEW, 1978).

[74]*Public Assistance Statistics* is published monthly by the Office of Research and Statistics in the Social Security Administration as part of its A-2 series.

[75]The National Center was formerly located within the Social and Rehabilitation Service in HEW. When SRS was abolished in March 1977, data collection functions of the Center were transferred to different offices with their corresponding organizational units. For example, responsibility for the AFDC Foster Care Program was transferred from SRS to the Social Security Administration, and monthly reports on participation in the program formerly prepared by the National Center are now prepared by the Office of Research and Statistics in SSA.

social services by type of living arrangements of the child,[76] but because this survey was voluntary, the data were virtually useless. In 1975, only about half of the state welfare departments responded completely to the survey; 19 states submitted no reports. Moreover, even if there had been complete reporting, nothing would be known about the length of time these children had been in care, their current legal status, their race or age.

- Reporting of adoption statistics is also voluntary and frequently incomplete.[77] As a result, national totals of the number of adoptions in the United States have not been published since 1971. In 1975, only about 30 states reported complete data even on the number of adoptions. Fewer than 20 included data on the functional condition of children, adoptive parents, and whether adoption subsidies were used.

The response by states to voluntary reporting efforts has been poor, but when states are required to report statistics upon which program allocations will be based, they produce figures. However, these figures may well be of questionable quality.[78]

- The annual formula count for allocations under Title I of the Elementary and Secondary Education Act calls for state-by-state breakdowns of the number of children aged 5-17 in publicly supported foster homes and local institutions for neglected children and for delinquents, including adult correctional facilities. Similarly, allocations for the Title I amendment programs are based on state-by-state figures on the average daily attendance of handicapped children in state-operated and state-supported schools, many of which are residential programs.[79] States are required to supply such information in order to be eligible for Title I funds, and seem to produce the figures when it is to their advantage.

The lack of routinely available racial data about children out of their own homes is particularly disturbing because it inhibits efforts to monitor discriminatory treatment of the children and families affected.

- None of the approximately 20 federal data collection efforts which include data on children out of their homes in various types of settings, with the exception of the ten-year census conducted by the Bureau of the Census, collects data on the children's race or ethnicity. Nor do the statistics tell us anything about the comparative lengths of placements for minority and nonminority children, or comparative rates for children being returned home or adopted.[80]

- There has also been little attention to data on Indian children in the child welfare system. For example, statistics published by the Bureau of Indian Affairs include no references to the extent to which Indian children are placed in non-Indian foster care homes and institutions.[81]

Reporting about individual federal programs is so poor that it is difficult—sometimes impossible—to know whether specific programs are accomplishing their goals or benefiting recipients. The fiscal information available often is not related to the numbers and types of services provided, much less to their outcomes.

- Title XX funds can be used for a continuum of services to children at risk of removal or in out-of-home care. But the way state plans are prepared and use of services is reported make it impossible to get an accurate picture of which services under Title XX

---

[76]The most recent report of this type, *Children Served by Public Welfare Agencies and Voluntary Child Welfare Agencies and Institutions, March 1975,* was published in March of 1976.

[77]The National Center for Social Statistics published annual adoption statistics in its E-10 report series; the most recent is *Adoptions in 1975* (Washington, D.C.: NCSS, Social and Rehabilitation Service, HEW, April 1977).

[78]Given our unsuccessful experience in trying to obtain data at the state and local levels, we are extremely skeptical of statewide and national figures which are portrayed as absolute counts.

[79]For Fiscal Year 1977, 318,849 children were counted as being in foster homes or institutions for neglected or delinquent children and 201,429 handicapped children were reported in state-supported programs, many of them residential programs. Office of Education, Department of Health, Education and Welfare, "Elementary and Secondary Education Act of 1965, As Amended, Title I, Assistance for Educationally Deprived Children in Programs for Neglected and Delinquent Children," Fiscal Years 1967-1977; "1977 Formula Children Count for Local Educational Agencies"; and Printout, "State Agencies Eligible to Participate Under P.L. 89-313, Amendment to Title I, Elementary and Secondary Education Act of 1975," August 3, 1976. These numbers do not include children under five or over 17 in publicly supported foster homes or local institutions for neglected or delinquent children, nor handicapped children in nursing homes or other residential facilities that are not state-supported schools.

[80]A national survey conducted by the National Urban League with a grant from the Administration for Children, Youth and Families in HEW requested racial data on children in foster care and adoptions from all 50 states and the District of Columbia. Although at least 20 states reported some racial breakdowns for adoptions, only nine of these reported similar breakdowns for children in foster care. National Urban League, "Preliminary Report for IAP Nationwide Survey on Adoption and Foster Care and the Black Child," New York, Fall 1977. (Unpublished.)

[81]The Task Force On Federal, State and Tribal Jurisdiction of the American Indian Policy Review Commission has expressed great concern about the adoption of Indian children by non-Indian families and the temporary and permanent placement of Indian children in non-Indian foster care homes and institutions. They state that in 1974 it was estimated, on the basis of the best available data at the time, that 25 to 35 percent of all Indian children were being raised by non-Indians. For further discussion of their findings and recommendations, see Task Force Four: Federal, State and Tribal Jurisdiction, *Report on Federal, State and Tribal Jurisdiction–Final Report to the American Indian Policy Review Commission* (Washington, D.C.: U.S. Government Printing Office, 1976), pp. 78-87.

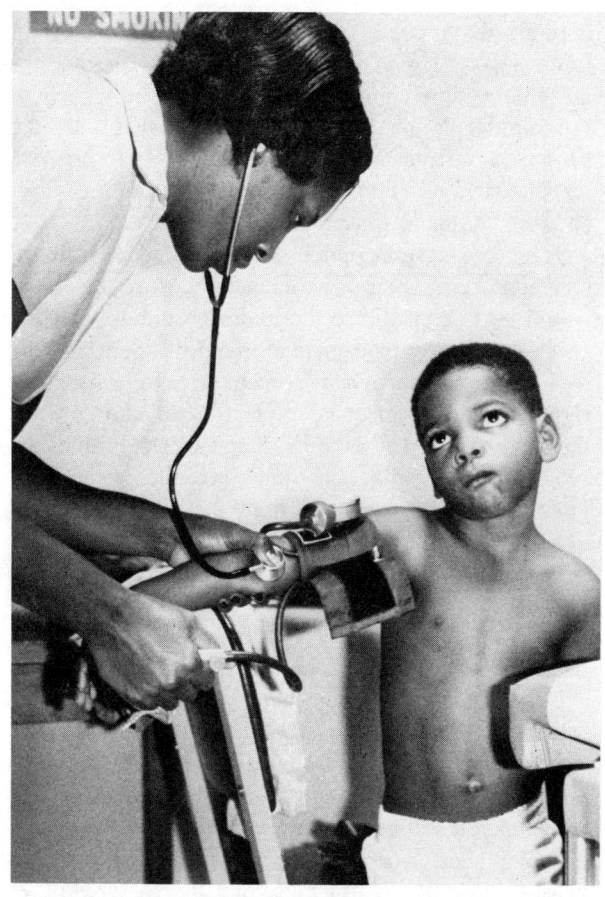

are for children and which are for adults.⁸² This lack of precision makes it almost impossible to contrast how states *plan* to allocate resources for services to prevent the out-of-home care of children, with how they actually *deliver* such services.

- Title XX training funds can be used for training foster parents to care for children with special needs, but it is not possible to determine to what extent states are using the funds for this purpose.⁸³

---

⁸²For example, in Fiscal Year 1977, over half of the 31 states indicating in their state services plans that they were going to use Title XX funds to provide day treatment services to children and adults, gave no breakdown of expenditures for the two groups. Even when a separate count of child and adult recipients is required, as in data collection forms for the Social Services Reporting Requirements, the figures, when analyzed and aggregated, are not useful because reporting is done in terms of the primary recipient of the service. Thus, for example, the January through March 1976 report showed that 66 percent of the recipients of "day care—children" were adults and only 34 percent were children. See, Social and Rehabilitation Service, Department of Health, Education and Welfare, *Social Services U.S.A. (January-March 1976)* (Washington, D. C.: HEW, 1977), p. 51.

⁸³Figures are available on the types of staff development activities funded, i.e., salaries, training, etc., but there are no data on the content of the training.

- HEW has attempted to develop a reporting system which will include data on individual youths served by projects funded under the Runaway Youth Program. Although the system is designed to include useful information on dispositions as well as previous court involvement of the youths, a recent GAO review of the program reported that the system is plagued with thousands of incomplete or inaccurate forms from the projects which require manual editing.⁸⁴

- Figures are available on the number of children on whose behalf Medicaid payments are made. However, with the exception of services under the EPSDT Program and other services targeted only to children, there are no data to indicate the number of children receiving other services, such as outpatient mental health services under Medicaid.

- No data have been systematically provided on evaluations of federally funded research and demonstration efforts. It is only recently that the Administration for Children, Youth and Families in HEW has made a concerted effort to replicate successful demonstration projects.

- Although programs funded under the Juvenile Justice and Delinquency Prevention Act are supposed to promote the diversion of youths from the juvenile justice system and development of community-based alternatives to juvenile detention and correctional facilities, virtually no data are available to evaluate the impact of these programs.

Few federal laws require the administrative agencies responsible for children at risk of removal or in placement to report to Congress and the public on the status of these children or their families or on the impact of federal programs. When program data are available, they frequently are not comparable to those from other programs.

- In a 1975 study, the GAO concluded that virtually nothing was known about the impact of child welfare programs on the well-being of children. It recommended that Congress consider requiring the Secretary of HEW to submit a report periodically on the well-being of children that could be used in assessing the need for various program and budgetary decisions.⁸⁵ To date, there has been no progress in

---

⁸⁴Statement of G. J. Ahart before the House Subcommittee on Economic Opportunity on the Runaway Youth Program, March 7, 1978, pp. 12-13.

⁸⁵See, General Accounting Office, *More Can Be Learned and Done About The Well-Being of Children.*

implementing this recommendation.

- Although HEW administers numerous federal programs affecting handicapped children, it is not required to evaluate the overall impact these programs are having on the needs of these children.

The lack of attention to the impact of federal programs on vulnerable children and families and on the efforts of states to comply with federal legislative requirements are in part indicative of "the new federalism"—an approach which emphasizes self-monitoring of programs by the states. It also reflects the relatively low priority of children's issues within the federal government. Above all, it is another example of the general regulatory failure of the federal government in regard to children without homes.

What Can Be Done?

Redirection and integration of the myriad pieces of legislation, regulations, programs and agencies comprising the federal role regarding children out of their homes is long overdue. The problems of children out of their homes have been repeatedly and thoroughly documented—and the inadequacy of federal leadership is clear. The time for action is now.

Although we recognize that direct responsibility for these children and families lies with the state, we believe the federal government has a crucial role in ensuring that:

▶ Appropriate substantive and procedural protections accompany the use of federal funds.

▶ Federal resources are used to prevent unnecessary and inappropriate out-of-home placements.

▶ Quality care is provided to children placed in out-of-home care.

▶ Timely decisions are made about which children can be reunited with families and which must be provided alternative permanent settings.

▶ Federal initiatives and financing are used to enable states to improve their child placing systems so as to provide necessary services, reviews, protections and data.

Federal leadership will evolve only as the fragmentation that affects the current limited federal effort on behalf of children at risk of removal or in placement is minimized. A central focus at the federal level for leadership and oversight responsibility on behalf of these vulnerable children is therefore urgently needed. Program regulations must be designed so that states can pool money from multiple federal sources to create a responsive continuum of services. Both administrative and programmatic consolidations are necessary.

There are several options for such federal reform. One approach, which is perhaps the most far reaching, would be to consolidate the major programs affecting children at risk of placement or in out-of-home care and to incorporate sufficient procedural and substantive rights to ensure adequate protection of children and their families.[86] The Title IV-B and AFDC Foster Care programs, the child abuse and juvenile justice programs, as well as a portion of the services monies available under the Title XX program, might be integrated into one program using a single state plan. Such a comprehensive program would require a strong statement of objectives, uniform definitions, a consolidated fiscal structure, and a maintenance of effort provision.

The achievement of any such consolidation would be extremely complex. Jurisdiction for these programs is scattered among several Congressional committees; and their administration divided among two Departments and numerous offices within HEW. And these obstacles do not include, for example, the political difficulties involved in splitting off a piece of Title XX for children without corresponding awards for the elderly and other groups. Similarly, such a consolidation might not make sense unless it were part of a reorganization of all children's services, including general health and education programs having a broader scope than the population focused on here.

Other options for federal reform involve working for specific changes in the authorizing legislation and in the regulatory and administrative frameworks of existing programs to ensure that each has: sufficient targeted resources, regulations clearly specifying state obligations, strong reporting requirements, adequate federal, state and citizen mechanisms for monitoring compliance, and strong enforcement efforts. We believe that these are the most politically viable options at this time.

Changes are needed in many areas. The complexity of the task will vary depending on the agency and

---

[86]Such an approach has been proposed by Elizabeth Wickenden, a consultant to CDF, with longstanding expertise in welfare matters.

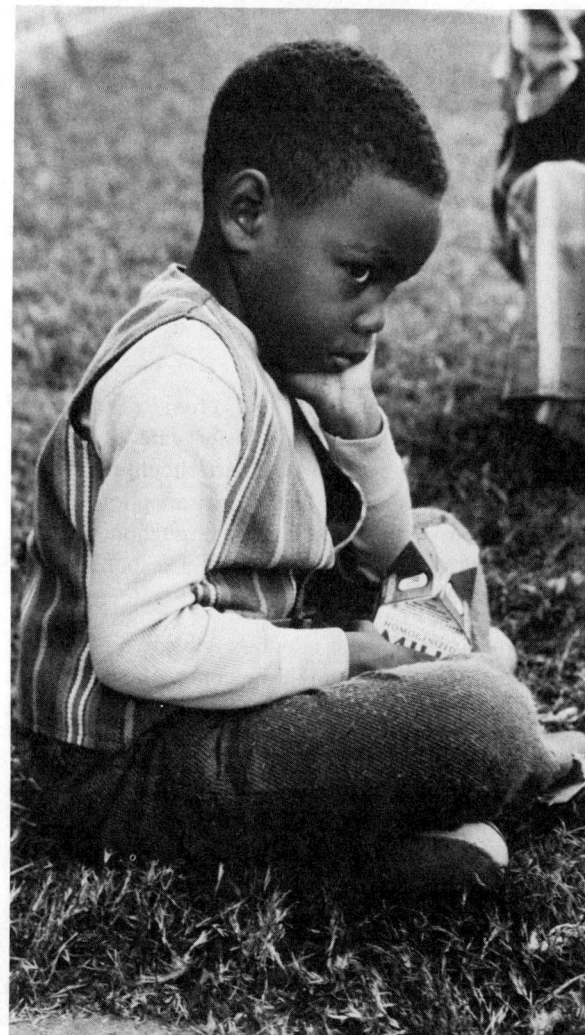

program involved. We believe, however, that the most urgent need for immediate reform is in the two major child welfare programs, the Child Welfare Services Program funded under Title IV-B and the AFDC Foster Care Program.[87] As presently constructed, these two programs offer few protections to children and taxpayers, although they affect—either directly or indirectly—many of the children in out-of-home care.

With this as a context, we outline below seven major recommendations for federal action, each with detailed sub-recommendations addressing legislative reforms, regulatory revisions, and administrative changes across agencies and programs.

[87]During the 95th Congress significant attention was given to the problems of children without homes. See, for example, H.R. 7200 (Titles IV and V, House passed version) and S. 1928.

Fiscal Incentives—Preventive Services

1. **Resources for the development of family support services to prevent unnecessary and inappropriate out-of-home placements should be increased and redirected.**

   a. The Title IV-B Child Welfare Services Program should be amended to provide for increased targeted funding by:

   - Converting it to an entitlement program at the current authorized level of $266 million, so states will be able to establish strong service programs and be assured continued funding for them.

   - Prohibiting increased funds over the current appropriation of $56.5 million from being used for maintenance costs. They should instead be targeted for family support services to prevent children at risk from entering care unnecessarily, and for ensuring that, where appropriate, children will be reunited with their families. Such services should include homemaker services, emergency respite care, day treatment, family and individual counseling, 24-hour crisis intervention services, and case advocacy services. Funds should also be available for the establishment of review mechanisms and case tracking systems.

   - Requiring states to maintain their current funding effort for child welfare services, so that increased federal funds will result in increased and improved services.

   b. In order to ensure that funds available under Title XX are utilized for family support services to prevent inappropriate placements of children, options for targeting and/or earmarking Title XX funds should be considered. In the absence of a total restructuring of the revenue sharing program, which would make program funds available for defined populations (a change we believe is ultimately needed), portions of the Title XX funds should be earmarked for children's services, including services to prevent unnecessary placements. As an interim measure, Title XX legislation should be amended to allow federal matching at 90 percent for services directed at preventing unnecessary family break-up and returning a child to his own home.

c. A portion of the training funds available under Title IV-B and Title XX should be earmarked for in-service training programs, with a requirement that these funds be targeted toward educating workers about preventive services and adoption techniques for hard-to-place children. Funds available for such training should be provided at a higher federal match than other training monies.

Fiscal Incentives—Permanence

2. Fiscal disincentives which prevent children who have been removed from their homes from being returned home or placed in another permanent living situation, including adoptive homes, should be eliminated.

Limitations should be placed on the length of time federal reimbursement will be available for children in "temporary" out-of-home care.

a. The rate of reimbursement that a state may claim from the federal government for the maintenance of a child in care should be reduced when the child is in care over 18 months. Exceptions should be allowed in special circumstances in which an agency documents at the time of the dispositional review that continued temporary care for a specified time period is necessary; or in special cases when there is a determination that a permanent living arrangement, other than adoption, is the only alternative for a child and funds for the continued long-term care of the child are not available from other federal programs. Decreasing federal reimbursement should apply to the AFDC Foster Care Program and to any maintenance payments reimbursed by the federal government under the Title IV-B Program.

b. To encourage reunification, maintenance under the AFDC Foster Care Program should be defined to include expenses for transportation for parent-child visits while the child is in care, and for transition services. These should include trial visits home for which special emergency allowances may be necessary, and additional necessary services when a child leaves care to facilitate his adjustment at home and reduce his chances of re-entering care.

Federal funds should be targeted for adoption services and subsidies.

c. Adoption subsidies for children with special needs should be reimbursable as maintenance payments under Section 408 of Title IV-A of the Social Security Act. Eligibility should continue until a child reaches age 21 as long as need for the subsidy continues.

d. Any federal program that provides funds for services to children in foster care or for the maintenance costs of their care should require the state to develop an operational adoption subsidy program and to implement it throughout the state within a period designated by a responsible federal authority.[88]

e. No state or federal adoption subsidy received by adoptive parents should be counted as income in determining eligibility for any federal financial assistance programs.

f. The Medicaid Program should be amended so that a child with a specific handicapping condition who was eligible for Medicaid while in foster care will continue to be eligible for Medicaid after adoption—regardless of the income of the adoptive parents.

Adequate Protections

3. Procedural and substantive safeguards for children at risk of removal or in out-of-home care should be required as a condition for receipt of federal funds.

a. Any legislation making federal funds available to states, either directly or through purchase-of-service contracts, for services to children at risk of removal or in placement, or for maintaining children in foster care should require states to provide the following protections to the children in care or receiving services.

---

[88] As of June 1978, 44 states and the District of Columbia had enacted adoption subsidy legislation, but a smaller number had actually implemented the laws.

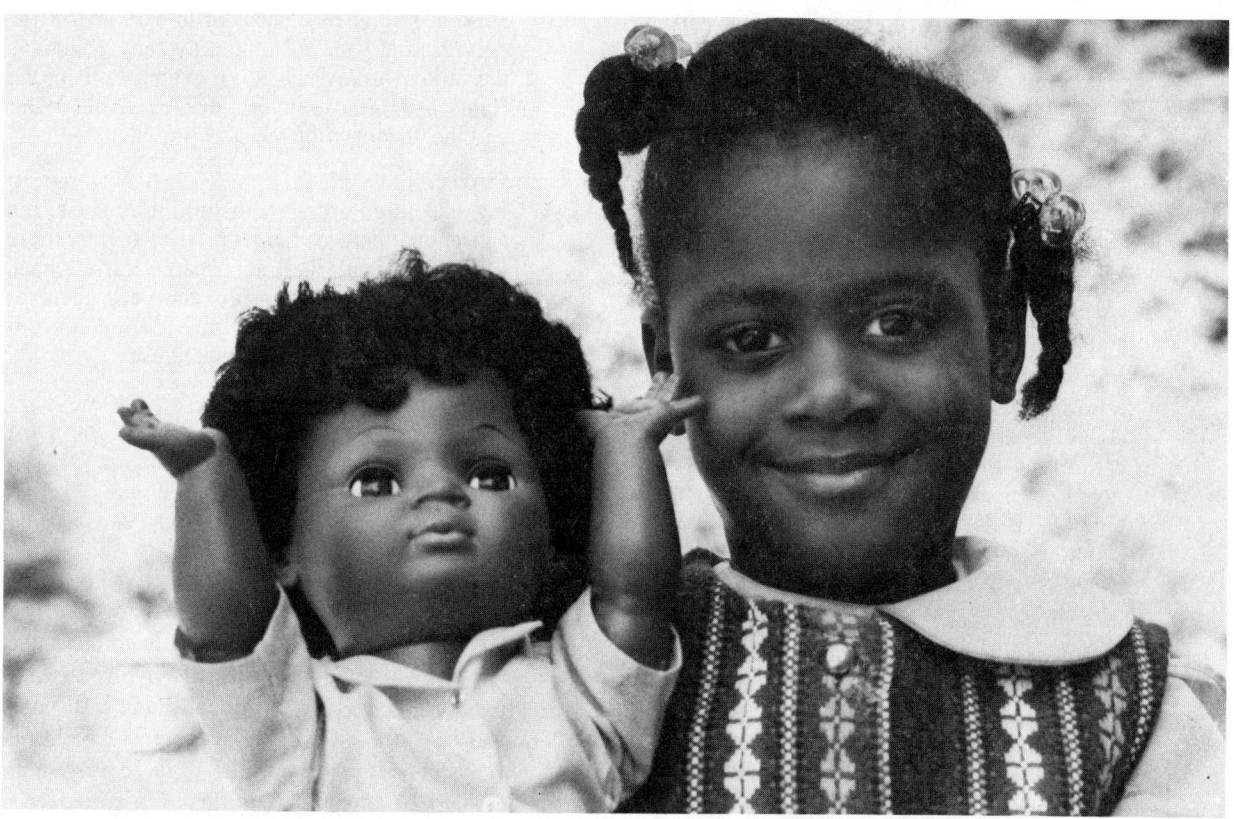

- Prior to the child's entry into care, preventive services should have been made available to the family and have failed to alleviate the need for care or been refused by the family. Exceptions should be made only when a court determines that the situation in a home presents a substantial and immediate danger to a child and orders the child removed from the home without such services first being made available, or when there is a judicial determination that a child who has committed a delinquent offense requires removal from home.

- Voluntary placement of a child in care should be made pursuant to a voluntary placement agreement signed by the parent or guardian placing the child and the placement agency. The agreement should specify: the legal status of the child; the rights and obligations of the parents and the agency, including the parents' right to have the child returned within a reasonable period unless parental rights have been terminated or a dependency or neglect petition has been filed; and the procedure that parents must follow to have the child returned.

- Placement in the least restrictive setting in accordance with the child's needs.

- Placement within reasonable proximity to the child's family and home community in accordance with the child's needs.

- Preference to the formal placement of a child in the home of an interested relative willing to provide care.

- Provision of family reunification services to a child in care and the child's family, including transportation, transition services and follow-up services once the child is returned home.

- Development of an individualized case plan for each child coming into care. The plan should include, but not be limited to, a description of the services to be provided to the child and his parents in order to allow the child's return home as rapidly as possible.

- Transfer of a child from one placement to another only when the move is to a less restrictive setting or the prior placement is inappropriate, with proper written notice to all parties prior to the transfer, unless such notice would endanger the child.

- Periodic reviews of the status and progress of each child in care. These must include:

    - An administrative or judicial review of the child's status at least once every six months, by an experienced person not directly involved in the provision of services to the family. The natural parents, foster parents and child should be notified in writing of their right to be present and to participate with representation of their choice. The review should assess progress toward family reunification and include a determination of additional services required. The child's natural parents, foster parents or other caretaker should be notified in writing of the outcome of the review.

    - A judicial review or review by a specially designated board independent of the agency having responsibility for the child (appealable to a court), no later than 18 months after placement. At this time, there should be a determination of the disposition of the case, i.e., whether the child should be returned home immediately; continued in care for a specified period; referred so he can be legally freed and placed for adoption; or, in special circumstances, placed in permanent long-term foster care. The natural parents, foster parents and child should be provided written notice of any such review and advised of their due process rights to representation, examine evidence, cross examine witnesses, and present testimony. Subsequent to a determination, there should be continuing periodic reviews to ensure compliance with the required disposition.

- The right to counsel should be extended to a child and his parents in any judicial proceeding where there is the likelihood that a child may be involuntarily removed from home, and at subsequent proceedings once a child is removed from the home. In proceedings in which termination of parental rights is at issue, the child and his parents should be accorded the right to separate counsel, including court-appointed counsel, if counsel is otherwise unobtainable.

- Provision of a fair hearing procedure whereby a child at risk of placement or in care and/or the child's family or foster family may challenge the failure of any agency to extend to them the rights and benefits to which they are entitled, and the adequacy of services provided.

- Provision of a mechanism to enable the reporting and monitoring of institutional abuse and subsequent enforcement activities against those individuals and facilities charged. Any such mechanism should ensure that all agencies using a particular facility are advised of confirmed reports of institutional abuse.

Steps should be taken to incorporate these protections in the numerous federal programs affecting children in out-of-home care. States should be required to phase in the protections pursuant to a timetable developed by a federal authority.

b. At a minimum, current regulations for the AFDC Foster Care Program should be expanded to incorporate provisions for periodic administrative reviews by a person not directly involved in the provision of services to the child and a dispositional hearing, as well as the protections addressing the child's placement. All of these provisions will help to expedite reunification, a goal currently referred to in the statute.

c. In order to expand the universe of children to whom the AFDC Foster Care protections will apply, eligibility requirements in Section 408 of the Social Security Act should be amended to include:

- AFDC-eligible children who have been voluntarily placed in care pursuant to a written voluntary placement agreement signed by the parent or guardian placing the child and the placement agency. The agreement should specify: the legal status of the child, the rights and obligations of the parents and the agency, including the parents' right to have the child returned upon request within a reasonable time period unless parental rights have been terminated or a dependency or neglect petition has been filed; and the procedure the parents must follow to have the child returned.

- AFDC-eligible children placed in public facilities housing 25 or fewer children.

Quality Care

4. Federal support to ensure quality care to children out of their homes should be strengthened, and a consistent federal policy toward deinstitutionalization developed.

Deinstitutionalization efforts across systems, agencies and programs should be coordinated and their impact on children analyzed.

a. All relevant Congressional committees[89] should jointly request the General Accounting Office to trace the impact of federal deinstitutionalization efforts on children across systems. Specific attention should be given to tracing the federal dollars flowing into specific group care facilities to determine what differential impact the various programs have on individual children. The program analysis should address, at a minimum, Medicaid, SSI, AFDC Foster Care, Title XX, the Title I Programs for institutionalized children, the Juvenile Justice and Delinquency Prevention Program, and the Indian Child Welfare Assistance Program.

Efforts must be undertaken to ensure that federal funds will be used for care in the least restrictive setting possible.

b. A review should be conducted by an interdepartmental task force within the federal government to determine the most administratively efficient way for states to document their efforts to ensure that children are placed in the least restrictive setting appropriate to their needs. In addition to focusing on the out-of-home care provided with federal funds administered by HEW under Titles IV-A, IV-B, and XX, the Emergency Assistance Program, Medicaid and SSI, the task force should look at the Indian Child Welfare and CHAMPUS Programs.

Efforts must be made to ensure that programs are available to address the needs of children as they are moved from institutions to community-based facilities.

c. As reconsideration is given to extension of the Community Mental Health Centers Program, special attention should be given to earmarking funds for services to children and adolescents.[90] Priority in funding should be given to those public or private nonprofit agencies which have in place a mechanism for coordination with other service agencies—social services, education and health.

d. Immediate attention should be given to developing appropriate services to meet the needs of status offenders who are being removed from detention facilities pursuant to the deinstitutionalization requirement in the Juvenile Justice and Delinquency Prevention Act. Demonstration projects for this purpose should be jointly funded under Section 426 of Title IV-B and the Special Emphasis Grants portion of the Juvenile Justice and Delinquency Prevention Act. Such projects should be administered jointly by child welfare agencies and probation departments in local communities.

e. Demonstration projects should be undertaken to determine ways in which the Foster Grandparent Program and Retired Senior Volunteer Program, administered by ACTION, can be used to promote services to families and children that would eliminate the need for children to be unnecessarily removed from their homes. Consistent with an effort begun by ACTION in 1974, further attempts should be made to expand the placement of foster grandparents in non-institutional settings. Program regulations should be revised to ensure that a foster grandparent who has worked with a child in an institution will be allowed to maintain contact with the child when he returns to the community.

The federal government must give increased attention to the quality of care provided with federal funds. For example, efforts must be taken to ensure greater utilization of federally funded health services by children in out-of-home care. Similarly, greater attention must be given to the appropriateness of educational programs and to mechanisms by which improved serv-

---

[89] These might include the Senate Finance Committee, House Ways and Means Committee, and House Interstate and Foreign Commerce Committee, together with the Senate Judiciary Committee and the House Education and Labor Committee, the Senate Select Committee on Interior Affairs, and House Committee on Interior and Insular Affairs.

[90] For further recommendations related to mental health, see *Report to the President from the President's Commission on Mental Health.*

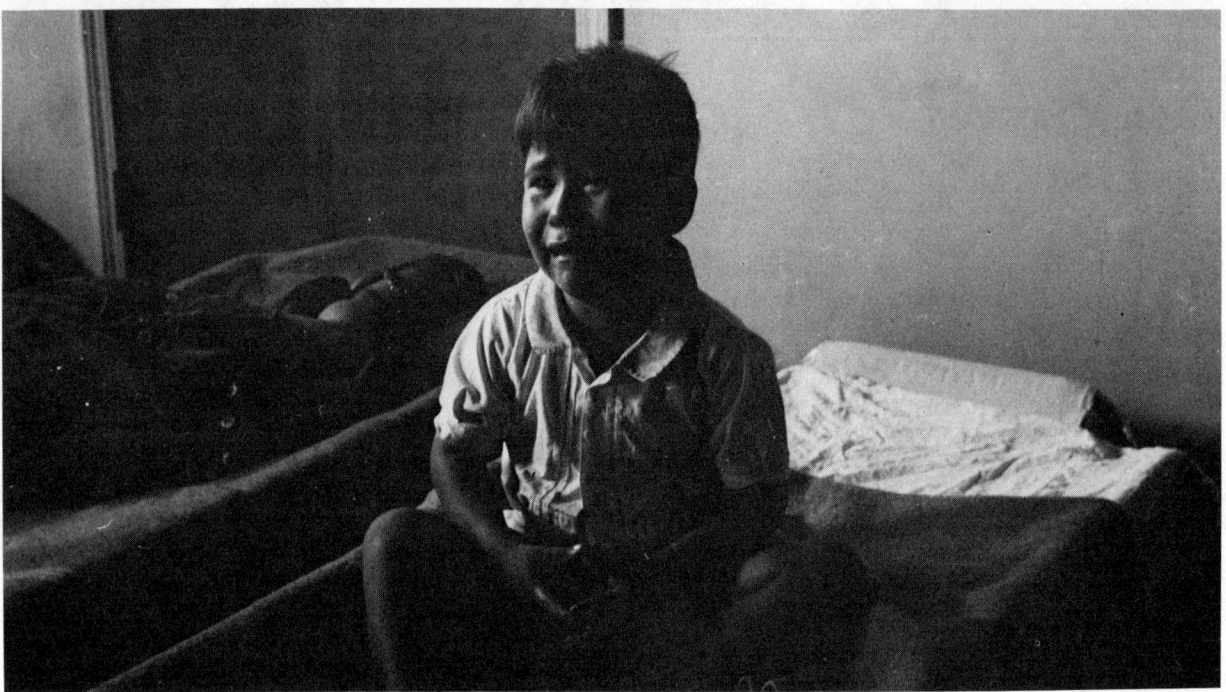

ices can be obtained.

    f. Regulations for the penalty provision applicable to the EPSDT Program[91] should specify procedures for ensuring that children in the AFDC Foster Care Program are informed about and have an opportunity to receive EPSDT services. Notification should be provided to each foster family home or nonprofit private child care institution in which AFDC Foster Care children are placed.

    g. Title XIX of the Social Security Act should be amended to mandate Medicaid eligibility for all individuals under age 21 who are financially eligible under the state welfare or Medicaid standard, but do not meet the categorical requirements. Until such time as Medicaid coverage is so extended, states should be allowed to continue to extend Medicaid coverage to subgroups of financially eligible children under 21, including those for whom public agencies are assuming at least partial financial responsibility in foster homes, psychiatric hospitals, intermediate care facilities, and in subsidized adoptive homes.[92]

    h. Welfare agencies should be required to notify the foster parents and institutions where they place children with AFDC Foster Care funds of the provisions of P.L. 94-142, specifically the provision for the appointment of a surrogate parent to advocate on behalf of the child in the special education process if the child's parents are unknown or unavailable.

    i. States should be provided technical assistance and special funds to encourage development of a mechanism for appointing surrogate parents for institutionalized children with special education needs to ensure that they are provided the education program to which they are entitled under P.L. 94-142. Legislation for programs providing funds for the care of children in institutions should include a set-aside for establishment of such protections.[93]

---

[91] 45 C.F.R. §205.146(c).

[92] See Appendix R. for a listing by state, of the subgroups of children to which Medicaid eligibility was extended as of December 1977.

[93] Such a provision might be attached to the requirements in the statutes which address the coordination of service programs. Examples of pertinent legislation would include Titles XVI, XIX, and XX of the Social Security Act.

Federal funds for training programs affecting children in or at risk of placement should be used explicitly to improve the quality of care children receive.

j. There should be systematic and increased emphasis on in-service training for persons working with children at risk of placement. A portion of the federal training money available under Title IV-A, Title IV-B and Title XX of the Social Security Act, the Child Abuse Prevention and Treatment Act and the Juvenile Justice and Delinquency Prevention Act, should be earmarked for interdisciplinary in-service training for persons working in the fields of child welfare and juvenile justice. Such training should emphasize provision of preventive services as an alternative to placement, development of appropriate community-based programs, identification of appropriate permanent placements for children in care with special needs, and continuing evaluation of case plans.

k. The regulations for the Title XX training program specifically provide for the use of funds to train foster parents to provide special services to children in their care. As an immediate initial step, efforts should be made to determine what portion of this money, if any, is used by states for such training.

l. A portion of the training funds available under the Education for All Handicapped Children Act should be targeted for training child welfare and juvenile justice workers about the rights of handicapped children, including their right to a surrogate parent when their own parents are unknown or unavailable.

Meaningful Compliance Efforts

5. Specific administrative and procedural mechanisms should be created to ensure compliance with federal program requirements and to ensure that the federal dollar is used to best serve the needs of children without homes.

Steps must be taken by the federal government to ensure that children are afforded the rights and protections contained in state laws, federal laws and the Constitution.

a. Technical assistance should be provided to help states put in place the substantive and procedural protections which we have recommended for children at risk of and in placement.[94] Assistance should also be available to evaluate the implementation of such techniques in both state and local agencies.

b. HEW should develop a system for monitoring compliance with requirements in federal child welfare legislation. It should include a range of mechanisms: mandatory periodic reports on the numbers of children and families served and the services received; periodic site visits by the regional offices; and a fair hearing procedure whereby recipients of such services or persons eligible for such services can appeal a denial or discontinuance of a service, or can complain when adequate services are not available.

c. Legislation authorizing service funds should include set-asides earmarked for technical assistance and for the monitoring of compliance.

d. The effectiveness of the state plan as a compliance tool should be reconsidered.[95] Although simplified state plans (often little more than checklists) are easier for the states, they tell the federal government, state officials and interested persons within the state little about how a state is fulfilling its obligations under federal law. Moreover, there is no systematic effort to hold the state accountable for failing to perform according to the state plan.

e. Specific regulations should be drafted by HEW which outline the responsibility of state welfare agencies for monitoring purchase-of-service contracts with other public agencies and private nonprofit agencies. State agencies should be required to ensure that contractees provide children and families the rights established by law and regulations. Further, state agencies should be required to make contracts available for public review.

---

[94] For example, the federal government should develop model procedures which can be adapted by the states for voluntary placement agreements, individual case plans, and periodic review procedures, both administrative and judicial.

[95] State plans have been reevaluated in an effort to reduce the paperwork burden on the states, but attention to date has focused on the quantity rather than the quality of the data requested from the states.

Federal agencies should move diligently to enforce the protections for which they are responsible.

 f. The Office for Civil Rights within HEW should immediately establish a system to determine whether state and local welfare authorities, mental health and mental retardation agencies, and juvenile justice authorities receiving federal funds, as well as the placement facilities and community-based programs that receive referrals from these sources, are in compliance with Section 504 of the Rehabilitation Act of 1973 which prohibits discrimination on the basis of handicap. A similar effort must be made with regard to Title VI of the Civil Rights Act of 1964, outlawing racial discrimination.

 g. Legislation should be enacted affirming that the Department of Justice has standing to bring action against a state when it has evidence that a state has failed to meet its responsibility for the welfare of a child in its care. The Department should also be given standing to bring litigation when it has evidence of institutional abuse and inadequate treatment of children placed outside of their homes.

 h. The Bureau of Consumer Protection in the Federal Trade Commission, pursuant to Section V of the Federal Trade Commission Act, should monitor the promotional literature of private child-caring facilities, including residential treatment facilities, to uncover deceptive and misleading advertising.

Monitoring and evaluation are of limited value if they are not accompanied by follow-up and the imposition of sanctions when compliance is not forthcoming.

 i. In developing a system of compliance sanctions, consideration must be given to both penalties and incentives. Penalties should include a percentage reduction in a state's share of federal payments under a program which is of significance to the state: revenue sharing funds, for example. There should be a provision for court action whereby a court could order a state to transfer funds from another program for the purpose of carrying out the requirements of the program. Attention should also be given to positive incentives for good performance. For example, a higher rate of federal reimbursement for the AFDC Foster Care Program might be given to states that have instituted independent review procedures.

Congress should take a more active role in carrying out its oversight role for programs affecting children without homes.

 j. The General Accounting Office should be requested to conduct a study every three years and to issue a report to the relevant commmittees in Congress on the well-being of children at risk of placement and in out-of-home care, and their families. The first report of this type, to be submitted in December 1980, should specifically address the extent to which states are using preventive services, periodic independent reviews, adoption subsidies and grievance procedures, and the effectiveness of these programs and procedures.

Administrative and Programmatic Coordination

6. A body should be designated within HEW with clear centralized administrative responsibility for major programs affecting children at risk of or in placement, and a mechanism developed for cross-agency programming, monitoring and reporting.

Attempts to end programmatic fragmentation must be initiated if there is to be a consistent federal policy toward children at risk of placement and in out-of-home care.

 a. The Secretary of HEW should consider ways to further consolidation of child welfare programs begun by the 1977 reorganization orders, by transferring administration of the AFDC Foster Care Program to the Office of Human Development Services.[96] Until legislation to effect such a transfer is passed, we recommend that the Social

---

[96]The AFDC Foster Care Program was moved to the Social Security Administration with other income maintenance programs in March, 1977. While we are not concerned with the Social Security Administration distributing maintenance payments to states, we believe an adequate federal effort to fulfill the mandate of the program and afford necessary substantive and procedural protections to children requires more than distribution of funds. It requires, for example, careful coordinated federal monitoring to ensure that mandated periodic reviews are conducted, and preventive services have, in fact, been offered to those eligible for federal reimbursement.

Security Administration contract with the Office of Human Development Services to carry out the necessary programmatic and monitoring functions of the program.

b. Encouragement should be given to legislative efforts that would consolidate authority for the AFDC Foster Care Program, currently authorized under Section 408 of Title IV-A and the Child Welfare Services Program authorized under Title IV-B, in a new section of the Social Security Act focused solely on child welfare matters, including foster care and adoption.

c. Administrative authority for many of the programs directly affecting children at risk of removal or out of their homes has been centralized within the Office of Human Development Services. Programmatic responsibility within that office at both the national and regional levels also needs to be consolidated in order to make the federal administrative role less cumbersome for states and local communities.

- Confusion in the administration of training funds under Section 426 of Title IV-B of the Social Security Act, between the Administration for Public Services (APS) and the Administration for Children, Youth and Families (ACYF), needs to be resolved.
- A formal mechanism must be created to ensure coordination of child welfare services funded under Title XX and administered by APS, and child welfare services funded under Title IV-B and administered by ACYF.
- Coordination must also be maintained among Title XX, Title IV-B, and the Administration for Handicapped Individuals which administers the Developmental Disabilities Program.
- Responsibilities of particular bureaus within each of the Administrations also need to be coordinated at both national and regional levels.

d. To further programmatic coordination, the Child Abuse Prevention and Treatment Act should be repealed and discontinued as a separate authority. Legislation should be introduced to transfer the funds currently available under the Act to the Child Welfare Services Program, earmarked for services for abused and neglected children. States should be required to maintain their current spending effort for child abuse and neglect programs, and to incorporate planning for these children in their larger child welfare services plan.

Sufficient staff resources are essential to meaningful federal program administration.

e. Staff resources within the Children's Bureau should be increased at both the regional and national levels to enable that office to more adequately monitor state plans; collect and analyze child welfare services data; provide technical assistance to the states; monitor compliance; and provide coordination of child welfare related activities with other federal agencies.

Coordination among the numerous programs affecting children without homes within HEW alone is not sufficient. Coordination efforts must extend across federal departments.

f. There should be a clear delineation by statute of the powers and responsibilities of an office with coordination and monitoring authority for all federal programs affecting children at risk of removal or out of their homes. Such authority might be centered in the Office of the Assistant Secretary for Human Development Services within HEW, but it should extend across agency lines and include maintenance and service programs, research and demonstration projects, and training monies. Coordination will be required with the Departments of Agriculture, Defense, Housing and Urban Development, Interior, Justice, and Labor, and the ACTION agency.

National Data

7. **States should be required to develop an integrated data collection system that provides meaningful, timely data to state and local officials on the status of children in their care, and provides useful data at the national level, comparable to the extent possible across systems, for ensuring compliance with federal policies and programs and for planning future program directions.**

Federal agencies which provide funds to the states for services to children at risk of placement or in care should require the states to report on the status of the children and families.

a. HEW should require states receiving federal funds for child welfare services (including foster care and adoption services) to develop tracking systems whereby they can maintain information on each child in the foster care system including, at a minimum: date of birth, sex, race, legal status and geographic location upon entry into care; date of entry into care; and services provided prior to entry. The system should also contain a record of case transactions including, at a minimum: dates of intake, first foster care placement, each subsequent placement, changes in legal status, return to natural parents, termination of parental rights, and adoptive or other permanent placement. Technical assistance should be provided to enable states to establish data systems that track the progress of children through and across child care systems.

b. Such data systems should also enable states to submit annually to HEW and to make public, aggregate statistical reports covering information on the number of children by age, race and sex in foster care; the length of time they have been in care; the type of placement in which they reside (foster home, group home, institution); their legal status and the reason for the initial placement; the number of children by age, race and sex moved out of foster care during the preceding year and the dispositions of these cases; the number of children placed in adoptive homes with adoption subsidies during the preceding year; and the number of children whose parental rights have been terminated but who have not yet been placed for adoption.

c. HEW should publish annually the aggregate data received and should publicize the availability of such data at the state and regional levels.

There should be a coordinated effort within the federal government to review existing data collection efforts for their relevance to children out of their homes.

d. The Bureau of the Census should coordinate a review by the Departments of Defense, Health, Education and Welfare, Interior and Justice of their data collection efforts to determine their relevance to children without homes. Data collection instruments should then be revised to identify more adequately the number and status of children out of their own homes. Coordination among agencies will ultimately require more uniformity in reporting, such as the use of identical age breakdowns and comparable definitions of facilities.

e. The Bureau of the Census should be required to include questions about the number of children in foster home care in the 1980 Census. At present, the Census Bureau in its decennial census collects data on children out of their own homes, but does not specify the number of children in foster home care either with relatives or non-relatives. In order to determine the number of children in foster home care, by state and county, as well as nationally, the questionnaire used in the 1980 Census should be revised to include this information.[97]

The quality of data reported by states should be given as much attention at the federal level as the quantity of reported data has been given. Too often little is known about whether the intended beneficiaries of programs are in fact benefiting from them.

f. Program reporting requirements for the programs described in this chapter should be reviewed to ensure meaningful outcome and fiscal data are included. Characteristics of those served by a program and a description of the services provided should always be included.

Data are also essential components of a meaningful civil rights compliance program.

g. The Office for Civil Rights in HEW should prepare and conduct a survey of long-term care facilities as well as welfare and social services agencies and other child-placing agencies that receive federal funds to determine their compliance with Title VI of the Civil Rights Act of 1964 and Section 504 of the Rehabilitation Act of 1973. Any such survey should provide data by which to assess discriminatory treatment of children and adults in these facilities and by the agencies. Specific age breakdowns should be included.

---

[97]More specifically, "foster child," defined as a child whose maintenance is being paid for by a public or private organization, should be added as a distinct subcategory under "other not related to head" and under "other relative of head," in Question 2 of the 100 percent population questions used in the 1970 Census.

Part III.
Effecting Change

**Chapter 6
Programs That Work**

**Chapter 7
Advocacy for Children
Without Homes**

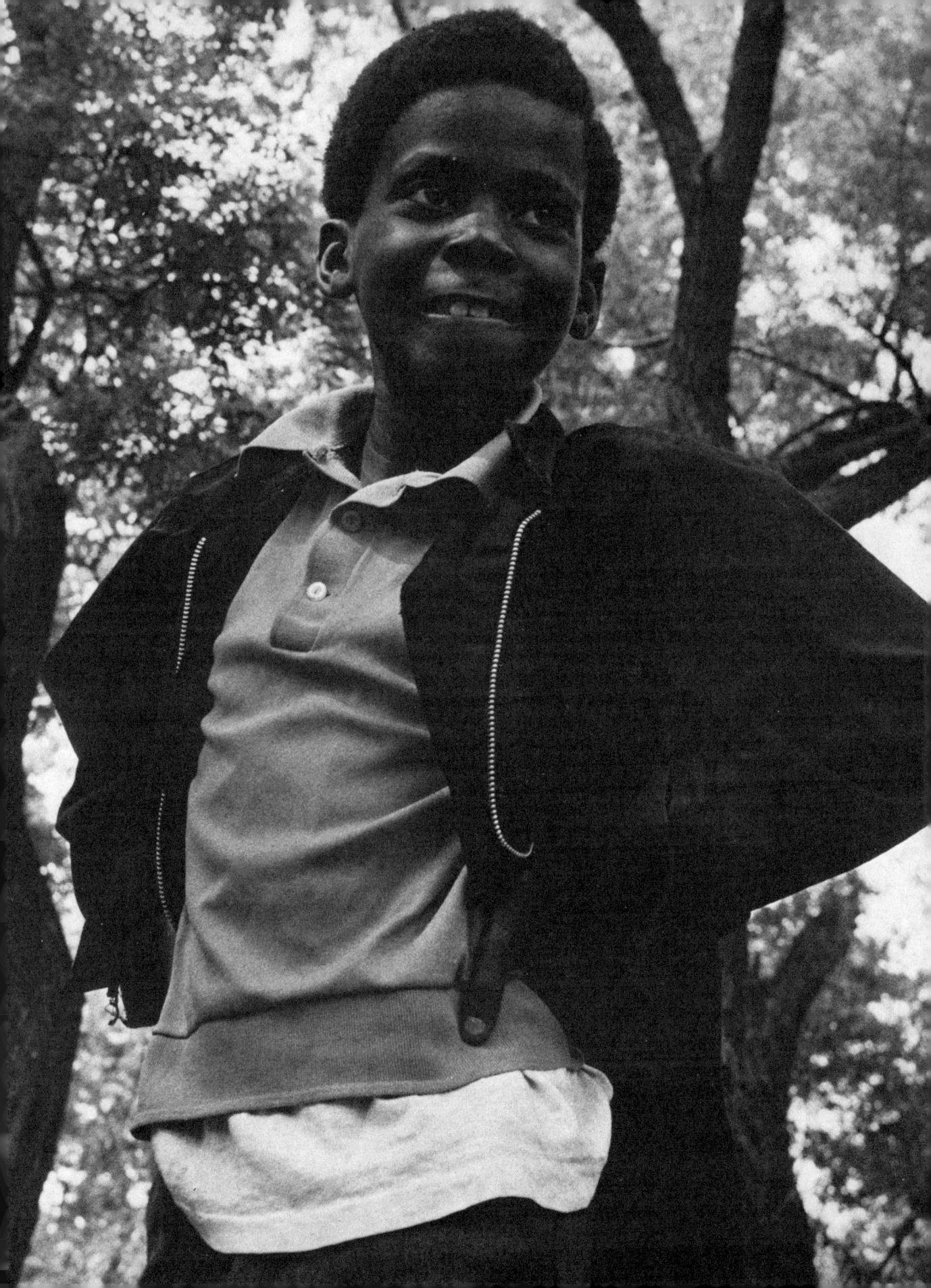

6 Programs That Work

Varied Approaches

Within recent years, purchased services, deinstitutionalization, improved regulations, legal reforms, and administrative reorganization all have affected patterns of banishment and state responsibility for children without homes. Each has promised significant change. But each has rarely lived up to its promise. We have learned that inadequate resources can defeat the best idea for reform and that children's service systems have their own ecology. Changing one part positively may have unanticipated negative consequences for others. Citizen advocates, policymakers and program developers need to be aware of these pitfalls.

But at the same time, there are also many examples of programs that "work"—that make a positive difference in the lives of children and families. Here we describe some of these efforts: direct service programs to prevent family disruption and provide quality care to children out of their homes and services to their families; innovative statutory and administrative efforts to correct system failures affecting large numbers of children; and the role of effective advocacy groups in stimulating change. Our list is not exhaustive,[1] but describes successful approaches that might be tried elsewhere.[2]

Direct Service Programs for Families and Children[3]

The Family Reception Center

The Family Reception Center (FRC) in Brooklyn, New York, is a mental health clinic, a settlement house and a community center all in one. The Center's goals

---

[1] Time and resource constraints limited the scope of our exploration of innovative efforts, and particularly our capacity to make site visits and talk with people in detail about how they have faced and often overcome barriers to change.

[2] The Child Welfare Resource Information Exchange compiles abstracts on innovative programs, methods or technologies relating to improved services to children and youth, and may be a useful resource for additional models. Copies of abstracts organized according to particular subject areas, e.g., adoption, foster care, and mental health services, can be obtained directly from the Exchange, Suite 501, 2011 Eye Street, N. W., Washington, D. C. 20006.

The National Institute of Law Enforcement and Criminal Justice in the Law Enforcement Assistance Administration in the Justice Department also operates an Exemplary Projects Program through which outstanding criminal justice programs are identified. As of September 1977, there were 25 exemplary projects, including five community-based juvenile programs. Informational materials on these projects and others designated "exemplary" are available through the National Criminal Justice Reference Service, Post Office Box 6000, Rockville, Maryland 20850.

In addition, states and localities sometimes compile descriptions of innovative programs. See, for example, *Peter's Cookbook—A Catalog of Model Youth Programs* (Albany: New York State Division for Youth, 1977).

[3] The names of project directors and addresses for all the projects discussed in this chapter are listed in Appendix S. Further information about individual projects can be obtained by contacting the projects directly.

are to prevent family breakup and to divert youth from the juvenile justice system. Since its beginning in 1972, the FRC has served the community through a direct service program, advocacy efforts, and mobilization of the community to meet the needs of its families and youth more effectively.

Operated under the auspices of the Sisters of the Good Shepherd, the FRC serves a primarily low-income community with a population of 120,000, over 43,000 of whom are under 20. When FRC opened, the rate of juvenile delinquency in the community was rising faster than in surrounding areas. A review of the zip codes of parents with children in out-of-home care throughout New York City indicated that a high percentage of those parents were among the community's residents.

Sister Mary Paul, the Center's driving force, was angry about these many "nomad" children and her helplessness in preventing their removal from their homes and community. Thus, the FRC began with a commitment to end family breakup.

An intensive outreach planning effort preceded the FRC's development, with eight months of street corner meetings involving local residents, merchants, police, judges and youth. A 30-member community board was established to guide the program's development and to ensure its responsiveness to the community.

The FRC has grown to include a wide range of programs. Initially, there was a small, bilingual staff and a "crash pad" for adolescents that at times also provided shelter for families undergoing a crisis. Now the Center provides direct services to over 300 families. Services include crisis-oriented counseling, individual and family casework, sustained family group therapy, family life education, peer group therapy, psychiatric consultation, legal and educational advocacy, temporary foster home care, referral services, and many social activities including weekly parents' nights, teen nights and drop-in nights.

The FRC is open from 8:00 a.m. to 11:00 p.m. daily. It serves a diversified population representative of the community. Two-thirds of the youths served are between 10 and 15 years old; 40 percent of the clients are white, 40 percent Spanish surnamed, and 20 percent black.

In addition, the FRC operates the Children and Youth Developmental Center (CYDC), a mini-school and a neighborhood group home. The CYDC is geared specifically to the needs of youths. It originated as a delinquency prevention effort designed to provide direct services to youth—walk-in counseling, crisis intervention at police precincts, job development and placement, and youth leadership training programs—and to increase the responsiveness of the systems that alienate and isolate youth—schools, courts, community agencies, and police. Like the FRC, the CYDC also reaches out to parents of youth using the services.

The mini-school was established in response to a desperate need for educational alternatives to reach children excluded from and/or turned off by the traditional school system.[4] A mini-school staff member, if necessary, goes to a child's home, helps him get dressed, and accompanies him to the mini-school. The neighborhood group home provides community-based care so that children who cannot remain with their families can still maintain family and community ties.

The FRC believes strongly in the power of the community and has created a system of community support services combining innovative and traditional strategies. The words of an early evaluation by an independent review team capture its uniqueness.[5]

> A strong tenet of the ideology of the Center is that it is not an island unto itself. Its purpose is not to supplant other organizations and services, but to supplement them and to make them more accessible to potential clients....
>
> The indomitability of the leadership appears to have infused staff with a courage and optimism that flavors the whole program. The prevailing attitude is that anything can be coped with. If you don't have a needed service, find one. If it doesn't exist, find the resources to develop it. A constantly evolving program has resulted to which staff reacts with excitement and enthusiasm.

Mother and Child Residence

In a recent report of teenage pregnancies in the United States, Planned Parenthood reported that:

> Each year, more than one million 15-19 year olds and

---

[4] A 1974 report by the Children's Defense Fund estimated that more than two million children were excluded from schools. The vast majority of them had not been involved in any acts of violence but rather were in some way "different." They were minority children, handicapped children, or sometimes, children too poor to pay textbook fees. See, *Children Out of School in America* (Washington, D. C.: Children's Defense Fund, 1974).

[5] A. Shyne and R. Neuman, *A Commitment to People–An Evaluation of the Family Reception Center* (New York: Research Center, Child Welfare League of America, 1974), p. 98.

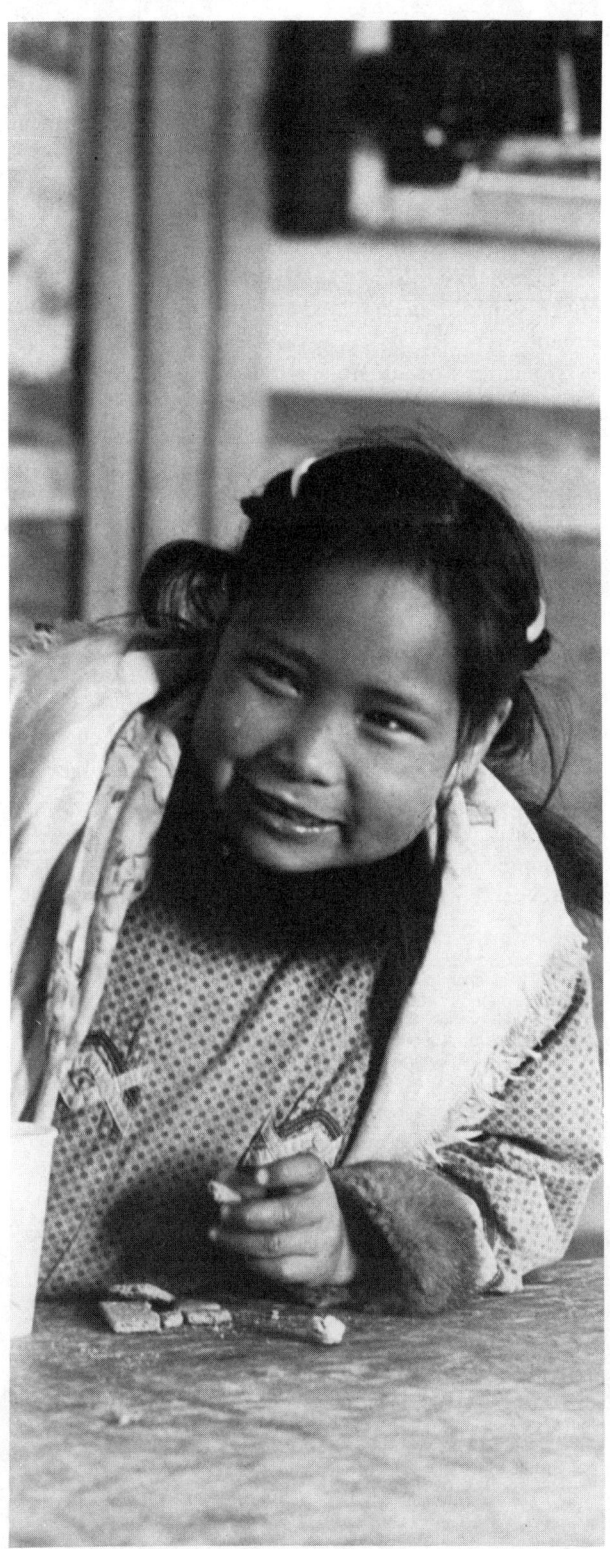

30,000 girls below age 15 become pregnant. This results in over 600,000 births each year: 247,000 to adolescents 17 and younger; 13,000 of these girls under 15.[6]

For teenage mothers there are many stresses—financial and otherwise—in caring for their children. Many of the mothers want to keep their children, but need help to do so: adequate, affordable housing, help in caring for the baby, day care so they can continue in school or get a job, friends and people who care. Most of these young mothers do not get what they need, and as a result, some of their children end up in out-of-home care.[7]

But others do not. A lucky few are the ten mothers at the Mother and Child Residence of Louise Wise Services in New York City, a group home for mothers 16 to 18 years old and their babies. Begun in 1972, the program is part of an organization that first opened its door in 1916 as an adoption agency. All the mothers in the program either have a job or are in school. The children are cared for in the residence while the mothers are away. The staff—committed to helping the mothers strengthen their child-caring skills, cope with the demands of a job or school and plan for the future—consists of eight residence counselors, a social worker, two part-time psychiatrists, and a pediatrician specializing both in infancy and adolescence. They work with the mother and other people close to her; her parents, a boyfriend, the baby's father. The mothers and their babies usually stay for one year, although some stay longer. After leaving the residence, most continue to care for their children.[8]

Project Ku-nak-we-sha ("Caring")

American Indian children face grave risk of separation from their families, extended families and their traditions. However, within the past few years, several projects developed and governed by Indians have been initiated to protect Indian children against banishment. We visited one, Project Ku-nak-we-sha serving the

---

[6]Planned Parenthood Federation of America, *11 Million Teenagers: What Can Be Done About the Epidemic of Adolescent Pregnancies in the United States* (New York: The Alan Guttmacher Institute, 1976), pp. 10-11.
[7]Surprisingly, no study has yet determined the number of children born to teenage parents who end up in out-of-home care.
[8]For another approach to responding to young single parents, see D. T. Heger, "A Supportive Service to Single Mothers and Their Children," *Children Today* 6 (September-October 1977): 2-4, 36.

Yakima nation, located near Seattle.[9] *Ku-nak-we-sha* means *caring*. The project explicitly seeks to revitalize old traditions and to involve the tribal extended family in nurturing and caring for children at risk of placement.

Yakima reservation children removed from their homes are usually placed off the reservation. For instance, at the time of our visit, more than 100 adolescents needing special services were in Bureau of Indian Affairs boarding schools—although everyone acknowledged that the schools did not provide the needed services. Other children were sent from the reservation because of alleged abuse and neglect by parents. Tribal officials estimated that 80 percent of the children removed from the reservation did not return.

Project Ku-nak-we-sha reflects tribal determination to end the removal of children from the reservation. Begun in 1975, with money from the Office of Child Development in the Department of Health, Education and Welfare, the project has established a group receiving home for children whose families are experiencing crisis. Even the physical location of the home is linked to traditions of the tribe, for it once belonged to a respected tribal officer. The location of a home on the reservation means that its school-aged occupants can continue in the schools they had been attending. The project also provides emergency caretakers on a 24-hour basis to give counseling and support to families facing crises in their own homes.

Homebuilders

The Homebuilders, begun in 1974 in Tacoma, Washington, under the auspices of Catholic Children's Services, is a unique family-oriented crisis intervention program designed to prevent the removal of a family member from the home. After there has been a determination that removal is necessary, but before the removal takes place, a Homebuilders team goes into the home to help the family deal constructively with the problems and behaviors that precipitated the crisis. The Homebuilders' team works individually and collectively with all family members. They remain in contact with the family for up to six weeks after the initial intervention and then refer them to other agencies as necessary.

The staff of the project is composed of therapists trained in a variety of techniques including: Parent Effectiveness Training, Crisis Intervention, Values Clarification, Rational Emotive Therapy, Assertiveness Training, Self-Reward and Relaxation Techniques, Situation Structuring, Behavior Contracting, Fair Fight Techniques, and Effective Advocacy. This broad range of skills enables them to respond flexibly to each family situation.

Evaluations of the Homebuilders' efforts have indicated the approach reduces placements and saves money.[10] Importantly, since a large proportion of those for whom placement is avoided are adolescents, it also represents a successful strategy for dealing with a population often described as difficult to serve.[11]

The Door—A Center of Alternatives

Over and over again in the course of our study, we heard in alternate tones of resignation, frustration, or anger that "there is nothing for adolescents."[12] There is nothing for adolescent status offenders; and there is nothing for adolescents who have not been involved in an offense but who need help with impossible family situations, with finding meaningful activities, or with finding people who care.

In New York City, a group of professionals from all

---

[9]Examples of other projects include the Urban Indian Child Resource Center (Oakland, California), the Choctaw Child Advocacy Program (Philadelphia, Mississippi), and the Native American Family and Children's Service in the Minneapolis Regional Native American Center (Minneapolis, Minnesota).

[10]One evaluation found that in 90 percent of the families served, removal of a family member was avoided at an estimated cost savings of $312,478 or $2,332 per person. W. Gschwend, "The Homebuilders Program of Catholic Children's Services, Tacoma, Washington," (Sacramento, California: Technical Assistance Project, American Justice Institute, undated), p. 5. (Mimeographed.)

A second study, conducted by Washington State, found that avoiding placement in 119 families during a 12-month period saved the state $645,312, $614,316 of which would have been for child placements. It further estimated that Homebuilder staff costs were less than 25 percent of projected placement costs. Washington State Department of Social and Health Services, Homebuilder Evaluation, November 3, 1976, pp. III(5)-III(7). (Mimeographed.) See also, J. Kinney, B. Madsen, T. Fleming and D. Haapala, "Homebuilders: Keeping Families Together," *Journal of Counseling and Clinical Psychology* (1976).

[11]The Gschwend study cited above found that 70 percent of the families in which placements were avoided included youth classified as runaways, incorrigible children or delinquents. Gschwend, "The Homebuilders Program," p. 24. Another study reported that 52 percent of the family members in the 119 families in which placements were averted were children between 11 and 15, and another 11 percent were 16-20 year olds. Washington State Department of Social and Health Services, "Performance Audit Report, Homebuilders Program" (Audit No. FC-P1-41-76), Attachment A.

[12]See, for example, J. Lipsitz, *Growing Up Forgotten: A Review of Research and Programs Concerning Early Adolescence* (Lexington, Massachusetts: Lexington Books, D. C. Heath & Company, 1977). A Report to the Ford Foundation.

disciplines, increasingly concerned about "non-service" for adolescents, came together to do something about it. Beginning with 12 planners, the group soon expanded to several dozen, all of whom worked on specific aspects of program development. The result, a year later: "The Door—A Center of Alternatives," a comprehensive, multi-service center for urban youth. For its first seven months of life, the Door was staffed entirely by volunteers—primarily professionals from the New York City community. While there is now a paid staff of over 60 part-time and full-time workers, many lawyers, physicians and mental health professionals, among others, continue to provide volunteer services.

Philosophically, the Door provides an open, accessible resource to adolescents by offering a wide range of activities, including traditionally defined "services."[13] Located near public transportation, it serves youth from all five boroughs of New York. There has even been an effort to make the physical structure responsive to the participants' preferences. Because the Door's clients say they feel more comfortable when counseling services are in open areas close to other activities, the few individual rooms designed as counseling areas are now used for storage. Problems and difficulties are treated within the context of normal, healthy activity, rather than as symptoms of pathology.

The Door is not just "a place to hang out." During a youth's first visit, a contract is made requiring involvement in one or more of the Door's programs. With a range of interesting activities and the commitment of the staff, this approach works.

The Door serves young people from all ethnic backgrounds. Forty percent are white, 34 percent are black; 25 percent are Puerto Rican or other Hispanic heritage; and one percent are Oriental, mostly Chinese. Their ages range from 12 to 20 years with a majority (70 percent) between 15 and 19 years old. Fifty-one percent are male; 49 percent female. Referrals come from schools and community programs, hospitals, courts, youth residences, youth centers and service agencies.[14] Some young people hear about The Door and come in on their own.

The Door respects the strengths of youth and builds upon the goodwill and genuine "helping" motivation of agencies, public service systems, and professionals. Its success is refreshing and powerful in view of the many ineffective services for adolescents.

The Children's Center

The San Antonio Children's Center in Texas is over 90 years old. It began its life as the San Antonio Home for Destitute Children in 1886, and today serves as a nonprofit psychiatric treatment center for emotionally disturbed children. At the core of its treatment philosophy is a belief that residential treatment should be for a short time only, should deeply involve the child's family, and should respect and protect the legal, civil and human rights of children and parents in practice as well as theory.

The Center, serving 38 children aged six to 15 years, provides comprehensive residential treatment.[15] There are three firm requirements for admission to the program: (1) parents must participate in the treatment program; (2) a child is accepted only if outpatient alternatives will not work; and (3) a child is accepted only if there is reason to believe the Center's program will help. Children requiring long-term placement are not accepted. At least two staff members must approve an admission. Ninety percent of the children come from within the county in which the Center is located; none are from out of state. Approximately 60 percent of the children served come from lower socioeconomic backgrounds.

In the residential unit, two beds are reserved for mentally retarded children whose families may place them for respite care for up to 14 days during a one year period. Families may use this respite care no more than

---

[13]These include family planning, sex counseling, therapy, social services, crisis intervention, and educational, vocational, legal and drug counseling services. The Door also has a learning center, holds youth awareness seminars, and offers creative and rehabilitation workshops in arts, graphics, poetry, dance and theatre. There are several ongoing structured programs including a multi-modality psychiatric treatment program, an adolescent health program, an adolescent family planning program, prenatal, post-natal and early child rearing programs, and a recently established court diversion and delinquency prevention program. There are also frequent special programs, workshops and activities.

[14]According to a survey of the Door's clients, 48 percent of the young people were living with one or both parents, 14 percent with friends, 13 percent in agency residences, 9 percent with relatives, 8 percent alone, and 8 percent had no place to live. Sixty-two percent were enrolled in elementary school, junior high school, high school or high school equivalency programs, 10 percent in college. Twenty-seven percent had dropped out before completing high school. "The Door - A Center of Alternatives:" A Report, January 1972 - January 1975, p. 4.

[15]Recently a day treatment program serving 16 school-aged and eight pre-school children was established. Over 54 percent of the children it serves are Mexican-American.

twice during a year. The remaining 36 spaces are for children who stay from six to nine months. The average stay is six months.

Program goals and objectives at the Center are carefully detailed and treatment plans are developed for each child and family. The purposes and approaches are discussed periodically with the families. All staff are closely involved in the program. Since 1974, the Center has had a Committee on Patient and Family Rights, composed of eight staff members. Parents have also been invited to join the Committee, which has developed thoughtful, detailed policies and procedures to protect patient and family rights. These are shared with families during the intake process. Both parents and the child, if the latter is old enough, are given copies of the policies with a full discussion of the procedures.

Unlike many other residential treatment centers we have described in this report, the San Antonio Children's Center is committed to supporting a child within a familial context and has built into its operating program specific provisions both to protect the rights of children and families and to ensure quality care. Each family is assigned a primary contact person responsible for periodically seeking familial opinions and questions and providing information to the family. Within three weeks of a child's admission, there must be an initial formal meeting with the family, with quarterly follow-up meetings. All treatment procedures, including the use of any drugs or unusual approaches, must be clearly explained.

The Children's Center also has a continuing patient care evaluation system that includes clinical case reviews scheduled 30 days after admission and every 90 days thereafter to determine the effectiveness of the treatment plan. The results of this review must, as a matter of right, be shared with the family and child.

A Center-funded follow-up study of children served by the program indicated a high success rate. Reports by parents and school personnel suggested that, of 76 children discharged from the Center between July 1974 and 1975, 70 percent continued to function effectively in the community. Although the program is costly—averaging $20,000 a year per child—it is cost effective. Few children remain for a full year. Moreover, after a short stay at the Center most return to their own homes and do not require costly, long-term out-of-home care.

Comprehensive Emergency Services

The direct service programs we have discussed so far operate under private, nonprofit auspices, although all receive public funds. Public agencies providing services directly can also counter the "families don't count" mentality and develop quality services for children. The Comprehensive Emergency Services Program (CES) in Nashville - Davidson County, Tennessee, initially developed as a two year demonstration project by the local Department of Public Welfare, provides one example.[16]

The CES program was designed to reduce the number of emergency removals of children from their homes, and the over-reliance on short-term but inappropriate institutionalization of these children. The program required the development of an integrated system of crisis intervention services designed both to create new resources to prevent unnecessary removals of children from their homes and to reduce the fragmentation of services.[17] The Nashville network grew to include emergency caretaker and homemaker services, emergency foster homes, 24-hour intake, outreach and follow-up, an emergency family shelter, and, most recently, an emergency adolescent shelter.

The results of the effort to increase and coordinate service resources, according to an evaluation, are impressive.[18] Between 1969-1970 and 1973-1974:

— The number of Nashville children removed from their homes and placed in substitute care decreased 51 percent from 353 in 1969-70 to 174 in 1973-74.

— The number of Nashville children for whom dependency and neglect petitions were filed was reduced from 262 to 35, a decrease of 87 percent.

— The number of children under age six who were institutionalized was reduced from 180 to 0 during the same time period.

---

[16] Although the program proposal was developed by the local welfare department, the Metropolitan Nashville Juvenile Court's Protective Services Program also had a key role in the emergency services program.

[17] The Children's Bureau is encouraging other localities to develop similar systems. Six states and the Hennepin County (Minnesota) Welfare Department currently have grants of approximately $130,000 each for projects providing intensive support services to prevent separation of families at risk. The six states are Arizona, California, Nebraska, New Jersey, New York and Virginia.

[18] For a comprehensive discussion of the evaluation of the program, see M. Burt and R. Balyeat, *A Comprehensive Emergency Services System for Neglected and Abused Children* (New York: Vantage Press, Inc., 1977) pp. xxiv, 49, 54.

THE RIGHTS OF CHILDREN AND FAMILIES AT THE SAN ANTONIO CHILDREN'S CENTER[1]

All patients and families served by the Center shall have and are encouraged to exercise:

- The right to be fully informed of all rights.
- The right of confidentiality of all records and personal information.
- The right to information regarding the training, professional credentials and agency affiliations of all service providers.
- The right to be fully informed and to consent before being recorded or observed.
- The right to frequent visitation unless specifically restricted.
- The right to maintain close telephone and letter contact unless specifically restricted.
- The right to information about treatment plans, goals and procedures.
- The right to information regarding the results of all evaluations and assessment procedures.
- The right to meaningful input in the process of treatment and discharge planning.
- The right to a forum by means of which different points of view concerning the rights of patients and families may be aired and reconciled.

In addition to the rights stated above, every child patient at the Center shall have:

- The right to treatment by the least restrictive methods consistent with therapeutic effectiveness.
- The right to unrestricted expression of religious belief and to participation in religious activities compatible with treatment programming.
- The right to express appropriate individuality in dress, speech and general demeanor.
- The right to be spared all unnecessary regimentation and interrogation.
- The right to the assignment of uncrowded sleeping quarters and sufficient space for personal belongings.
- The right to privacy and modesty in sleeping and toilet facilities.
- The right to be informed regarding any necessary searches of personal effects.
- The right to be informed when visitors will be touring the unit.
- The right to humane treatment in matters of discipline.[2]
- The right to consult an attorney.[3]

---

[1] The rights set forth below are cited in San Antonio Children's Center, "Policies on Patient and Family Rights," Revised June 1976, pp. 3-4.

[2] Implementation directives to the staff note: "No form of corporal punishment in any of its varieties (hitting, scratching, pinching, spanking, etc.) is acceptable at any time at the Center. Staff are subject to immediate dismissal for use of corporal punishment." "Policies on Patient and Family Rights," p. 18.

[3] Implementation directives to the staff note: "No agency staff member shall dissuade, prohibit or prevent any child from contacting an attorney. Children who express a desire for legal consultation shall be asked first to discuss the matter with the parents or guardians who shall bear the cost of legal consultation. At their request, parents or children shall be informed by the clinician with responsibility for their treatment of legal options open to them and of free or low cost legal services available in the community. Should a child wish to contact an attorney against the wishes of his parents, the child shall be so allowed though the agency thereby assumes no responsibility for the cost of the legal consultation." "Policies on Patient and Family Rights," p. 20.

— In 1969-70, 94 percent of the Nashville children in foster care remained in care longer than one year. In 1973-74, only 34 percent remained in care for over one year.

As another consequence of the project, a custodial institution, which previously had accepted many of the unnecessary emergency removals, redefined its program and became a badly needed treatment facility for adolescents.

Further, the project resulted in a net cost savings during a two-year period of $68,000. This figure does not take into account the additional costs which would have been incurred in the future, had the children diverted from care by the project entered and remained in care until their majority.

Administrative and Judicial Protections

System-induced neglect of children out of their homes is a predictable chronic condition. Systematic effective checks against this neglect are few, but there are some models. In Chapter 4 we described the most promising of the review systems in our study states. Recall that in South Carolina, the citizen review boards have a clear mandate and specific authority to influence what happens to children out of their homes for more than six months.[19] The Ohio system relies on a court or court-appointed body to review cases periodically and decide what should happen to children out of their homes. Both models have the potential to provide more than *pro forma* reviews. Here we briefly describe three additional efforts designed to ensure that children out of their homes are not abandoned by those with public responsibility, and a fourth which responds to the grievances of natural parents.

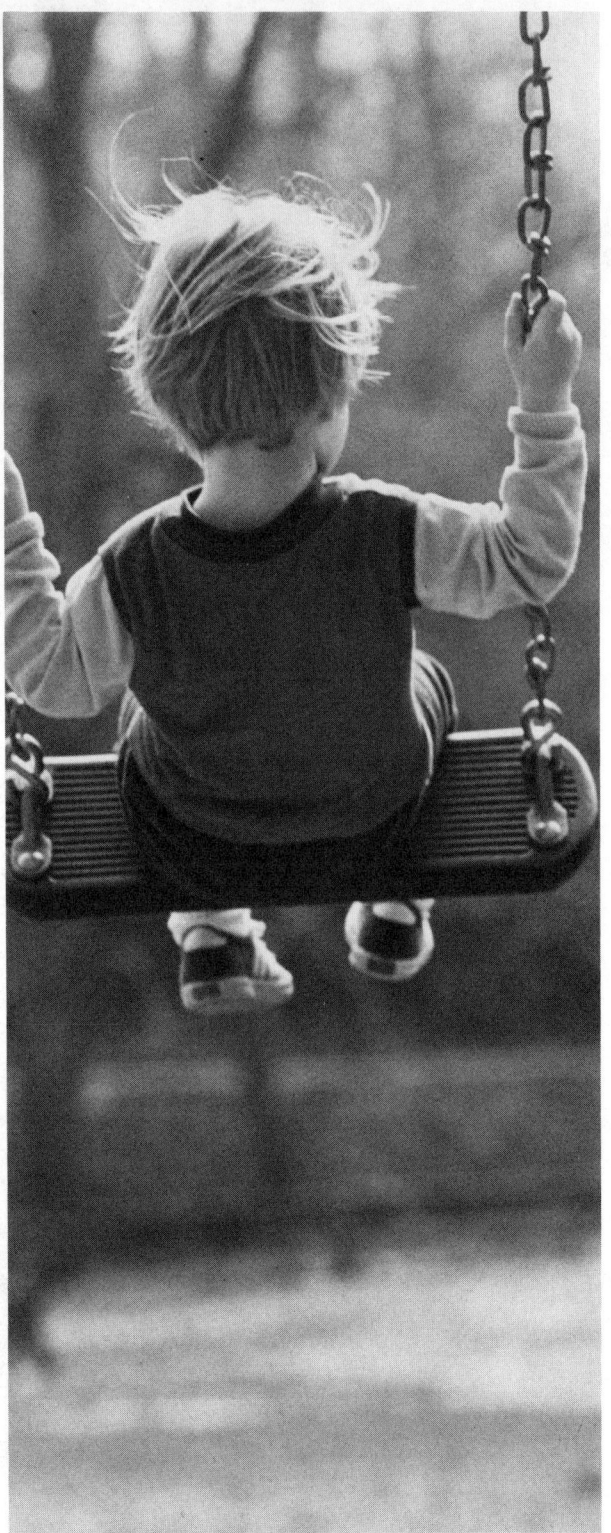

---

[19]The experience in South Carolina has been a positive one. Two years ago, when the review boards were established, only 5.8 percent of the children entering care left within one year. Now, 33 percent of the children entering care leave within six months. The movement of children out of care also has had a positive effect on caseloads in the child welfare system. Further, there has been a significant increase in the number of children in long-term foster care for whom parental rights have been terminated. South Carolina Office of Child Advocacy, "Children's Foster Care Review Board System, Progress Report," March 1, 1978. (Mimeographed.)

The New York State Court Review System

In 1971, the New York State Social Services Law was modified to require a periodic court review of the status of any child voluntarily placed in foster care under child welfare auspices, and remaining in such care for 24 months or longer.[20] In 1975, the length of time in care was reduced to 18 months, making it consistent with already required reviews of children placed involuntarily.[21]

The New York law was the first of its kind.[22] It requires that the agency caring for the child petition the court for a review. At a hearing, the court then determines whether the child should be: continued in foster care; returned to a parent, guardian or relative; legally freed for adoption; or, if already freed, placed in an adoptive home. All parties—the agency, the foster and the biological parents—must be notified of the hearing and of the dispositional alternatives before the court. Children may be present at the hearing. In cases in which children are continued in care, the court must re-hear the case at least every 24 months, or more frequently if the court believes it is necessary or is petitioned to do so by one of the parties.

The impact of this review system on agencies and on the outcomes for the children has been carefully evaluated by Dr. Trudy Festinger. In 1974, comparing a sample of cases reviewed by the court by December 31, 1973, with cases that were not reviewed, she found that agencies were more likely to move toward permanence for a child (either by obtaining a voluntary relinquishment or by initiating termination proceedings) if there was a court review.[23] In 1975, Festinger re-examined the sample of court-reviewed children comparing actual outcomes for the children with the orders from the initial reviews. She found that by 1975, 77 percent of the children for whom discharge was initially ordered had been discharged, and 91 percent of the children for whom adoption was ordered were in adoptive homes. Of the children for whom the initial order was continuation in foster care, 46 percent had either been discharged or adopted by June 1975. In all, between 1972 and 1974, 46 percent of the sample children entering care in 1970 had left. By 1975, 71 percent of the children had left.[24] This is a clear reversal of the usual pattern that the longer the child is in care, the more likely that the child will remain until the age of majority.[25] Thus, Festinger's studies provide some empirical support for the positive impact of periodic judicial review systems that set forth specific dispositional alternatives and include mechanisms for ensuring compliance with those dispositions.[26]

The Concern for Children in Placement Project

The Concern for Children in Placement Project (CIP) represents another approach to ending the banishment of children now in the system. Initiated in 1974, under the auspices of the National Council of Juvenile and Family Court Judges, the project relies on volunteers sworn to an oath of confidentiality. It is their responsibility to review court records on children out of their homes and to initiate, where appropriate, follow-up judicial reviews and action.[27]

In the first phase of the project, more than 4,000 cases were reviewed in 12 courts across the country by 250 volunteers. In a number of places, the reviews have resulted in changes within the service systems and consequently, positive changes in the lives of the children.

— Rhode Island reported a 50 percent increase in the filing of termination petitions, a 100 percent increase in adoption petitions, and a new request in the family court budget for a permanent care review monitor.

---

[20]New York Social Services Law §392.

[21]New York Family Court Act §1055(b).

[22]For a state by state analysis of statutory provisions for reviews of children in foster care, see Appendix L.

[23]T. B. Festinger, "The New York Court Review of Children in Foster Care," *Child Welfare* 54 (April 1975): 237.

[24]T. B. Festinger, "The Impact of the New York Court Review of Children in Foster Care: A Follow-up Report," *Child Welfare* 55 (September-October 1976): 538-539.

[25]It is also true that during the period that the review system was implemented, New York established an adoption subsidy program. This too, no doubt, facilitated the movement of children out of foster care.

[26]In 1974, the Family Court set up a system to notify agencies if reports were overdue, and assigned a staff member in the Office of Probation to review reports for substantive compliance with the court orders. The failure of agencies to carry out court orders, however, remains a continuing problem. The New York State Temporary Commission on Child Welfare plans to develop some new recommendations to strengthen the follow-up of court orders. Temporary New York State Commission on Child Welfare, Memorandum on Children's Defense Fund Recommendations re: *Children Without Homes*, undated. (Mimeographed.)

[27]Virginia Cain, Project Director, The Concern for Children in Placement Project, Testimony Before the House Subcommittee on Select Education and the Senate Subcommittee on Children and Youth, Joint Congressional Hearing on Foster Care, September 8, 1976.

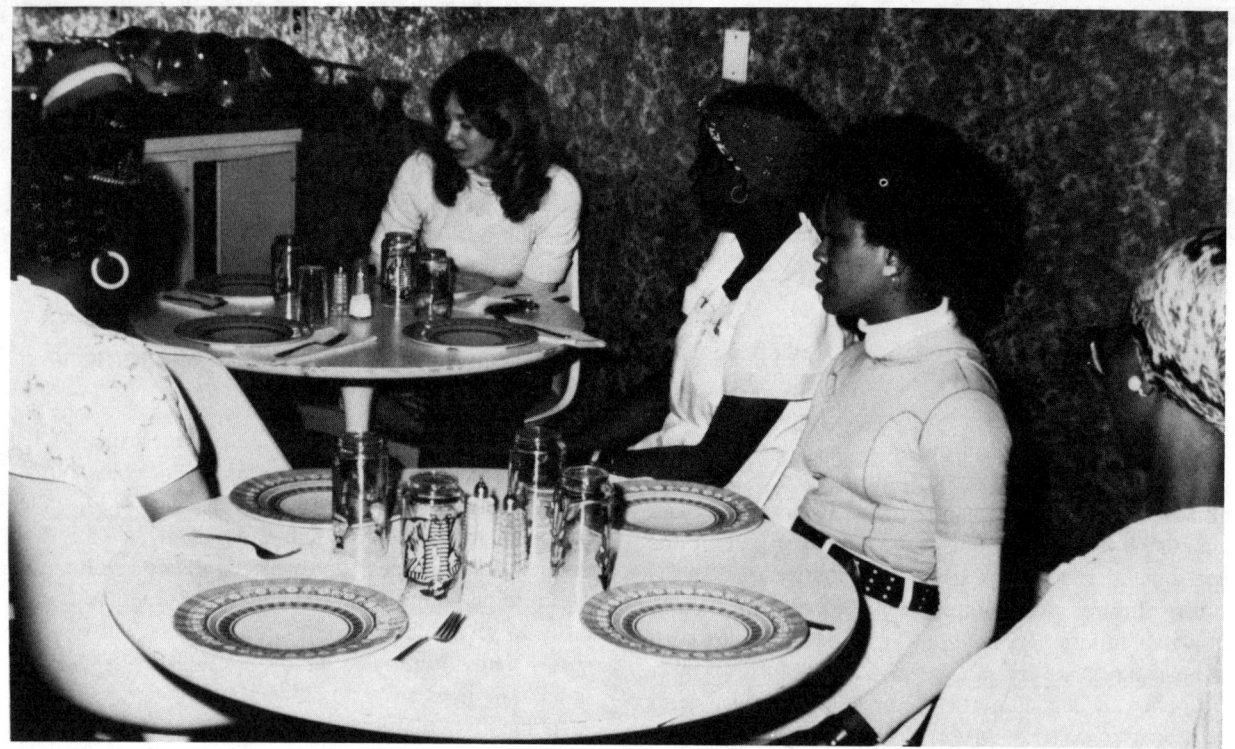

— In Ohio, 26 out of 99 children reviewed were moved out of foster care.

— In Oregon, 671 out of 1,006 children reviewed—67 percent—were removed from foster care.

— In Texas, 136 of the 222 children reviewed—61 percent—were removed from foster care.[28]

A second phase of the project is now underway, involving implementation of the review procedure in 25 additional courts, the development of training materials, a follow-up study of a sample of the children initially reviewed, and the orientation of at least 150 additional juvenile and family court judges to CIP techniques.[29] The project will also pilot test a guardian ad litem[30] program in selected courts.

[28]The general characteristics of the children involved in the reviews revealed familiar patterns. Twenty-four percent had been in foster care 5-10 years. Thirty-one percent had had no court review in 3-10 years; 49 percent had little or no contact with biological parents; and 56 percent of the sample had been moved three or more times (223 children were moved 7 to 18 times, and 10 moved 19 times). *CIP Alert*, Vol. 1, (February 1977).

[29]Children in Placement Project, Loose Leaf Training Manual, National Council of Juvenile Court Judges.

[30]"Guardian ad litem" generally refers to a party appointed by the court to determine the interests of a young child or an incompetent adult in a court proceeding. Its specific use varies from state to state.

Freeing Children for Permanent Placement

The New York court reviews, the South Carolina Foster Care Review Boards and the Ohio reviews provide for periodic reviews of children out of their homes. They are required by statute and are conducted or approved by persons who have no direct service or administrative responsibility for children. The Children in Placement Project derives its authority from the concern of local judges. But public agencies providing services to the children have also initiated review efforts targeted on a specific group of children. The Freeing Children for Permanent Placement (FCPP) project is an example of such an effort.

Conducted by the Children's Services Division of the Oregon State Department of Human Resources, the FCPP project was funded in 1973 for three years by the Children's Bureau in the Department of Health, Education and Welfare.[31] The purpose of the project was to identify children in unplanned long-term foster care and provide the intensive services necessary to

[31]The project subsequently received funding for a fourth year to continue following the children's placements.

reunite them with their families or ensure their adoption. Over 2,200 cases were screened in 15 Oregon counties. The screening indicated that 40 percent of the children had been in care more than three years; 40 percent had been in three or more homes; and 58 percent were 12 or older. The average time in out-of-home care for the group was four and one-half years.[32] These statistics reflect national patterns. Of the group screened, 509 children were selected for intensive casework. They represented children who had been in foster care one year or longer, who were regarded by their caseworkers as having little chance to be reunited with their own families, and who seemed adoptable.

The results were dramatic. As of October 1976, 26 percent of the children had been returned home (despite the initial selection criteria); and another three percent placed with relatives. Thirty-six percent of the children had had parental rights terminated and were living in adoptive homes (19 percent with their foster parents); and seven percent were in formalized long-term foster care. Final action had not been taken for the remaining 29 percent, although adoption was planned for many of them.[33]

Cost data from the project indicate that over 4,000 months of foster care were saved during the project period alone when the children were returned home or adopted. This resulted in a savings to the state of $1,082,695 in direct maintenance payments, excluding the cost of follow-up services (usually provided for approximately four months).[34]

A project staff of 11 caseworkers, each with caseloads of about 25 children, provided the actual services. Legal assistance for children was purchased with project funds from the Metropolitan Public Defenders Office. The lawyers provided technical assistance to the casework staff in bringing termination actions, as well as representation for the children. Project funds were also used for psychological and psychiatric evaluations and expert testimony related to court action. The easy access to legal assistance helped to remove some of the usual barriers to termination.[35]

The FCPP project demonstrates what an intensive, coordinated legal and social service effort can accomplish toward ending the banishment of children.[36] State agencies around the country have been responsive to this approach. When the Office of Child Development in HEW requested proposals from the states to replicate and/or adopt key aspects of the project, 36 states responded. Ten of these states and Puerto Rico were given grants for specific projects to ensure permanence to children now in foster care or to prevent unnecessary foster care.[37] The Oregon project, under a grant from the Children's Bureau in HEW, is also now providing technical assistance to states interested in providing permanence for children in long-term care.

The Parents' Rights Unit

One of the repeated themes throughout this report is that parents have few, if any, opportunities to challenge decisions about their children or to express in any meaningful way their continuing concern about what happens to them. In the course of our study, we learned of a program within a large public bureaucracy designed to break the "families don't count" pattern.

In 1975, the New York City Office of Special Services for Children (SSC), which is responsible for more than 28,000 children in foster care, established the Parents' Rights Unit (PRU). A unique ombudsman program, the PRU provides a resource for natural parents of a child in care having difficulty with a public agency or an agency under contract to the city. Once contacted, the staff of five experienced social workers and a supervisor first encourage the parent to try to settle the matter directly with the facility. If that fails, the PRU becomes involved.

---

[32] Regional Research Institute for Human Services, *Barriers to Planning for Children In Foster Care: A Summary* (Portland: Portland State University School of Social Work, 1976), p. 1.

[33] For further discussion of the project, see V. Pike, "Permanent Planning for Foster Children: The Oregon Project," *Children Today* 5 (November-December 1976): 22-25, 41.

[34] A. Emlen, J. Lahti, G. Downs, A. McKay and S. Downs, *Overcoming Barriers to Planning for Children in Foster Care* (Portland: Regional Research Institute for Human Services, Portland State University, 1977), pp. 6, 89-110.

[35] See, for a discussion of the barriers to termination in Oregon, Regional Research Institute for Human Services, *Barriers to Planning for Children in Foster Care: A Summary*.

[36] A handbook based on the project's experience is now available. See, V. Pike, et al., *Permanent Planning for Children in Foster Care: A Handbook for Social Workers* (Washington, D.C.: DHEW, Children's Bureau, 1977).

[37] Grants of approximately $90,000 each were awarded for demonstration projects in Alabama, Arizona, Maryland, Michigan, Minnesota, Nebraska, New York, Puerto Rico, Virginia, Washington and Wisconsin. In September 1977, the projects were funded for a second year.

The PRU's role is that of ombudsman, not advocate.[38] A PRU social worker investigates the complaint by exploring the problem, first from the parent's point of view, then as perceived by all other participants such as caseworkers and foster parents. In addition, there may be a reading of case records and a field investigation of the parent's complaint. After this evaluation of the situation, recommendations are formulated, and all parties informed. The parent is told about the possibility of legal alternatives if the PRU cannot resolve the problem satisfactorily.

The Parents' Rights Unit recently received a positive evaluation from the Citizen's Committee for Children of New York (CCC).[39] The CCC study, based on interviews with parents, agency workers and directors, PRU workers, and in some instances children, recommended expanding outreach efforts to parents, strengthening and formalizing follow-up procedures to ensure implementation of the PRU recommendations;[40] and developing a specific mechanism to provide feedback on the systemwide policy implications of the individual problems identified. In addition, it suggested that the PRU's mandate be broadened to respond directly to complaints of children, particularly adolescents,[41] and to include more specific responsibility for problems related to services to children in their own homes and to children discharged from foster care needing aftercare services.

The study found most of those interviewed supportive of the PRU. Approximately 70 percent of the natural parents interviewed said they would use the PRU again and recommend it to others. This is particularly interesting in view of the fact that 85 percent of the parents said that before using the PRU, they had discussed their complaints with the agency concerned and found workers unhelpful or overtly hostile.[42] The majority of the agency social workers interviewed felt, in turn, that the PRU handled investigations fairly, some noting that the PRU provided an alternative to litigation and enabled parents to become more involved in their child's care.[43]

The PRU's role as a counterforce to the anti-family bias within the foster care system also has cost-saving implications. While the CCC study does not address the cost effectiveness of the unit, the Office of Special Services for Children has noted elsewhere that during the period from September 1975 through October 1977, 95 children were reunited with their families through PRU efforts at an estimated cost saving of $1,432,410.[44]

The Parents' Rights Unit is not now mandated by statute. It is the result of internal administrative action by the SSC and depends upon the commitment of the agency head. There is no requirement that parents whose children are in foster care be notified in writing about the project. It is, however, the only systematic official attempt we found to acknowledge that efforts to work with natural families often fail because of chronic problems in the system, not because of the families.[45] It is also the only systemwide vehicle we learned of that provides redress, short of court action, to natural families whose children are in out-of-home care.

---

[38] While an "ombudsman" investigates all sides to a complaint and reports his findings in order to arrive at a fair settlement, an "advocate" pleads a case in favor of one side in an attempt to arrive at a settlement that is in that side's favor.

[39] Citizen's Committee for Children of New York, *The Parents' Rights Unit* (New York: Citizen's Committee for Children of New York, Inc., October 1977).

[40] In the sample of cases reviewed, the PRU recommendation clearly supported the parents' request in about 30 percent of the cases; did not support it in about 30 percent; and was a compromise recommendation in about 15 percent of the cases. For a variety of reasons—e.g., the complaint had been withdrawn, litigation was pending or the matter was referred to a more appropriate body—there were no recommendations made in the remaining 25 percent of the sample cases. Citizens' Committee for Children of New York, *Parents' Rights Unit*, pp. 13-14.

[41] Interestingly, an analysis of the ages of 225 children involved in 123 cases (those closed by mid-March of 1976, plus 50 percent of the active cases) revealed 28 percent were under six and 68 percent under 11. The age distribution of children in out-of-home care throughout the child welfare system in New York City reflected a different pattern. Nineteen percent of the children were under six; 26 percent under 11. Citizens' Committee for Children of New York, *Parents' Rights Unit*, p. 21.

[42] The report of the evaluation notes: "Some examples of parents' recollections of Agency responses are: (1) Agency worker kept saying I was emotionally ill—she'd see me in Court. . . .(2) The head manager told me it was foolish to have my children back. I wasn't married and my neighborhood was bad. . . .(3) I have been telling those people that I want my children for ten years. No one listened." Citizens' Committee for Children of New York, *Parents' Rights Unit*, pp. 15-16.

[43] Citizens' Committee for Children of New York, *Parents' Rights Unit*, pp. 17-18.

[44] This calculation was based on a reduction of 1.68 years in care for each of the 95 children reunited with their families. The mean length of time the 95 children spent in care (2.55 years) was subtracted from the mean length of time in care for New York City children (4.23 years). New York City Department of Social Services Special Services for Children, "PRU Information Sheet," November 29, 1977. (Mimeographed,)

[45] As we indicated in Chapter 4, the Massachusetts HELP Program, which also reflects a response of the system to predictable system-induced service failures to children and families, has a broader mandate and is not specifically directed to children in out-of-home care.

> ### THE PARENTS' RIGHTS UNIT COMPLAINTS AND OUTCOMES[1]
>
> From August 1975 to June 1976, the PRU handled 228 complaints. One hundred and seventy of these were resolved with the following outcomes:
>
> 25 cases — full support for natural parent
>
> 41 cases — full support for agency decision
>
> 45 cases — compromise solution
>
> 59 cases — complaint withdrawn (usually the result of informal resolution when the agency learned the parent had registered a formal complaint)
>
> It is clear that the types of complaints received indicate a "families don't count" syndrome:
>
> 33 cases — involved problems in scheduling visits or situations in which parental requests for increased visiting were blocked by the agency.
>
> 29 cases — involved services to natural parents (e.g., complaints by parents that promised aftercare to children in their own homes was not forthcoming).
>
> 3 cases — involved issues of termination of parental ties, including one case in which, as a result of the PRU's action, one child for whom the agency had sought termination will be returned home within the year.
>
> 44 cases — involved complaints about discharge planning.
>
> 15 cases — involved complaints about lack of services to children in foster care.
>
> ---
> [1]Interview with Linda Greenman, Supervisor, Parents' Rights Unit, New York City, July 13, 1976.

Advocacy Groups

The structural and political forces that shape public responses to children at risk of removal or removed from their homes are complex. Policies that ignore families, funding formulas that encourage long-term out-of-home care at the expense of preventive services, restorative services or services ensuring permanence to children, statutory inadequacies, and compliance failures at all levels of government reflect deeply embedded patterns and practices. Effective advocacy is needed to support policymakers and administrators concerned about the problems, and to insist that those with responsibility refocus local, state and federal efforts to remedy the problems.

Advocacy in the Seven Study States

In at least four of our seven study states, advocates have had a visible impact on the state's response to children at risk of public abandonment and their families. In South Carolina, the Foster Care Review Boards[46] are a product of outside groups working for change. Similarly, the creation of the South Carolina Office of Child Advocacy is a result of a process lasting several years. There, a coalition, including the South Carolina Civil Liberties Union, League of Women Voters, and Council for Human Rights, worked for passage of a revised termination statute; then (as it became obvious that the new statute was having no impact) for creation of two additional monitoring mechanisms.

In Ohio, which ranks low on indices of state responsibility to its children, the Citizen's Committee for Ohio Children's Services has tried to develop political support for change. Composed of concerned citizens and professionals, the Committee's first task was to urge the state to make a commitment to child welfare by allocating state funds specifically for that purpose. In 1971 they succeeded. At the time of our visit, the Committee was gathering data (which the state should have been gathering) on the number of children out of their homes, some basic characteristics of county services, and the legal status of these children. Other groups in Ohio[47] have worked for passage of reform legislation

---
[46]See Chapter 4 for a detailed description.
[47]Since the time of our visit, the Institute for Child Advocacy in Cleveland has been established to focus on problems and to press for change on behalf of children without homes.

providing for changes in the state's adoption law, as well as creation of the periodic review mechanisms described earlier.[48]

In New Jersey, the New Jersey Citizens' Committee for Children (now called the Association for Children of New Jersey) monitors the activities of the New Jersey Division for Youth and Family Services, focusing particularly on problems relating to children out of their homes. The NJCCC, through public conferences and legislative activity, tries to increase public concern about state neglect of children in out-of-home care. It has trained volunteers to visit facilities used by the state and issued a public report. It has also actively monitored the state's response to large numbers of New Jersey children sent out of state.

In California, advocacy has taken a different form. California is one of several states with an organized lobby on children's issues that works primarily on legislation and related matters. As part of its legislative agenda, the Children's Lobby worked for the passage of the Child and Family Protection Act.[49]

In addition, we learned of advocacy efforts in other parts of the country. To illustrate the range of advocacy possibilities, we describe some of them.

For Love of Children

For Love of Children (FLOC) in Washington, D. C. is a program committed to making life better for children in foster care, as well as ensuring permanence for foster children.

FLOC was organized in 1965 by concerned volunteers from socially active churches in the Washington area. At that time, there was virtually no foster home care in the District of Columbia: children were institutionalized in "Junior Village," which then warehoused 900 children (capacity 700).

FLOC's initial goal was to get all of the children out of Junior Village within one year. Small groups of volunteers were assigned to explore alternative placements for groups of four or five children. This strategy failed, and the programmatic and political growth of FLOC began. The local goverment told FLOC that there were no homes for the children. However, when FLOC recruited 175 foster parents, the Department of Welfare processed only 35 applications and failed to place any children with the recruits. FLOC then embarked on a plan to establish group foster homes, and in five years developed homes for more than 90 children.

A different group of FLOC volunteers organized a learning center for children in foster care. That learning center has expanded and now serves children in their natural families as well. Most recently, FLOC has been involved in running a wilderness program for adolescents.[50]

Concerned not only about direct services to children at risk of or in placement, FLOC was instrumental in establishing the Child Advocacy Center to act as a focal point for systemwide reform. The Center, with a salaried attorney as director and the assistance of many volunteers, has worked on a series of issues related to child welfare. Initially, it was involved in a lawsuit to close a mini-institution established by the Department of Human Resources after Junior Village was emptied. Since then it has conducted a study of foster care practices in the District of Columbia and worked, often by organizing coalitions, for the passage of legislation relating to subsidized adoption, child abuse, and termination of parental rights. The Center is now committed to monitoring regulations to ensure adequate implementation of the new legislation. The Center demonstrates the important role a broad-based, local child advocacy effort can play in making systems accountable.

The Illinois Foster Children's Association

Advocacy efforts involve parents, professionals, other interested citizens, and sometimes the children themselves. In Illinois, for example, a group of foster children, with some adult assistance, has formed the Illinois Foster Children's Association (IFCA) to focus

---

[48]See Chapter 4 for a detailed description.

[49]At the time of our visits to the other states, we did not find advocacy efforts specifically focused on either the child welfare system or the problems of children out of their homes. The Massachusetts Advocacy Center was monitoring the implementation of the Massachusetts Special Education Law. South Dakota had a Committee for Children and Youth which addressed the problems of all children and youth. We found no focused advocacy in Arizona on behalf of the population with which we were concerned, although since our visit, the Arizona 4-C Committee, which initially focused on day care issues, has become involved in the problems of children out of their homes.

[50]Initially, the project was designed for adolescents experiencing difficulty in foster family care. It was hoped that participation in the program would enable the youth to remain in their current foster homes rather than be transferred to a new home or institution. That idea failed because the D.C. Department of Human Resources would not hold the space in the foster homes during the time the youth were to participate in the wilderness programs. The program now recruits a different group of adolescents.

specifically on the special problems of children in foster care. According to its bylaws,[51] the IFCA works to:

— "Improve the image of Foster Children in the eyes of the community
— Improve the quantity and quality of foster homes
— Enhance communication among Foster Children
— Provide recreational activities for Foster Children
— Advocate the legal and natural rights for Foster Children
— Promote the development of programs and resources for Foster Children"

The group has encountered and still encounters difficulty in achieving these objectives. Some foster parents feel threatened by the organization and do not want their foster children to attend. The county agency was initially reluctant to share the names of foster children so the IFCA could recruit members. But the youth persevered, and now have about 20 active members. This small, but committed group conducts a number of activities including:

— Holding monthly meetings to which all foster children are invited
— Consulting with other communities to help new associations get started
— Participating on the Illinois Council of Youth (part of the Illinois Commission for Children)
— Recruiting and conducting training sessions for foster parents
— Developing a handbook for foster children explaining their rights and advising them about where to go for help
— Taking a position on corporal punishment and trying to influence regulations currently being drafted by the State Department of Children and Family Services[52]

The IFCA wants to become a nonprofit corporation and seeks support for expanded activities, including a hotline, a peer counseling service, and technical assistance to others who want to start similar groups.[53]

Other Organized Advocates

Across the country, associations of foster parents, including the National Foster Parents Association, and organizations of adoptive parents, such as the North American Council on Adoptable Children, have formed to focus on specific problems. There is also a network of Action for Foster Children Committees, part of the National Action for Foster Children Program, a citizen effort first developed in 1972 on behalf of foster children.[54] Some of these groups work for change in the child-placing systems and can provide valuable information to others.

Groups traditionally not involved with the problems of children out of their homes also have begun to mobilize advocacy efforts. For example, the National Association of Junior Leagues is sponsoring a child advocacy project and encouraging the Leagues to move from direct service/volunteer activities to advocacy. The local Leagues are free to choose the area of most concern to them, and a number have selected foster care as their area of concentration. They are studying the problems within their communities and working with others to ensure that corrective action is taken and reforms are monitored.

A National Commission for Children in Need of Parents, consisting of representatives of industry, business and public affairs, has also recently been formed to identify obstacles to finding permanent homes for children and to encourage and help implement reforms.

---

[51] Illinois Foster Children's Association, Bylaws, Article II.
[52] Illinois Foster Children's Association, Description of Composition, Purpose and Program, September 1976. (Mimeographed.)
[53] For a fuller account, see W. T. Perozzi, "Speaking Out for Their Rights. The Illinois Foster Children's Association," *Children Today* 6 (November-December 1977): 16-17, 34-36.

[54] The impetus for this effort came in part from the Children's Bureau in the Department of Health, Education and Welfare. In Fiscal Year 1977, the National Action for Foster Children Committee was awarded $90,000 to train local action committee chairmen to improve services to foster children, and the grant was extended on February 1, 1978, for an additional 12-month period.

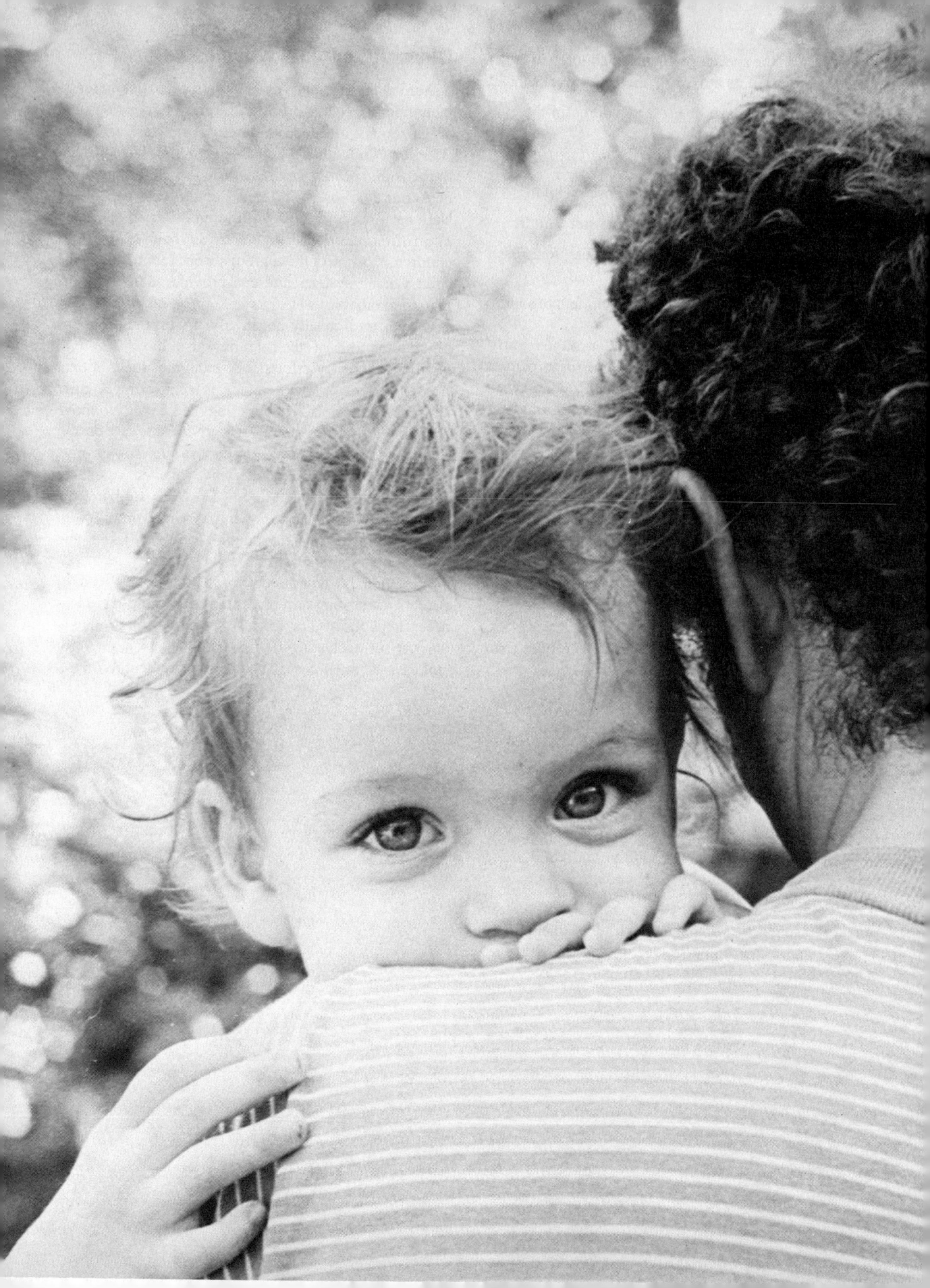

7 Advocacy for Children Without Homes

Strategies for Change

Advocacy for children without homes means many things. It means seeing that an individual child is not a victim of abuse in an institutional setting. It means speaking out on behalf of a group of children and families who now too often lack a sustained voice to ensure attention to their needs. It means helping foster parents get decent rates for the work of caring for children and extra training and support if the children have special needs. It means working with a state legislator to pass legislation creating a strong independent periodic review system. It means helping to start a preventive service project. In short, it means learning about what happens to children and families and trying to do something to correct the kinds of problems we have identified in this report.

Advocates for children without homes and their families come in many different styles. Some are professionals—lawyers, social workers, psychologists—fed up with the ways this vulnerable group of people are treated. Some are legislators concerned about the non-accountability of public systems. Others are concerned volunteers. Some advocates are parents, foster parents and foster children who want to improve the quality of care for individual children or make the system work better for all children. But all are people who share a sense of outrage and urgency. Advocates know change is needed now.

The hardest part about being an advocate is getting started. The problems we have been describing may seem overwhelming—so that even if you care, you may not be sure how or where to begin. You don't have to take on all the problems. In a small community, one or two foster parents asking questions about why children are not being adopted may start the ball rolling. A newspaper article about children in one institution may trigger the interest of a local civic group which can then begin to ask questions about institutions in which other children are placed.

In this chapter, we offer some guidelines for both *case advocacy*—advocacy on behalf of individual children and families, and *class advocacy*—advocacy on behalf of groups of children and families.

Case Advocacy

Case advocacy is a way of ensuring necessary services to and protecting the rights of individual children and families. It is a way of making the service systems work for and not against them. Parents typically are case advocates for their children. But for many children without homes, parents are either unavailable or beset by too many pressures. And so foster parents, child care workers or others with concern must ask the persistent questions about what is or what is not being provided for one child—and must put pressure on those in a position to respond.

There is no one way to be an effective case advocate. Sometimes the first step is getting information to parents about what services are available, or what their rights are. For example, it would help foster parents, anxious to adopt a 12-year-old child they have cared for for five years, to know if their state subsidized adoption law gives priority to long-term foster parents. A mother, concerned about her son's letter from a residential facility telling her that he was only in school for an hour a day, might be helped by information on her son's right to an appropriate education and how to see that he receives it.

Some of the children mentioned earlier in this report have benefited from the efforts of case advocates. Others might have benefited. Recall, for example, the plight of Cindy and Alvin. Cindy is a seven-year-old retarded child whose mother was charged with neglect and forced to institutionalize her after the school system refused to provide appropriate educational services. A case advocate knowledgeable about the Education for All Handicapped Children Act could have helped Cindy's mother try to get the school to comply with the law. Moreover, a case advocate could have seen to it that Mrs. G. was represented by counsel in the neglect proceeding. This might have resulted in a far different disposition than the actual judicial order that Cindy be placed in a state institution; or it might have resulted in an appeal of that order.

Alvin is the 15-year-old who has been in out-of-home placements for seven years, three of them out of state. His mother cannot find the caseworker assigned to Alvin, get any information on his progress, or find anyone to help her get Alvin back home. A case advocate familiar with the state bureaucracy might, by persistent efforts such as contacting the case supervisor and if necessary the welfare commissioner, get a caseworker assigned to Alvin promptly and then see that necessary further action is taken.

Gathering accurate information, arguing a position persuasively, and negotiating firmly are fundamental tools of case advocacy.[1] Beyond that, strategies vary with the particular situation.

Case advocacy for children at risk of or in placement has unfortunately not been developed to the extent that case advocacy has for other vulnerable groups of children. Children with special educational needs, for example, now have a statutory right to an appropriate education—a right guaranteed through explicit state and federal regulations. The existence of these laws and regulations has generated a large variety of training materials and programs for parents, other advocates, and professionals.[2] There is no comparable statutory right to appropriate care for children in out-of-home placement. Indeed, as we have shown, the parents of these children are frequently unaware that they or their children have any rights at all. Case advocacy efforts are often time-consuming and difficult even where a statutory right exists, more so without it. But there is also no question that a resourceful advocate can make a difference in the lives of at least some of the children without homes.

Class Advocacy

While each case has its own unique characteristics, there are frequently common patterns of experiences that reflect systemic failures or abuses. It is often more effective, therefore, to deal with these common problems of systems than to focus on resolving the painful circumstances of one family's or child's situation. This is the essence of "class advocacy." Like a "class action" in the legal world, it goes beyond the protection of individual children and families to attack systemwide barriers affecting groups of children in need, thereby increasing the impact of any reform.

Steps To Take

Class advocacy typically requires that advocates:

1. *Analyze local needs to identify priority problems.* Particular problems and needs vary from community to community and state to state. In some states, for example, existing statutes may be vague; in some adequate appropriations will be needed to implement existing programs; in others advocates may need to investigate destructive practices such as placing children long distances from home, over-institutionalizing

---

[1] For a useful discussion of the role of case advocacy in child welfare, see B. McGowan, "The Case Advocacy Function in Child Welfare Practice," *Child Welfare* 52 (May 1978): 275-284.

[2] See, for example, Children's Defense Fund, *94-142 and 504: Numbers That Add Up to Educational Rights for Handicapped Children* (Washington, D. C.: CDF, 1978).

large numbers of children, or failing to pay foster parents adequate rates to provide care to children. Identify the problem on which you want to focus.

2. *Learn the facts of the local situation.* Find out who is involved and talk with them. Talk with the staff of local child welfare and probation offices, the schools, and the local community mental health center. Meet with juvenile or family court judges and lawyers. Talk with local officials who have fiscal responsibilities[3] and talk with local governmental representatives.

Ask the people you talk with for specific information such as:

— How many children are in institutions?

— How long have they been there?

— What are the institutions like? How do they know?

— How do existing review systems work? How do they compare with review systems in other states?

— How many children are represented by lawyers in court proceedings? How many are not?

— What formal ombudsman mechanisms or vehicles for case advocacy exist?

In addition, try to meet with the people directly affected. Talk to groups of foster parents and foster children.[4] Try to learn about the experience of parents who have sought services to keep the family together or whose children have been placed voluntarily and involuntarily in foster care. Talk to people who are seeking to adopt, or who have adopted foster children.

Talk to parents and foster parents of children who are handicapped or who are status offenders. Find out about their concerns. Find out what obstacles they have faced in trying to get services or effect change. Find out why their efforts have succeeded or failed.

3. *Identify sources of authority.* Examine budgets, licensing regulations, administrative procedures, laws and statistical and program reports.[5] Learn who makes which decisions, who is accountable to whom, and where the authority to make changes lies. This may involve meeting with state officials, mayoral staff or county councils, and child advocacy groups, and with regional officials of the federal government, especially those within the Department of Health, Education and Welfare.

4. *Decide what corrective action is necessary.* Advocates must be specific—global calls for change won't work. Formulate realistic remedies that will alleviate the problem. This may require setting both long and short-term goals. Suppose, for example, that children remain in care for a longer time in your community than in neighboring communities. The immediate remedy might be to work for a local citizen's review board; the long-term remedy might be to work for major revisions in the child welfare code so periodic reviews are mandated by statute throughout the state.

5. *Mobilize support for the desired change.* You might start by encouraging local civic and church groups to become familiar with the problems of children without homes, and to understand why corrective action is needed. Encourage them, for example, to visit local institutions in which the children live, or to have community meetings on the problem. You might try to form an ad hoc coalition or special task force, drawing on different community groups.[6] Often, it will be helpful to use the media to focus public attention on the human, social and fiscal costs of inappropriate care. Encourage news articles or testimony which bring the stories of these children to the attention of councils,

---

[3]Often in the course of our study, we found that those involved with the budget were able to provide the most factual answers to our questions. Indeed, many of the strongest criticisms of the failure of child caring systems to provide adequate care for children have resulted from fiscal audits. See, for example, New York City Comptroller's Office, *The Children Are Waiting* (New York: Institute for Public Affairs, 1977); General Accounting Office, *Children in Foster Care Institutions: Steps Government Can Take to Improve Their Care* (Washington, D. C.: General Accounting Office, February 1977), and HEW Audit Agency's Reports of State AFDC Foster Care Program Audits. (Individual state audits are identified in Appendix B.)

We have also learned of at least one advocacy effort that is based on training advocates to analyze budgets for services to children and families. JAC, Joint Action for Children, a coalition of seven children's groups in New York City has developed a project to help community planning boards examine total local expenditures for children and families and determine the proportion of administrative vs. direct service costs. For further information about the materials developed through this project, contact Interface, 95 Madison Avenue, New York, New York 10002.

[4]The privacy and confidentiality of families involved with the child care systems must be protected. But in many communities, there are organized groups, such as foster parent associations and individuals willing to tell their experiences to advocates.

[5]If access to information to document the problems is difficult, many states have freedom of information acts, which define the information that must be available to the public by request. In addition, there is a federal Freedom of Information Act. Under the Act, the public is entitled to certain information concerning federally funded programs maintained by federal agencies. See 5 U.S.C. §552.

[6]Possible groups include church groups, Junior Leagues, the YMCA and YWCA, League of Women Voters, the American Friends Service Committee, Rotary Clubs, local and state chapters of the American Civil Liberties Union, groups particularly concerned with the needs of minority children, and local associations of professionals.

county boards of supervisors, and state legislators.[7] Sometimes, lobbying will be necessary. Other times, you may choose to negotiate with officials to change a regulation or administrative procedure.

6. *Use as many strategies as necessary*. Often, an advocacy effort will involve all of these strategies at different times. Occasionally, when none of these works, it may even require bringing a lawsuit. The difficulty involved and the time consumed in mobilizing support for change varies with the task and the level of government involved. Passage of federal or state child welfare reform legislation may be a long process, involving several sessions of the legislature. On the other hand, if the goal is to change existing regulations and the administrator with responsibility and authority recognizes the need, the advocacy effort may lend the support needed to act quickly.[8] If the administrator does not admit the need for change, more adversarial strategies may be necessary. In general, it is best to try persuasion first, and only if that fails, to resort to efforts such as concentrated lobbying, publicity and litigation.

7. *Monitor the change*. Effecting change is only half the task. Making sure the change is carried out is the other half. This requires monitoring. Monitoring is a means of ensuring that laws, systems, programs and professionals serve children and families in the ways that they are intended to, and that changes are meaningful, not merely symbolic. It is vital to ensure that the spirit and not just the letter of new statutory or regulatory requirements is complied with, and to see that targeted funds are spent as intended.

Monitoring of both ongoing programs and demonstration efforts is important. Numerous federal and state programs affecting the delivery of services to children and families should be scrutinized locally to ensure that statutory and regulatory requirements are met, and funds are used for the maximum benefit of children without homes and their families. Development and execution of various state plans (under Title XX for example) should also be monitored by advocates to ensure they do not become meaningless pieces of paper.

Public agencies *must* be held accountable to the children and taxpayers. Monitoring provides one mechanism for ensuring this accountability.

8. *Don't lose sight of the overall picture*. Change is needed in many parts of the child care system. There are complex problems within and across the different systems. So, for example, it will not be enough for advocates to work for funds and mechanisms to facilitate adoption, without also increasing funds to prevent the unnecessary use of out-of-home placement and increasing the protections afforded to families at risk of separation. The politics of change may require attention to limited aspects of the problem initially, but it is important to see the whole problem.

9. *Keep records*. In all stages of the advocacy process, it is important to keep written records of discussions and telephone calls, as well as more formal meetings. Keep copies of statistics and other data you receive, and a log of the stages in your progress so you can be accurate when you remind people of past promises or decisions. Request that officials give you decisions and timetables for change. Get it in writing. Verbal promises often carry little weight.

10. *Be patient but persistent*. Advocacy is often a slow process. Be enthusiastic but also be prepared to be patient and to follow each advocacy effort with another. Consider what happened in one South Carolina advocacy effort to ensure permanence for children. In 1972, that state's termination statute was revised to facilitate the adoption of children. But its staunchest backers soon discovered that getting a new law on the books was not enough. One and a half years after its passage, parental rights had been terminated in only 38 cases. A study initiated by the Department of Social Services estimated that 75 percent of its workers were not even aware of the contents of the new law or the legal procedures involved. Studies conducted by the South Carolina Civil Liberties Union and the South Carolina Council for Human Rights further highlighted the problem by adding more detailed information on the number of children in the foster care system for whom termination was thought to be appropriate. The impact of these facts, coupled with intensive lobbying by committed advocates, led to the creation of a foster care review board system and a subsidized adoption program.

But even this was not enough. It became clear that there was a crucial need for some centralized focus of

---

[7] The recent passage of legislation authorizing periodic reviews of children in foster care by citizen boards in Arizona followed a hard hitting series of articles in the *Tucson Daily Citizen* entitled "Children Adrift—An Arizona Crisis." Copies of the articles were made accessible to all state legislators.

[8] As we have noted, many of those who are part of the child caring system are frustrated with the ways they must function. They welcome outside support to help them to make desired internal changes.

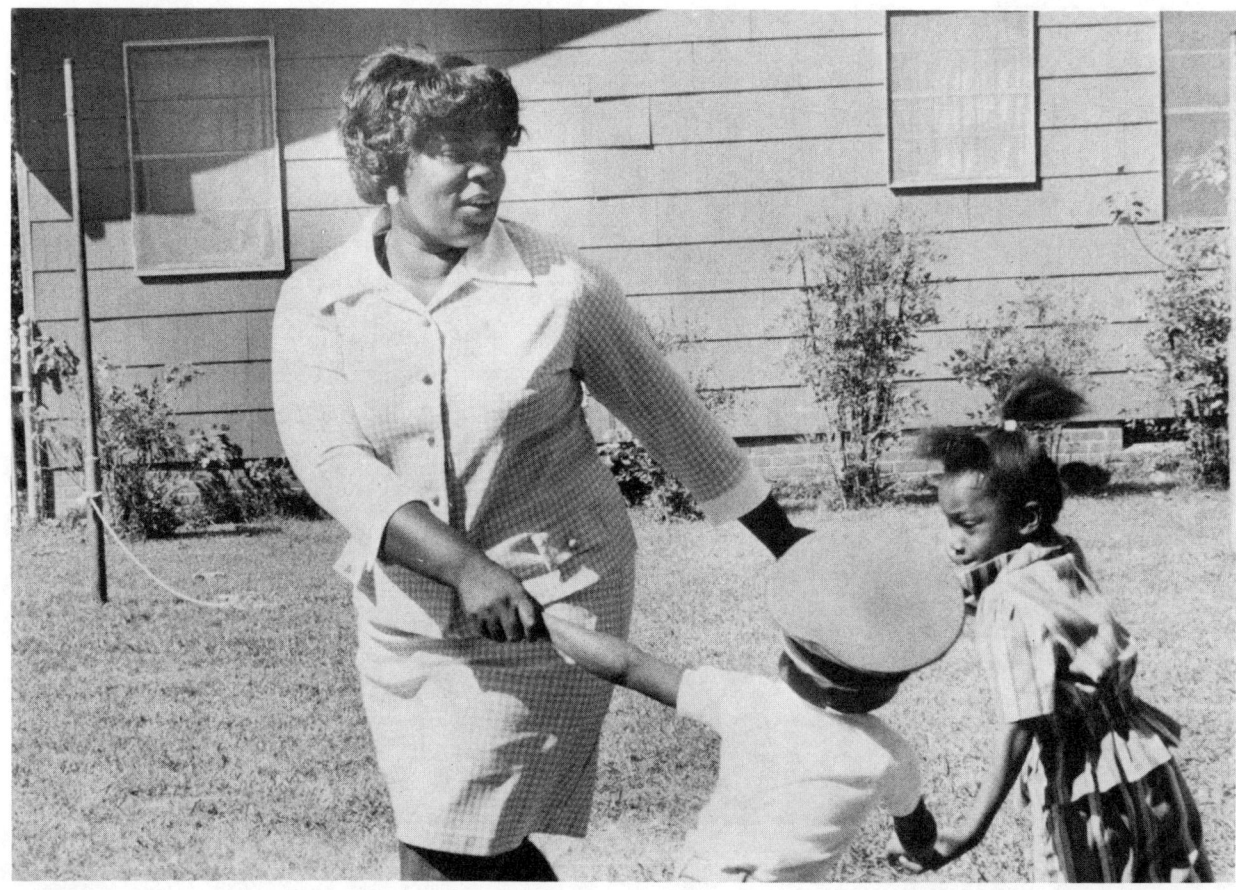

responsibility to monitor state policies and insist they be carried out. This led in 1975 to an Executive Order of the Governor establishing an Office of Child Advocacy.[9]

This account is too smooth. Interspersed throughout the effort were struggles and setbacks. But the South Carolina experience illustrates the need for advocates to be flexible—to shift from statutory to administrative to practical efforts and back again, when necessary. And, it highlights the need to get the *facts* about what really is happening to children and families to justify change and enlist others in supporting specific remedies.

Questions to Ask

The following questions may be helpful to advocates seeking to identify, document and act on problems of children without homes.[10] They are organized according to the major categories of information in which you may be interested.

To have a general overview of what is happening to children at risk of placement and in care in your community and state:

Studies. Have any studies been done of the child care systems in your community?[11] In your state?

Systems. What are the particular child care systems through which children are placed in out-of-home care?

---

[9] For a fuller discussion of the events in South Carolina over the three year period, see B. Chappell, "Organizing Periodic Review in Foster Care: The South Carolina Story," *Child Welfare* 54 (July 1975): 477-486.

[10] For additional questions to ask, see U. S. Department of Health, Education and Welfare, Office of Human Development, Children's Bureau, *Action for Foster Children Community Self-Evaluation Chart* (Washington, D. C.: U. S. Government Printing Office, 1974). Note, however, no specific questions are addressed to children in group settings or in out-of-state placements.

[11] For a helpful manual that can be used in assessing child welfare services in your community, see The Urban Institute, *Local Child Welfare Services Self-Assessment Manual* (Washington, D.C.: U. S. Department of Health, Education and Welfare, Office of Human Development Services, Children's Bureau, 1978).

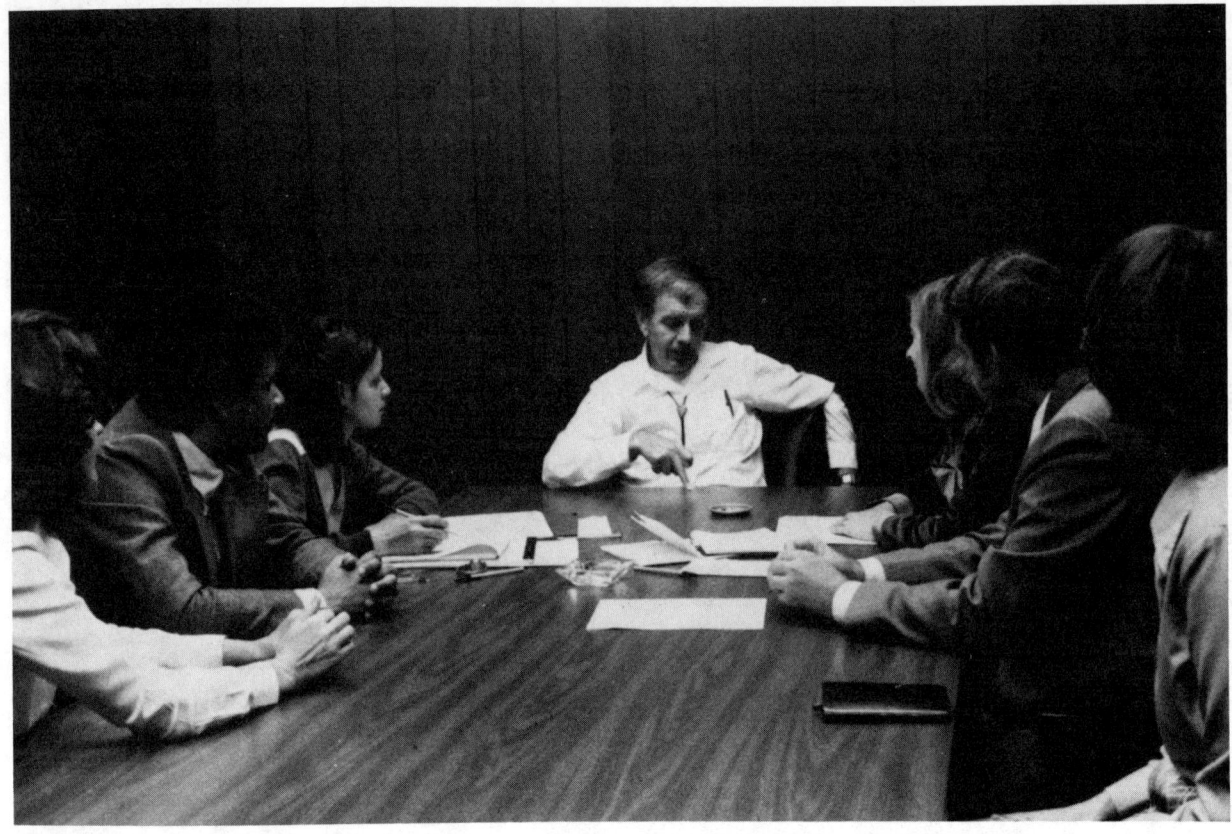

What are the procedures by which children are placed out of home?

Preventive Services. What services are available to prevent the removal of children from their families and to strengthen the family? How are such services funded? How many children received preventive services last year? What are specific barriers to increasing the availability of preventive services?

Voluntary Placements. What are parents told and given to sign when they place their children voluntarily? Is the material in a form and language parents can understand? Does it say how to request their children's return?

Due Process. Who has a right to be represented by counsel at various points in judicial proceedings involving neglect and abuse? In delinquency proceedings? In proceedings involving status offenders? What really happens in practice?

Relatives. What are the local child welfare policies and practices regarding placement with relatives? Are relatives eligible for foster care payments? If not, why not? If so, do they receive the same level of payment as non-relatives?

Parent Visits. What are the local child welfare and probation policies and practices regarding parent-child visiting? How are parents notified of such policies? What funds, if any, are available for transportation for parent-child visits?

Foster Parent Eligibility. What are the eligibility requirements for foster parents? Do they vary according to each child-placing system within the community? What rates are paid to foster parents? Do they vary by agency? Are they sufficient? What training and support do foster parents receive?

Foster Parent Training. How many specialized foster parents are available? How are they recruited? What training do they receive? Whom do they serve? Adolescents? Handicapped children? What types of foster homes are needed?

Residential Facilities. What are the different residential facilities in which children are placed? Which officials regularly visit the children? Who in the community visits the children? Do rates and reporting procedures vary depending upon which public agency is responsible? What are they?

Right to Information. What information is routinely provided to parents about their children's placements and progress? About grievance procedures? Are foster parents told about the educational rights of foster children if their parents are unavailable? Do foster parents know about the EPSDT and WIC Programs?[12] Is such information provided to institutionalized children and their parents? If not, why not?

Reunification Services. What services are available in your community to help reunite children with their families? How are they funded? How many children were reunited with their families last year?

Deinstitutionalization Services. What services are provided to children who are returned from institutions to their own families or transferred to less restrictive settings? Who provides them? What is the role of the community mental health center? The schools?

Case Reviews. How frequently are case reviews for children out of their homes conducted? Who conducts the reviews? Are they required by statute? Are they independent of the agency providing or funding the services? How thorough are they? Who is notified? Do parents, foster parents and children (when appropriate) participate? Are statistics on the outcomes of reviews made public? Have there been any studies to see if decisions resulting from these reviews are carried out?

Termination Proceedings. What training or guidelines are caseworkers given about when to institute termination proceedings? How many children have had parental rights terminated during the past year? What has happened to these children? How many of these children have been adopted? How many by foster parents with whom they were living? For how many were subsidies provided? Who has a right to be represented by counsel in termination proceedings?

Adoptions. How do foster care and adoption staff coordinate efforts? How are potentially adoptable children identified? How are adoptions handled? Are adoption subsidies available? Who is eligible for them? How many foster children were adopted during the past year? By foster parents? How many with subsidies? How many of these were children with special needs? Is there an adoption exchange in your state? Do the agencies in your community use it?

Children With Special Needs. What happens to status offenders? To mentally ill or retarded children needing out-of-home care? To other handicapped children needing foster care? Where are they placed? What special services are available to them?

Training. What training is available to caseworkers? To supervisors? What substantive areas are covered? Are local universities involved? What is the role of the state? How much public money is spent for training?

Data. What aggregate data are available about children out of their homes who are the responsibility of the child welfare system: age, race, length of time in care, number of moves, etc.? Is the information available locally? At the state level? What information is available from other systems: i.e., the juvenile justice, mental health, mental retardation and special education systems? How much of it is comparable across systems?

To determine the scope of out-of-state placements:

Numbers, Rates and Selection. How many children are placed out of state? In which facilities are they placed? In how many states? Which public systems place children out of state? Why? What rates are paid to the out-of-state facilities? Which children are sent out of state?

Determining Appropriateness. What, if any, state or locally mandated procedures exist for ensuring an out-of-state placement is necessary and appropriate for a particular child?

Visits. What, if any, state or locally mandated procedures exist for ensuring that children out of state are visited periodically by parents and caseworkers?

Case Reviews. What procedures exist to ensure that individual cases are periodically reviewed to determine whether continued out-of-state placement is necessary? Is the periodic review procedure different from that required for children placed in state? When was the last time the cases of the children now out of state were reviewed?

Evaluations of Out-of-State Facilities. Is a site visit to the out-of-state facility required prior to its use? By whom? How frequently is the program reviewed? By whom? Who has access to the information?

---

[12]The Early and Periodic Screening, Diagnosis and Treatment Program under Medicaid, and the Special Supplemental Food Program for Women, Infants and Children. See Chapter 5 for a fuller description of these programs.

In-State Facilities. What in-state resources are available for children now sent out of state? What must be done to create more adequate resources?

To assess the adequacy of the state statutory and administrative framework to protect children and families:

State Statutes. How adequate are existing statutory protections? Are preventive services mandated? Do children and parents have a right to representation by counsel in court proceedings? By separate counsel in termination proceedings? Must children be placed in the least restrictive setting consistent with their special needs? Close to the community? Is an independent periodic review of a child's progress and status required by statute? How could such a review be strengthened? How do administrative guidelines or regulations address periodic reviews, appropriateness of placement, or preventive or reunification services?

Comparing State Statutes with CDF Recommendations. How do state statutes, regulations and policies compare with the CDF recommendations outlined in Chapter 4? (It would be particularly appropriate for a team including legal aid lawyers, caseworkers, citizen advocates and legislative aides to undertake such an analysis)[13]

Funding Resources. Are there sufficient resources so that the statutory requirements, when adequate, are carried out? What more is needed? Money? Training? Staff?

Licensing. Do licensing regulations address the quality of programs in facilities? What facilities are exempt from licensing? How can the licensing and program review functions be strengthened? More staff? Better training? Public reports?

---

[13]The New York State Temporary Commission on Child Welfare chaired by Senator Pisani prepared a detailed analysis comparing New York State statutes and policies with CDF recommendations, and outlining steps the Commission could take in areas of state statutory weaknesses. The Commission conducted the analysis based on a summary of our study findings and recommendations prepared for limited distribution prior to the publication of this report.

To assess the capacity of different child care systems to monitor what is happening to children individually and collectively, and to ensure children equal treatment across systems:

Exchangeable Children. What groups of children are shuttled from one system to another? To what extent are children from different systems placed in the same facilities?

Purchase-of-Service Contracts. What is the extent, across systems, of reliance on purchase-of-service contracts? Are these between public agencies or between public and private agencies? How specific are the agency requirements detailed in the contracts? How are the contracts monitored?

Cross-System Coordination. What coordinating mechanisms exist at the state level and locally across child welfare, juvenile justice, child mental health and special education systems? Are these adequate? How should they be improved?

Ombudsman, Grievance Procedures. What ombudsman programs exist within public agencies? Are parents told of any grievance procedures? Are children? If not, why not? Do other case advocacy mechanisms exist? How do parents and children learn about them? How effective are they?

To monitor implementation of federal programs at local and state levels:

Title XX. How are the needs of the children and families at risk of separation and in placement covered under the Title XX services plan? How is the Title XX plan coordinated with other state plans for children (e.g., Title IV-B, Juvenile Justice)? Can the state differentiate federal moneys spent for children from those spent for adults?

Are Title XX funds used for day care and/or homemaker services for families with handicapped children; for parents experiencing such severe mental or emotional stress that the child is at risk of placement? If so, what proportion of day care funds are used for these purposes? Is this adequate?

What adoption services are provided with Title XX funds? What proportion is this of the child welfare services funded under Title XX?

How are Title XX funds used to prevent institutionalization and develop community-based

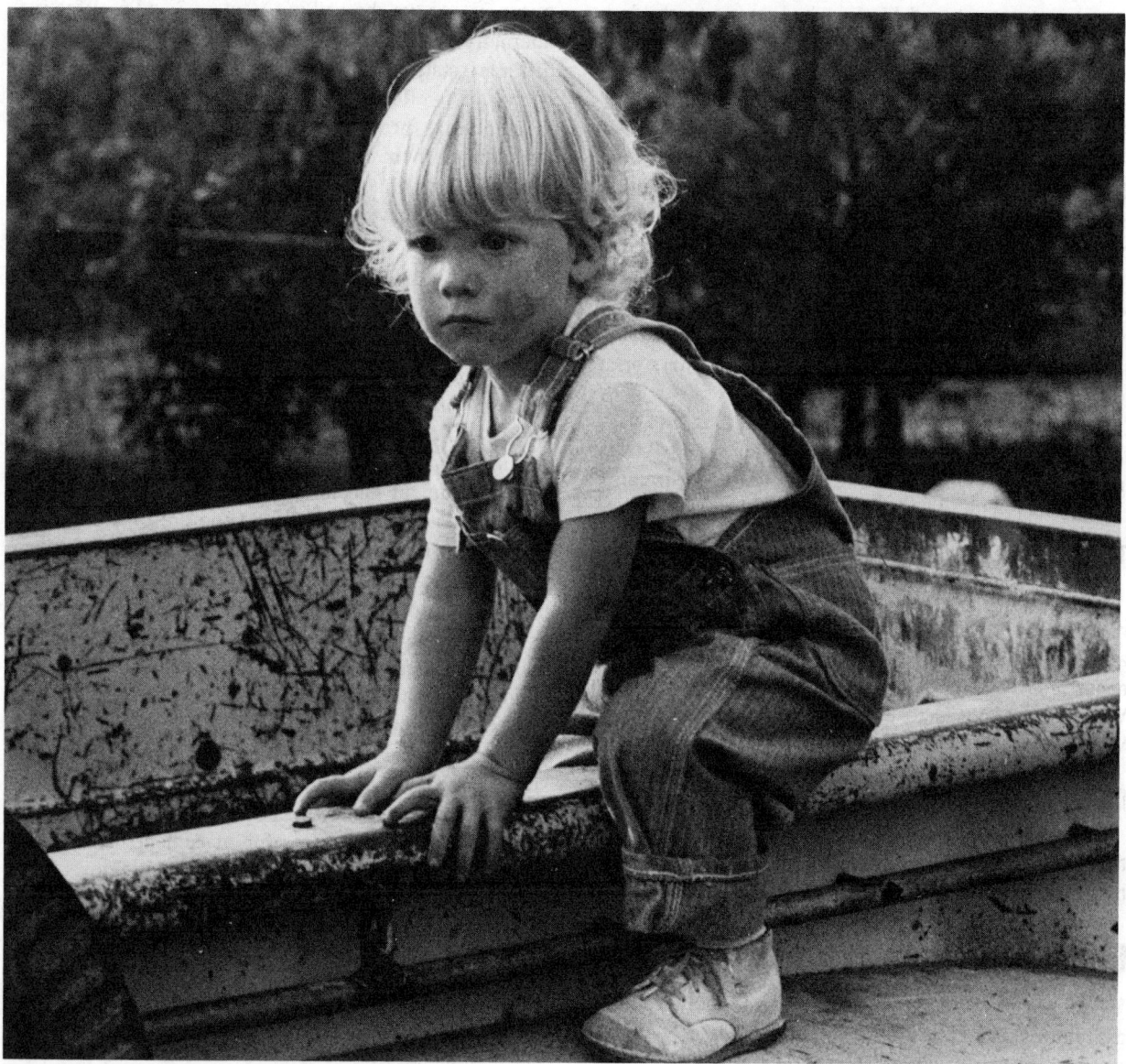

facilities for children? Which children are included? Children in institutions for dependent or neglected children? Children in nursing homes? Children in institutions for the physically or mentally handicapped?

Title IV-B. What proportion of state Title IV-B funds is used for out-of-home care as opposed to preventive services? How can these moneys be reallocated?

SSI. What services are provided for handicapped children receiving federal benefits under the SSI program? How do parents learn about these services? Do child welfare workers know about the SSI program?

Juvenile Justice. To what extent has your state complied with the deinstitutionalization requirement in the Juvenile Justice and Delinquency Prevention Act? Are status offenders held in detention facilities? Dependent or neglected children? Are children held in local jails and correctional facilities? To what extent do they have contact with the adult prisoner populations?

Medicaid. Are children remaining in hospitals, where their care is reimbursable under Medicaid, even though they no longer require hospital care? To what extent are children being cared for in nursing homes?

Does your state extend Medicaid coverage to children in foster care? In subsidized adoptions? Have foster parents and child care workers been notified of the eligibility of children in their care for the EPSDT Program?

Community Mental Health Centers. To what extent do community mental health centers in your community provide services to children? What has their role been in providing aftercare to children released from mental hospitals and other psychiatric inpatient facilities? What mechanisms exist for utilization of these centers by children in the juvenile justice system? Are children screened by the community mental health centers prior to their admission to institutions?

Training Funds. What, if any, federal funds are used for training child welfare staff and foster parents? How are they used? What federal funds are used for training others involved with children out of their homes?

To be effective advocates:

Existing Groups. What community groups are already working on these problems or could be encouraged to do so? Are new coalitions or organizations necessary? Which decision makers are sympathetic? Which are opposed to change? Which professionals? Why?

Priorities. What change is most crucial? What problem should be tackled first?

Strategies. What strategies are required? Investigation? Coalition building? Negotiation? Publicity? Lobbying? Litigation? All?

Responding to Excuses

Attempts to change well-entrenched policies and procedures affecting children without homes will inevitably be met with resistance. Confusing federal, state and local laws, official apathy, public ignorance about the facts, and parental inexperience in challenging public bureaucracies will all contribute to reluctance to press hard for answers.

But answers and solutions are possible. Advocates must be prepared to counter some of the most frequent excuses for inaction.

"There is no money for preventive services."

While it is true that federal dollars, as presently allocated, provide little targeted money for these services, federal and state funds can be used for these purposes, As we showed in Chapters 5 and 6, effective alternatives to removal have been implemented in different states using a variety of funding sources. Moreover, while the initial costs of refocusing services to emphasize prevention may be high, there is little question of their cost effectiveness over time. Don't give up. Insist that any funds saved by decreasing the need for expensive out-of-home care (using perhaps a base line year, or a similar measure) be "recycled" back into children's and family services. Monitor to ensure that such funds do not become absorbed in general revenues.

"We do not need any mandated protections for children and families. They will create too much bureaucratic red tape. Besides, good professional practice already embodies these principles."

The argument that the principles embodied in these protections are already part of good professional practice is true. But it is also true that the kinds of barriers we have described can defeat the intentions of even the best professionals, as well as those who are less conscientious. The child care systems must respond to many pressures. A system of checks to ensure that children's needs for adequate care and permanence are met is not too much to ask.

If there were no need for such protections, the situation today would be very different from what we describe in this report. Implementing mandated protections such as requirements for placement in the least restrictive setting close to home, periodic reviews, and dispositional hearings will not require an increase in red tape. It will require substituting meaningful case documentation and reviews for meaningless paperwork and procedures. Some in-service training may be required at the start, but this will enable workers to make more effective decisions about children and families, and help to eliminate inappropriate placements. This, in turn, is likely to reduce the cost of maintaining children in out-of-home care, and should free some money for the provision of needed services.

"We have a computerized data system; we do not need statutory independent periodic reviews."

As we have pointed out elsewhere in this report, data systems may provide (depending on the accuracy of the data fed into them) an effective means of knowing what is happening to groups of children. They may also be an efficient way of summarizing important information about what has happened already to individual children. But they can only record what has happened in the past, and if there is a good tracking system indicate when it is time for another decision. For this reason, it is crucial to combine computerized tracking systems with periodic reviews of the status and progress of each child, independent of those providing or purchasing the services.

"Reviews of children in out-of-home care by citizen review boards would violate family privacy."

Any independent review mechanism, as is true of any administrative review procedure by the agency providing or purchasing services, must safeguard a family and child's right to privacy. Standards of confidentiality for those who have access to case records must be rigorous, with clear sanctions for violations. But if such protections are explicitly stated in statutes or regulations and if appropriate training is provided for review board members, citizens reviewing the progress of children in out-of-home care (functioning either as an arm of the court, or independently of it) can play a valuable role in reducing the harm to children from needlessly lingering in care.

"We can bring home all the out-of-state children within six months."

While this may sound like an easy victory for advocates, it may not be. The real question is what will happen to the children when they are returned home. For those still needing placement, are there appropriate in-state facilities? What must be done to create such facilities, to negotiate new contracts, to set up group homes, etc.? Insist on a timetable, reviews of children and facilities, and hard evidence showing that the mere return of children to the state will not simply represent a new version of abandonment. Meanwhile, a system must be established to ensure that inappropriate out-of-state placements are not made in the future.

"No one really wants to adopt kids like these."

All the evidence indicates that when special efforts to ensure the adoption of so-called "unadoptable" or "hard to place" children are made, they work. Find out about these efforts, and encourage public officials to learn with you. Find out what efforts have been made in your community and what specific barriers exist. While some public systems are making serious efforts, far too many are not and must be pressured to do more.

Action at the National Level

The federal role, as we showed in Chapter 5, is extremely significant for what happens to children at risk of or in out-of-home care and their families. While much advocacy needs to be carried out at the local level, advocates have a special obligation to keep informed about what happens at the federal level. Meet with your Congressional representatives. Find out what they know about the issues and where they stand. Share information with them and their staff so they can be more knowledgeable when they vote on legislation affecting these children and their families, and so they understand that their position does make a difference to their constituents.

Do the same with your Senators. Become familiar with Congressional committees that have jurisdiction over relevant legislation.[14] Find out what, if any, relevant national legislation is pending, and make your views known to committee members and your representatives. Let them know how different outcomes will affect children in your community. And don't forget that there are national organizations following federal efforts which can be a resource to local advocates.

. . . .

The forces sustaining destructive patterns affecting children without homes are complex. Resources are and will continue to be limited, and advocates will have to make hard choices about priorities. No advocacy efforts will be without mistakes. But no group of children and families is more in need of the attention and commitment of advocates than the children and families this report is about. They need your help now.

---

[14]See Appendix P. for a list of some of the key committees with jurisdiction in areas affecting children without homes.

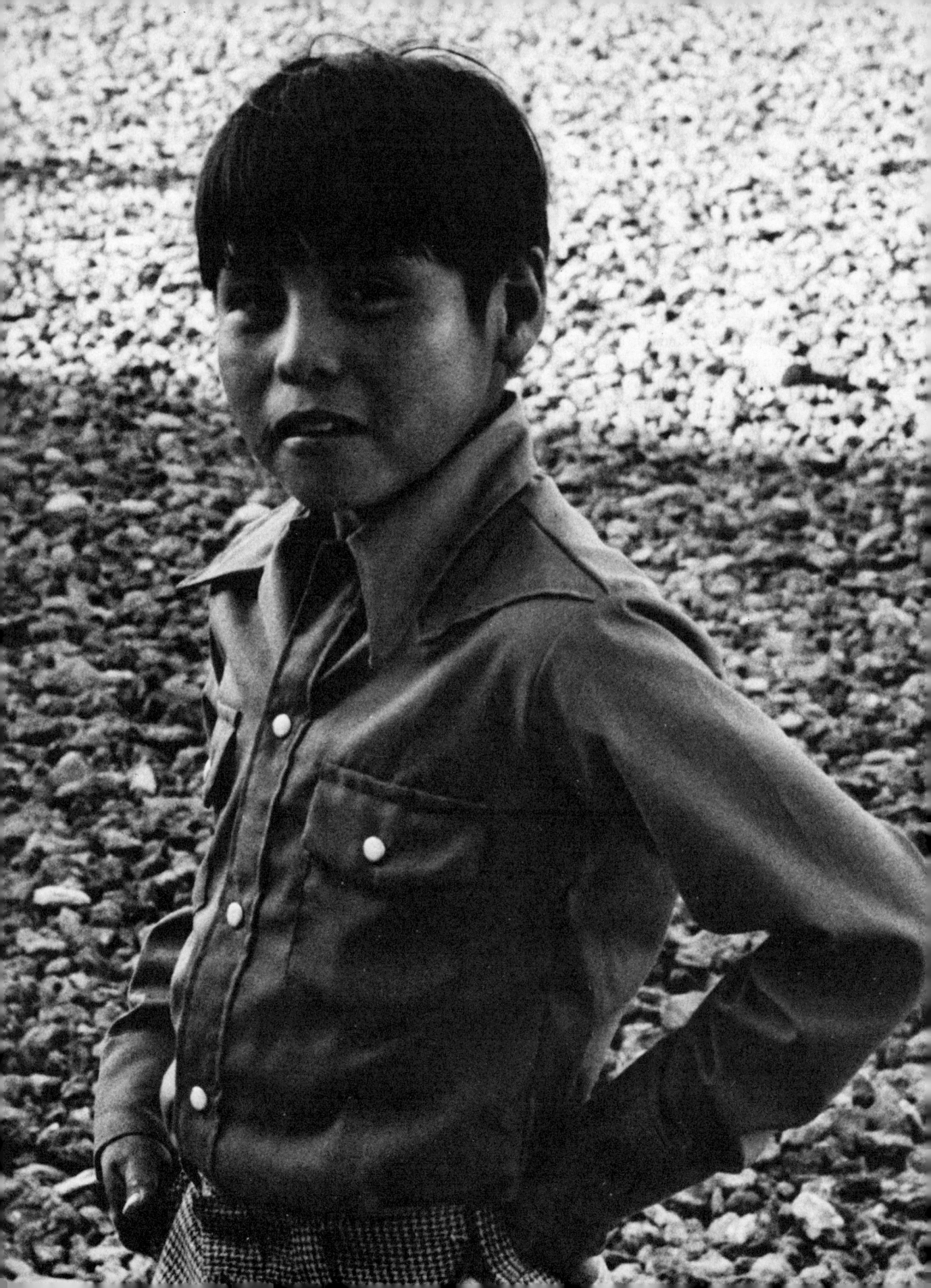

Appendices

Appendix A.
THE STUDY METHODOLOGY

I. The County Survey
II. The Seven State Study
III. The Out-Of-State Study

I. The County Survey of Child Welfare and Probation Agencies

Selection of Counties. In order to have a representative, random sample of counties, we: (a) developed separate lists of counties or independent cities with populations over and under 300,000[1]; (b) computed the population of children under 18 in each; (c) determined the total child population in both types of counties; (d) generated a table of random numbers; and (e) based on the table, selected 113 counties of under 300,000, and 27 counties of over 300,000.

The Survey Questionnaires. Questionnaires for local child welfare and probation officials were developed by the CDF staff. These were pilot tested in 15 probation offices and 13 county welfare offices. On the basis of written and oral comments, the final instrument was developed. The questionnaires were mailed on November 10, 1975. Follow-up letters were sent to offices not responding in January 1976, with a February 15, 1976, deadline for response.[2]

Coding and Analysis. Code books were developed; data were coded[3] and keypunched; and the computer programs were run between April and December 1976, using the Statistical Package for Social Sciences.

II. The Seven State Study

Selecting the States. In order to select the seven study states, we developed a set of comparative social indicators for 16 states geographically distributed across the country. The indices included the following: total population; percentage of black, native American, Spanish-speaking, and under 18 populations; total population under 18; personal per capita income rank; percentage of rural population; percentage of children at or below the poverty level; number of AFDC and AFDC Foster Care recipients; AFDC and AFDC Foster Care payments; rate of children per 100,000 receiving social services; expenditures for child welfare in 1972; number of children in foster homes and institutions,[4]; percentage of blacks in institutions; membership in Interstate Compact On Child Placement.

Based on these comparative data and our budget, Arizona, California, Massachusetts, New Jersey, Ohio, South Carolina, and South Dakota were selected as the most representative on a cross-section of the indicators.

New Jersey: The Pilot State. Once the seven states were selected, we developed timetables for visits. Because of the proximity of New Jersey to the CDF staff[5] conducting the project, we decided to use New Jersey to test some of our questions and approaches, but did not try to study the state in as concentrated a time period, or as systematically as we did the six other states. The result was that we talked with more people in New Jersey, but studied the New Jersey counties less systematically.

The Six Other States. Except in New Jersey, we contacted by letter the heads of all the appropriate state agencies, informing them of the purpose of our study. We then selected the counties to visit, seeking a mix in each state of rural and urban, of varying percentages of minority populations and of varying income levels. In making the selections, we also considered travel time, and the accessibility of the local staff. We did not try to identify the most representative counties within each state.

The Site Visits. In total, we visited 22 counties in the seven states[6], as well as the state capitals. The equivalent of at least two full weeks were spent in each state except New Jersey. In each, we spoke with a range of officials, service providers and advocates, although in a few counties, our coverage was less comprehensive.[7] Prior to our visits, we prepared lists of people to contact, and added new ones as we learned of them during the site visits. In total, we talked with over

---

[1] The source for the county lists was U.S. Bureau of the Census, *County and City Data Book,* 1972 (Washington, D.C.: Government Printing Office, 1973).

[2] All the questionnaire forms and letters used are on file at CDF.

[3] Ten questionnaires, five child welfare and five juvenile court questionnaires, were recoded to check the reliability. The error rate for the child welfare questionnaires was .01, and .009 for the juvenile court questionnaires. The reliability quotient reflects the number of errors divided by the number of coding decisions on each question multiplied by the number of questionnaires coded.

[4] These figures were based on voluntarily reported federal data and were not very reliable.

[5] CDF had a Juvenile Justice office in New York City at that time. Since then that office has been closed and the staff centralized in Washington.

[6] *Arizona:* Cochise, Graham, Maricopa; *California:* Merced, Los Angeles, San Francisco, San Mateo, Santa Clara; *Massachusetts:* Barnstable, Middlesex, Worcester; *New Jersey:* Monmouth, Union; *Ohio:* Athens, Cayahoga, Delaware; *South Carolina:* Lee, Richland, Sumter; *South Dakota:* Hughes, Minnehaha, Pennington; *Indian Reservations:* Yakima, Washington; Cheyenne River, South Dakota

[7] This was particularly true in Arizona, where we were not given access to the field offices, and as noted above in New Jersey.

250 people.[8] In our interviews with state and local officials, we tried to get answers to a basic set of questions about the types of services provided, administrative organization, placement, review and discharge processes, relationships with private and other public agencies and other levels of government, funding problems, service gaps, staff levels, and indications of the groups of children considered most difficult to serve.

We also requested specific statewide statistical information, but with some exceptions, such information was not provided. Sometimes the data were given to us in different forms. Sometimes there were no data available.

III. The Out-Of-State Study

In order to gather systematic data concerning what state officials knew about the out-of-state placement of children, we conducted three separate surveys: one by telephone, two by mail. Our surveys focused only on children placed in out-of-state group residential facilities. It excluded children placed out of state in foster or pre-adoptive homes.[9]

The Telephone Survey. Using the 1975 APWA *Child Welfare Directory,* we contacted, by telephone, officials[10] identified as having responsibility for interstate placements. The officials were asked about:
— the number of children placed out of state, and the states to which the children were sent;
— the number of children entering the state from other states, and the states from which the children came;
— the name of the agency, if other than the one called, responsible for the out-of-state placement of emotionally disturbed, retarded or delinquent children;
— the licensing procedures for in-state and out-of-state facilities; and
— the review procedures for individual children in state and out of state.

Responses to these questions were recorded on a special form, along with notes about other comments the officials made on the out-of-state phenomenon. In addition, we requested lists of both in-state and out-of-state facilities used by the state.

The Mail Surveys. Administrators in juvenile justice agencies and mental health/mental retardation agencies with responsibility for interstate placements were contacted by letter. We requested information about:
— the number of children placed out of state, and the states in which they were placed;
— the number of children entering the state from other states and the states from which they came; and
— the in-state and out-of-state facilities approved for out-of-state use by the agency.

The data from the three surveys were gathered between March and July 1976 and were analyzed manually.

---

[8]In addition, we reviewed as much written material as was available concerning the various states, as well as state statutes and regulations.
[9]For the results of the surveys, along with summaries of the data collection procedures, see Appendices H and I.
[10]We are grateful to the many administrators who responded to our inquiries, often thoughtfully and at great length. We are particularly grateful to those few officials who conducted special studies to answer our questions.

Appendix B.
STATUS OF AUDITS OF THE AFDC FOSTER CARE PROGRAM BY THE HEW AUDIT AGENCY AS OF JUNE 1, 1978

State	Planned Not Yet Underway	Underway	Completed	Audit Control Number[1]	Date Issued
Alabama			•	04-80257	3/8/78
California			•[2]	09-70272	5/31/77
San Bernadino Co.			•	09-70282	9/23/77
Santa Barbara Co.			•[3]	09-80259	3/30/78
San Diego Co.			•	09-70264	11/29/76
San Francisco Co.			•	09-60255	8/31/76
" " "			•	09-60259	9/22/76
Los Angeles Co.			•	09-70277	3/31/77
" " "		•			
Colorado		•			
Connecticut			•	01-70258	11/23/77
District of Columbia		•			
Illinois			•	05-60253	7/26/76
			•	05-60253 (follow up)	3/30/78
Iowa			•	07-60252	9/8/76
Kansas			•	07-60251	6/16/76
Maryland			•	03-70256	2/11/77
Massachusetts			•	01-70256	1/27/77
Michigan			•	05-80252	1/20/78
Mississippi	•				
Missouri			•	07-70257	6/27/77
Nebraska			•	07-70251	9/22/77
New Jersey	•				
New York		•[4]			
North Carolina			•	04-70255	12/17/76
North Dakota			•	08-60250	9/22/76
Ohio			•	05-80257	2/3/78
Oregon			•[5]		
Pennsylvania			•	03-60254	5/17/76
Rhode Island			•	01-80255	12/8/77
South Carolina			•	04-70256	12/17/76
Texas		•			
Utah		•			
Virginia			•	03-60253	6/10/76
Wisconsin			•	05-80260	3/6/78

Source: Interview with D. E. Ryder, Office of Inspector General, HEW Audit Agency, Washington, D.C.; June 21, 1978.
[1] Copies of audit reports may be purchased from the Office of the Associate Director, Division of Audit Coordination, Office of Inspector General; HEW Audit Agency, Washington, D.C.
[2] Audit of foster care rates in 16 northern California counties.
[3] A second audit has been completed but a final report had not been released as of June 1, 1978.
[4] The Audit Agency is planning to issue at least three reports in New York State.
[5] Audit completed but final report not released as of June 1, 1978.

Appendix C.
FINDINGS FROM THE CDF SURVEY OF COUNTY CHILD WELFARE AND PROBATION OFFICES

This Appendix summarizes the data from the county survey of child welfare and probation agencies. The findings are based on the questionnaires returned by the 140 counties sampled. For the child welfare questionnaire: of 140 counties sampled, 88 returned the child welfare questionnaires; 33 counties did not respond; and 19 counties either told us they could not participate or said they returned questionnaires which we did not receive. For the juvenile court questionnaire: 58 questionnaires were returned; 62 were not returned; and 20 were not usable. For both sets of returned questionnaires, the response rate varied by question. The summary tables throughout this Appendix are based on the number of counties responding to each question.

TABLE 1
Response Rate

	Small Counties		Large Counties		Total	
	No.	Percent	No.	Percent	No.	Percent
Child Welfare						
Questionnaires Returned	72	64	16	59	88	63
No Response or Not Usable	41	36	11	41	52	37
Total	113	100	27	100	140	100
Juvenile Justice						
Questionnaires Returned	43	38	15	55	58	41
No Response or Not Usable	70	62	12	45	82	59
Total	113	100	27	100	140	100

We analyzed the responding and non-responding counties to see if there were any systematic differences as a function of total population, minority population, child population or density. The x^2 were non-significant for both questionnaires.

The Children Unaccounted For

The most consistent and shocking finding was the inability of public agencies to provide the most basic information on children in out-of-home care for whom they have responsibility. Thirteen of the county child welfare offices providing total numbers of children in placement could not provide *any* descriptive information (e.g. age, race or sex) about the children in placement. Forty-five child welfare offices could provide descriptive information for only half of the breakdowns which we requested. For instance, they provided information on the race of children in care, but not the age or sex. Only one county reported descriptive information on almost all of the breakdowns. The other counties reported lower percentages.[1] Table 2 summarizes, for each variable, the percentage of the 59,638 children reported to be out of their homes for whom the county child welfare offices could not provide descriptive data.

---

[1] These percentages are based on "discrepancy scores" calculated for each county. To generate these scores, using the total number of children reported, we calculated the percentage of that total described in terms of age, race, etc.

TABLE 2
Children Reported To Be In Placement Under Child Welfare Auspices For Whom No Descriptive Information Was Available

Descriptor	No. Unaccounted For	Percent Unaccounted For
Sex	34,721	58
Race	32,324	54
Age	29,492	49
Type of Placement	16,259	27
Placement Location[2]	38,369	64
Length of Time in Care	31,825	53
Number of Moves	52,213	87
Type of Custody[3]	43,578	73

The Juvenile Justice questionnaires were equally discouraging. Seven counties reporting information on numbers of children in placement could provide no descriptive information about any child in their care. The county providing the most information completed 80 percent of the requested breakdowns. Table 3 summarizes, for each variable, the percentage of the 24,809 children reported by probation offices to be out of their homes, but not accounted for by any descriptive information.

TABLE 3
Children In Placement Under Juvenile Court Auspices For Whom No Descriptive Information Was Available

Descriptor	No. Unaccounted For	Percent Unaccounted For
Sex	11,852	48
Race	14,552	59
Age	16,304	66
Placement	10,541	42
Geographic Location	16,011	65

The Child Welfare Survey
Characteristics of the Placed Children

Our analyses of the data returned to us, summarized in Table 4, reveal patterns that are consistent with other studies. Counties reported slightly more males than females in out-of-home care. Minorities were greatly over-represented, comprising 52 percent of the out-of-home population. Fifty-one percent of the children in out-of-home care in our sample were 12 or older, 31 percent were 15 or older.

TABLE 4
Characteristics of Children in Out-of-Home Placement Under Child Welfare Auspices

Sex	Number	Percent	Counties Reporting
Male	13,510	54	58
Female	11,452	46	58
Race			
White	13,150	48	63
Black	8,827	32	63
Spanish-speaking	3,669	13	63
Indian	193	1	63
Other	1,520	6	62
Age			
Under 2	2,247	7	61
3–5	3,137	10	61
6–8	4,330	14	61
9–11	5,081	17	61
12–14	6,046	20	61
15–17	3,964	13	61
18 +	5,386	18	61

---

[2]The placement descriptions used were in-county, in-state, out-of-state.
[3]Permanent or temporary custody.

Where Are The Children?

Sixty-three percent of the children were in foster homes; three percent were with relatives; four percent in adoptive homes; three percent in group homes; 15 percent in institutions; and the remainder in detention, shelter, or "other" types of facilities. (See Table 5.) Not surprisingly, counties provided the most complete data on this question, for it is a question tied to fiscal accountability. Counties know *where* to send payments, although they may not know *for whom* they are sending them.

In response to our question about where the placements were located: 91 percent were in-county, 8 percent out-of-county but in-state; and 1 percent out-of-state. (Table 11 summarizes both juvenile justice and child welfare out-of-state placements reported in the survey.)

What Happens To The Children?

As a group, the children spend long periods of time in foster care: over 52 percent were in care for more than two years; over 33 percent from four to six years. Yet, of the children for whom custody information was available, 77 percent were in temporary custody of the child welfare agency or court, 23 percent in permanent custody.

The children moved frequently. Only 43 percent had no moves; 38 percent moved once or twice; and 18 percent moved more then twice. Of the 17,849 children known to be discharged, 63 percent returned home; 7 percent were adopted or in adoptive homes; 11 percent left foster care upon reaching the age of majority. We do not know the status of the remaining 19 percent of the children discharged.(See Table 6.)

TABLE 5
Type and Location of Child Welfare Placements

Type of Placement	Number	Percent	Reporting Counties
Relative's Home	3,857	9	71
Adoptive Home	1,576	4	80
Foster Home	27,391	63	79
Group Home	1,384	3	78
Institution	3,833	9	79
Residential Treatment Center	1,681	4	77
Psychiatric Facility	532	1	75
Institution for Retarded	439	1	78
Detention	407	1	76
Shelter	655	1	80
Other	1,669	4	79
Location of Placement			
In-county	19,392	91	71
In-state	1,649	8	71
Out-of-state	273	1	74

TABLE 6
Length of Time, Number of Moves, Custody and Discharge Status, Child Welfare System

Time in Placement	Number	Percent	Reporting Counties
Under 3 months	2,530	9	62
3 months - 1 year	5,310	19	62
1–2 years	5,659	20	62
2–4 years	5,177	19	62
4–6 years	3,564	13	62
6 years +	5,618	20	62
Number of Moves			
None	3,217	43	49
One	1,754	23	55
Two	1,149	15	55
Three	641	9	54
Four	388	5	54
Five or more	321	4	51
Custody			
Temporary	12,326	77	61
Permanent	3,779	23	61
Discharge Status			
Returned Home	11,333	63	72
Adopted	1,237	7	72
Reached Majority	1,898	11	70
Other	3,481	19	69

TABLE 7
Summary of Reported Child Welfare Policies Regarding Caseworker Contact

Child In:	Foster Home		Group Home		Institution		Out of State Placement	
Policy on Worker/Parent Contact	No. of Counties	Percent	No. of Counties	Percent	No. of Counties	Percent	No. of Counties	Percent
No Written Policies	50	36	55	39	58	41	66	47
Yes—Periodic Visits Required	36	25	29	21	26	19	14	10
No Answer	54	39	56	40	56	40	60	43
Policy on Worker/Child Contact								
No Written Policy	24	17	39	28	45	32	59	42
Yes—Periodic Contact Required	64	46	42	30	35	25	17	12
No Answer	52	37	59	42	60	43	64	46

Policy Questions

In addition to the statistical data, we requested information on written policies regarding required parent-caseworker contact, caseworker-child contact, parental visiting and transportation. These data are summarized in Table 7. The pattern is striking: the less homelike the placement setting, the fewer the requirements for contacts between children and caseworkers and between parents and caseworkers. Sixteen percent of the counties reporting had no written policies on either parent-caseworker or child-caseworker contacts. With regard to visiting, 44 of the reporting counties reported a written policy and 44 reported no policy. Sixty-two counties reported written policies on transportation; 24 of the counties reporting stated they had no written policy.

The Juvenile Justice Survey

The Filter Process

The juvenile courts and probation offices deal in many different ways with children brought before them. Some counties have diversion programs or pre-petition programs so that only a small percentage of children are officially referred to the courts. Sometimes diversion efforts occur after a child is referred, so there is no adjudication. Thus, a relatively small group of children, when contrasted with the total number of children involved with the probation departments, are actually adjudicated delinquents or status offenders. Of these an even smaller number are placed out of their homes. We requested information on numbers referred, adjudicated and placed. We also requested information on children before the court for whom dependency, neglect or abuse petitions had been filed. Table 8 summarizes our findings.

TABLE 8
Children Having Contact With Probation Offices and Juvenile Courts

	Number Referred	Number Adjudicated	Number Placed
Delinquents	120,051	35,955	6,381
Status Offenders	37,288	7,791	2,117
Delinquents and Status Offenders[4]	1,994	975	2,256
Dependent and Neglected	12,562	6,374	1,625
Total Identified	172,895	51,095	12,379
Total Reported[5]	181,354	68,669	24,809

[4] Some counties did not report separate totals for delinquents and status offenders.
[5] The discrepancy between total identified and total reported reflects inconsistencies reported by counties; that is some counties reported larger totals than children accounted for in each category.

Five percent of the referred delinquents and 18 percent of the adjudicated delinquents were ultimately placed out of their homes. Six percent of the referred status offenders and 27 percent of the adjudicated status offenders were eventually placed. Thirteen percent of the children referred through dependency or neglect petitions and 25 percent of those adjudicated were placed.

Characteristics of Placed Children

Characteristics of children placed by the juvenile courts are described in Table 9. Almost 75 percent of the children placed were males. Sixty-four percent of those placed were white, 36 percent from minority groups. Seventeen percent of the children were 12 or under, 83 percent over 12. (See Table 9).

TABLE 9
Characteristics of Children in Out-of-Home Placements Under Juvenile Court Auspices

Sex	Number	Percent	Counties Reporting
Male	9,354	72	35
Female	3,603	28	34
Race			
White	6,546	64	26
Black	3,002	29	25
Spanish-speaking	608	6	21
Indian	36	-	21
Other	65	-	23
Age			
Under 5	369	4	25
5–9	345	4	25
10	147	2	24
11	184	2	25
12	387	5	24
13	830	10	25
14	1,329	16	24
15	1,792	21	25
16	1,723	20	24
17	1,286	15	24
18 +	113	1	24

Where Are The Children?

We found, based on our pilot questionnaires, that probation offices did not know the specific types of facilities (e.g., foster homes, group home, institution) in which the children referred by the court to other agencies were placed. Consequently, we inquired instead about the agencies or facilties to which the children were refered. State correctional facilities, including training schools and city and county correctional agencies, accounted for 56 percent of the children. Another 21 percent were placed in private agencies, and 19 percent were referred to departments of public welfare. One percent of the children were in facilities for the mentally ill or retarded. The remaining 3 percent were the responsibility of other state or local agencies. Seventy-three percent of the children were placed in their own county. (See Table 10.)

TABLE 10
Type and Location of Juvenile Justice Placements and Referrals

Type of Placement or Referral	Number	Percent
State Training School	2,342	16
Other State Correctional Facility	1,229	9
City or County Correctional Facility	4,379	31
Other Local Public Facility	243	2
Referred to Department of Public Welfare for Placement	2,672	19
Private Facility	3,029	21
Psychiatric Facility	211	1
Institution for the Retarded	9	21
Other State Agency	154	1
Location		
In-county	6,383	73
In-state	2,336	26
Out-of-state	79	1

Out-of-State Placements

Table 11 summarizes the number of counties in each state reporting out-of-state placements and the states to which children were sent. The Table reflects data reported by both child welfare and probation offices. In six states both the child welfare and probation agencies reported placing children out of state, sometimes in the same state.

TABLE 11
Children Reported In Out-of-State Placements By Survey Counties

Sending States (No. of Counties Reporting)	Receiving States Child Welfare Office Survey	Receiving States Probation Office Survey
AL (2)		
ARK (3)		
CA (4)		2*
CO (4)	TX, AZ, KA, FL	AZ, TX, NB
CT (1)		
FL (6)	GA	
HA (1)	CA	
IL (5)	TX	
IN (10)	KY, MI	OH, MI
IA (3)		
KA (1)		
KY (5)		
LA (1)		
ME (1)	NJ	
MD (3)	FL, PA, VA, OH, IL	FL, PA, VA, WV, CT, DC
MA (2)		
MI (8)	TX	
MN (2)		
MS (3)		
MO (3)		ARK
MT (1)	AZ, CO, ND	
NB (1)		
NH (1)		
NJ (4)		OH, PA, NY
NY (7)	CT, PA, FL, NJ, MA, NH, VA, SC, KA	AZ
NC (8)	GA, PA, TN, NJ	SC
ND (1)		
OH (8)	MI, PA, IN, WI, NB, NY	
OK (2)		
OR (2)		
PA (4)	OH, MI, NY	
SC (5)	GA, DC	
TN (5)		
TX (10)	CA, MI	MO, OK
VA (3)	PA, FL, MD, DC, NJ, GA, NY, NB	
WA (1)		
WV (3)		PA, OH, VA
WI (5)		
WY (1)		

*States not specified

Policy Questions

We asked a number of questions about who was responsible for limiting the time a child was in placement. However, the data were so inconsistent we do not believe they shed any light on the planning process for children in placement under juvenile court auspices.

National Projections

We made projections based on our data of the total number of children in out-of-home placement under child welfare auspices. The following ratio was used:

$$\frac{X}{\text{total U.S. child population}} = \frac{\text{children out of home in sample counties reporting}}{\text{total child population in sample counties reporting}}$$

Where X = total U.S. children out of home under child welfare auspices.

Using similar ratios, we also calculated the number of children entering into and discharged from care during the course of a year, as well as the number of children out of their homes at the beginning of the year. Our national projections are summarized in Table 12.

These figures suggest a yearly increase of eight percent in the rate of children in care.[6]

We did not similarly project the number of children in out-of-home placement under juvenile justice auspices because so few counties returned usable data.

TABLE 12
National Projections From Child Welfare Data

National Estimate of Children in Placement at Beginning of Year[7]	415,226
National Estimate of Children Entering Care	198,391
National Estimate of Children Discharged from Care	192,172
National Estimate of Children in Care at the End of Year	448,354

---

[6] Because of different reporting years, the rate of increase may be somewhat inflated.
[7] The year refers to either 1/74 - 12/74, 7/74 - 6/75, or 1/75 - 12/75

Appendix D.
POLICY STATEMENT ON PARENTAL VISITING[1]

Carol J. Parry
Assistant Commissioner
Department of Social Services, Office of
　Special Services for Children

"Like the frequent monitoring of body temperature information for assessing the health of patients in hospitals, the visitation of children should be carefully scrutinized as the best indicator we have concerning the long term fate of children in care".

This conclusion was drawn by Dr. David Fanshel, co-director of the five year longitudinal investigation of foster care in New York City, known as the Child Welfare Research Project. A key finding of the research is that the association between parental visiting and the discharge of children from care is a critical one. The more frequent the visitation, the more likely the child would return home.

The critical importance of parental visiting with their children in foster care has long been recognized in the child development literature. These visits are important for many different reasons:

— no matter how troubled or difficult the parents may be, the child may miss them deeply. They are his roots to his past. When he is separated from them, he feels that he has lost a part of himself;
— continuing contact with natural parents has an ameliorative effect on the otherwise detrimental consequences of long-term foster care;
— continuing contact with the natural parents gives the child opportunities to see his parents realistically and rationally and dispel highly irrational feelings and images;
— visits help calm some of the child's irrational separation fears; fears such as the parents are dead, the parents placed the child because they hated him or he was unimportant to them, etc.;
— visits may be therapeutic for the parents if the worker uses them to help the parents be better parents to the placed child, to bring out their "best" when they are with the child;
— if a child is to be returned to his family, visiting is absolutely essential. A child will experience innumerable problems if he is returning to a family where he has become a stranger.

The parent-child tie has deep emotional significance to both the parent and the child. It may be distorted by physical separation, but not eliminated.

There is yet another reason why parental visiting is so important. According to New York State law, failure by a parent to visit during a specified period of time without good reason could be grounds for termination of parental rights.

Some agencies have taken concrete actions to facilitate parental visiting. These include supplying carefare to parents, running special buses to agencies on a regular basis and setting aside a few days each year for special activity days for children and their parents. We recognize the value of these activities and wish to commend those agencies that engage in them. However, despite these gains, the area of parental visiting continues to be characterized by inadequate policies and practices. Too frequently

— during the early part of placement, when children need the support and encouragement of families, they are not permitted visitation. Studies have shown that the children do not "settle better" when their parents are forbidden to see them;
— workers fail to discuss with parents why visiting is so critically important while children are in care;
— agency visiting policies severely limit the number of visits possible;
— visits last for very short periods of time;
— visits take place in very unnatural settings which preclude natural interaction between children and parents;
— placement settings where visits take place are at great distances from the inner city, necessitating the expenditure of time and money;
— regularly scheduled visiting is discouraged;
— honoring requests for visitation by parents is contingent upon the convenience of the foster parent and the agency worker with little regard for the convenience of the family;
— the agency fails to facilitate visits by preparing children and foster parents for the visits;
— agencies fail to emphasize the relevance and importance of visits to the developmental needs of children of all ages, but especially those under six years of age;
— agencies unilaterally limit or terminate visits without adequate explanation based on consistent standards.

Clearly, our beliefs about the importance of parental visiting are not consistently supported by our practice and policy. This may, in part, be explained by the emphasis we place on another objective: to maintain children in stable situations, free from the trauma and damage that change inevitably creates. This objective

---
[1] Reproduced with permission from Department of Social Services' Office of Special Services for Children, New York City.

is sometimes thought to be inconsistent with an emphasis on parental visiting because visiting often generates problems which can jeopardize stability.

Parental visiting can be problematic. Visits may be characterized by interpersonal stress. There are children who are overwhelmed by anxiety each time they see their parents. Some are upset by their parents' unpredictable or disturbed behavior. Some children may become extremely unhappy and difficult to handle after visits. There are parents who may be hostile toward and critical of their children or the foster parents. Some will be argumentative, uncooperative or unpredictable. A few may even try to sabotage the work of foster parents and the agency.

Nevertheless, both despite these problems and because of them, I must stress how very important it is for agencies to strongly encourage parental visiting. We must weigh and give full value to the important benefits that derive from parent-child visiting against the various problems, ranging from administrative to psychological, that such visiting creates. A child who has recently been placed may become particularly upset after a parental visit. The response to this must be to work with the child and his parents, not to eliminate the visits. A parent may demonstrate his reluctance to visit by cancelling appointments or arriving late. The response to this must be reach out to these parents, to explain why their visits are so critical, to offer any assistance that will facilitate the visits, not to ignore the parents. A parent's manner or behavior may be considered dangerous to the child. The response to this must be a skilled explanation about why such behavior is unacceptable and the development of a contract between the worker and parent specifying what behaviors are not acceptable if visiting is to occur, not to unilaterally terminate the parent's right to visit. A parent may request longer visits, evening visits, visits outside of the agency office or foster home, visits on weekends and holidays to the parents' home. The response to these requests must be a serious discussion between the parent and the worker, where the benefits and problems are weighed and a mutual decision agreed upon, not a dismissal out of hand because "it's never been done before" or "it's against agency policy."

Over the years, restrictive visiting policies and practices, based more on the exceptional case rather than the rule, have developed. These policies and practices, where they exist, must be changed, in order to address the real needs of parents and their children. Special Services for Children is affirming the critical importance of parental visiting. As a very first step, all agencies shall be responsible for assuring that each of its congregate facilities and foster homes maintains a register in which the name and address of each person visiting the child can be entered with the date of each visit (existing SBSW rules require this). Extremely infrequent visiting or no visiting by the parent or guardian should trigger an appropriate response. There will be too many parents who will not visit. Whatever the reason, it is critically important that our reaction to this parental "giving up" is not "giving up" ourselves, but aggressive reaching out. Only in that way can we impress upon parents how very important their visits with their children are.

The following guidelines will help in the development of better visiting policies and practices:

1. An agency-wide policy which prohibits any parent from visiting during the "early part of placement" (up to 6 months) must be changed. Visiting during this time may be prohibited by a Judge. In specific cases, an agency may determine that visits would be dangerous and therefore favors elimination of the visits until the danger no longer exists. The decision must be discussed at length with the parent and be approved by SSC. A parent may request that the decision be reviewed by the Parents' Rights Unit at SSC.

2. At the time a child is placed in a foster care setting, the agency worker must discuss with the parents the critical importance of visiting while the child is in care. The worker should discuss with the parent both the likely positive and negative consequences of a visit. (S)he must stress the urgency of visiting during the early part of placement. Moreover, the worker should state that (s)he will facilitate visits in anyway possible.

3. An agency-wide policy which limits visits to once a month or even every two weeks must be changed. The frequency of visiting will depend upon a number of factors (e.g., location of agency, number of children at home, number of children in care in other agencies, reason for placement, etc.), but ultimately must be agreed upon by the parent and worker. The parent's desires and needs must take priority over the convenience of the foster parent and the agency. Weekly visits should be encouraged whenever possible for the parent, not prohibited.

4. An agency-wide policy which limits all visits to one hour must be changed. Again, the length of the visit should depend upon several factors, such as how long the parent traveled to the place of the visit, how much it cost, the age of the child and the length of time between visits. Once again, the parent and the agency worker must reach agreement on this matter.

5. Visits must not be limited to small, perhaps poorly equipped visiting areas in agency settings. Visits in the foster home, in the parent's home (where the child is brought by the agency worker) and outdoors should be considered. The location of visits should also be a "contracted" part of the plan.
6. Parents must not be prevented from visiting their children because they are unable to pay for the necessary transportation. Reimbursement to eligible families for transportation costs is covered by the per diem rate and is to be provided directly by the agency. When the children are cared for in SSC Direct Care programs, reimbursement to eligible families for transportation costs is available through the Imprest Fund. Families are eligible for reimbursement for these costs when:
   a. visiting is a part of the service plan which has been developed by the agency and the parent; *and*
   b. the family is receiving public assistance; *or*
   c. the financial evaluation that is done in accordance with the criteria of SSC Procedure No. 1 shows a budgetary deficit, or there would be such a deficit if the family was required to assume the transportation costs without assistance.
7. Parents must not be prevented from visiting their children when traveling is problematic for reasons other than expense. A parent may want to visit the child, but cannot do so for many different reasons. For example, the parent is ill and is not permitted to leave the home, there are other children in the home who require the presence of the parent, etc. Under such circumstances, consideration should be given to the worker's bringing the child to the parent's home, so that visits are not limited or prevented for those reasons.
8. If a parent wants to set up a regular visiting schedule, and this schedule is consistent with the child's best interests, the worker should incorporate it into the plan. The convenience of the agency or the foster parent can no longer be the determining factor. Moreover, workers must not "test" parental interest and concern by requiring that appointments be made prior to each visit, if the parent expressed interest in a regular visiting schedule.
9. The agency worker must discuss the matter of parental visiting with the child and his foster parent (or other surrogate caretaker). Skillful work in this area should minimize some of the problems created by parental visits.
10. Agencies should provide training for their workers, specifically related to child developmental issues. For example, the particular importance of frequent parental visiting for children at different stages of their development should be discussed and translated into agency practice.
11. An agency-wide policy that does not allow a child to visit home on weekends and holidays must be changed. Again, this is a decision that will be influenced by several factors and must ultimately be agreed to by the parent and the agency worker.
12. An agency-wide policy that does not allow evening visits must be changed. This, too, is a decision that will be influenced by several factors and must be agreed to by the parent and agency worker.
13. Limiting or terminating parental visits must be avoided whenever possible. A decision to limit or terminate visits must be carefully explained to a parent and approved by SSC. The agency must inform the parent that the decision can be appealed in the Parents' Rights Unit at SSC or appealed to a Judge.

It is time that all our actions become focused on our articulated goals for families involved in the child welfare system. I am sure that all agency child care staff at all levels share these concerns and goals with me. SSC staff is available to assist agencies in anyway possible to help facilitate parental visiting and to help achieve the reunion of families wherever this is possible.

Appendix E.
STATUTORY PROVISIONS FOR COUNSEL IN NEGLECT AND TERMINATION PROCEEDINGS

Appendix E sets forth a description of the statutory provisions for counsel and/or guardian ad litem in the 50 states and the District of Columbia in neglect and termination of parental rights proceedings.

The statutory provisions regarding such proceedings are complex, varied and often scattered throughout the state code. For example, there is a tremendous range in the specificity of the provisions. In some instances a right to counsel was inferred from a statutory reference to the requirement that notice of that right be provided, although there was no further mention of such a right. In others the statutory language was explicit.

Our analysis is based for the most part on statutes in effect as of December 1977. (Table III provides citations.) We have noted only what the statutes specifically provide, and have not examined either case law, or, except in one or two instances, court-rules, or the adequacy of the implementation of the statutes.

The coding scheme in Tables I and II indicates the general type of provision (e.g. a general right to counsel for parent and child, mandatory or discretionary separate counsel for the child), and the specific circumstances in which the provisions apply (e.g. the court shall appoint separate counsel for the child only when there is no parent, or when there is a conflict of interest between parent and child). If there are provisions for appointed counsel in the statute, we have used asterisks to indicate whether the appointment of such counsel is mandatory or discretionary, and for whom. In those instances in which the statutes specify that a guardian ad litem must be an attorney we have coded it as a statutory requirement for counsel.

Our primary purpose in compiling these tables was to determine the extent to which children are provided with separate counsel at these court proceedings. However, as can be seen from the tables, we found few clear-cut patterns, making it difficult to draw firm conclusions about how well a child's right to representation is protected in child welfare statutes.

As can be seen from Table I which summarizes the provisions for counsel in neglect proceedings, most states do make some mention of the circumstances in which counsel or a guardian ad litem must be provided; that is, they go beyond the mere indication of a general right to counsel for parents and children. The appointment of separate counsel or a guardian ad litem for a child is most likely to be required for the child either when there is no parent, or when the child has been abused. The appointment of a guardian ad litem to represent a child in a judicial proceeding in an abuse or neglect case is a requirement for receipt of federal funds under the Child Abuse Prevention and Treatment Act (42 U.S.C. §5103). Thus, many states have recently modified their child abuse reporting statutes to be eligible for those funds. Slightly under half the states also have provisions for representation of the child by counsel or a guardian ad litem, typically at the court's discretion, when there is a conflict of interest between parent and child or to protect the child's interest.

As can be seen from Table II which summarizes provisions for counsel in termination statutes, only seven states mandate, without conditions, separate counsel for the child, another five make counsel mandatory under limited circumstances. In eight states, we found no mention of counsel. Only seven states required the appointment of a guardian ad litem for the child. It should be noted that not all states have separate termination proceedings; in a number of states requirements for termination were incorporated into the adoption statutes and in others termination was a disposition in a neglect proceeding. It was particularly difficult to determine the applicability of counsel provisions to the adoption statutes.

Appendix E. continued TABLE I. Provisions for Counsel in Neglect Statutes

	No Mention of Counsel	Right to Counsel for Parent and Child	Right to Counsel for Parent and Child and *Discretionary* Separate Counsel for Child	
			No Conditions Specified	Conditions Specified
Alabama		X*		
Alaska				(2)¹
Arizona		X*		(1)
Arkansas				
California		X⊛		
Colorado		X⁸		(2)
Connecticut		X*		
Delaware	X³			
District of Columbia		X*		
Florida		X⊛		
Georgia		X*		
Hawaii				
Idaho		X*		
Illinois		X*		(1) (2)
Indiana				
Iowa		X*		
Kansas				
Kentucky		X**⁽***⁾		
Louisiana		X⊛		(5)
Maine				

Right to Counsel for Parent and Child and *Discretionary* Guardian Ad Litem for Child		Right to Counsel for Parent and Child and *Mandatory* Separate Counsel for Child		Right to Counsel for Parent and Child and *Mandatory* Guardian Ad Litem for Child	
No Conditions Specified	Conditions Specified	No Conditions Specified	Conditions Specified	No Conditions Specified	Conditions Specified
			(1) (2) (8)		
	(2)[1]				(5)[1]
	(4)[2]				(5)[2]
			(1) (5)		(5)
					(5)
			(2) (3) (5)		
	(5)	X			
			(1) (4)		(1) (2) (4)
	(2)[2]				(4)[2]
			(2)		
			(4) (5)		
			(4)[1]		
					(2) (4)
		X[4]			
					(5)[2]

197

	No Mention of Counsel	Right to Counsel for Parent and Child	Right to Counsel for Parent and Child and *Discretionary* Separate Counsel for Child	
			No Conditions Specified	Conditions Specified
Maryland		X ✸✸		
Massachusetts		X✸		
Michigan		X ✸✸		(6)
Minnesota		X*		
Mississippi		X		
Missouri		P-G. Ad L (8)²		
Montana		X✸		
Nebraska		X*		
Nevada		X ✸✸	X	
New Hampshire				
New Jersey		X✸		
New Mexico		X*	X	
New York		X*		
North Carolina		X		
North Dakota		X*		
Ohio		X*		
Oklahoma		X*		(5)
Oregon		X*	X	
Pennsylvania		X*		
Rhode Island		X*		

Right to Counsel for Parent and Child and *Discretionary* Guardian Ad Litem for Child		Right to Counsel for Parent and Child and *Mandatory* Separate Counsel for Child		Right to Counsel for Parent and Child and *Mandatory* Guardian Ad Litem for Child	
No Conditions Specified	Conditions Specified	No Conditions Specified	Conditions Specified	No Conditions Specified	Conditions Specified
			(2)		
			(5)		
				X[5]	
					(5)
					(5)[2]
X					
			(4) (6)		(4) (8) (2)
			(5)[1]		
			(5)		
	(1) (4)				
		X			
		X[6]			
			(1) (4)		(1) (4)
			(1) (4)		(5)
			(2)		
		X[7]	(1)[7]		
					(5)

	No Mention of Counsel	Right to Counsel for Parent and Child	Right to Counsel for Parent and Child and *Discretionary* Separate Counsel for Child	
			No Conditions Specified	Conditions Specified
South Carolina		X*		
South Dakota		X ⊛8		
Tennessee				
Texas		X⊛		(2)
Utah		X*		(2)
Vermont		X*		
Virginia		X*		
Washington		X*		
West Virginia		X*		
Wisconsin		X⊛		
Wyoming		X *		(2)

[1]No mention of right to counsel for parents was located.
[2]No mention of general right to counsel for parent or child was located.
[3]Family Court Rules (Rule 360) do provide that the Court may at any stage of a proceeding appoint a guardian ad litem for the child if he has no parent appearing on his behalf, or the interests of the parent appear to conflict with those of the child.
[4]The Kansas statute provides for the mandatory appointment of counsel for parents when they are minors and for parents when termination is a disposition in a neglect proceeding.
[5]Guardian ad litem requirement can be waived if counsel has been appointed or retained to represent the child.
[6]Court shall appoint a guardian ad litem (who shall be an attorney) to represent a child alleged to be neglected unless the court shall find as a fact that the child is not in need of and cannot benefit from such representation.
[7]If present in court, parent may waive child's right to counsel unless there is a conflict between parent and child.
[8]Right to mandatory appointment of counsel for parent and child when termination is a potential disposition in a neglect proceeding.
[9]Court shall appoint guardian ad litem *or* counsel under the conditions specified.
[10]Statute allows waiver of counsel if court approves and finds interest of child and parent or other party are not adverse.
[11]Statute specifies the court may appoint guardian ad litem in any case (for any party) in which it feels such an appointment is desirable.

Right to Counsel for Parent and Child and *Discretionary* Guardian Ad Litem for Child		Right to Counsel for Parent and Child and *Mandatory* Separate Counsel for Child		Right to Counsel for Parent and Child and *Mandatory* Guardian Ad Litem for Child	
No Conditions Specified	Conditions Specified	No Conditions Specified	Conditions Specified	No Conditions Specified	Conditions Specified
			(5)		(5)
			(5)		
					(1) (2) (4) (5)[2]
X					
					(5)
			(1) (2) (4)[9]		(1) (2) (4)[9]
		X[10]			
X					(5)
		X			
X[11]					
	(1) (4)		(5)		

Legend

(1) If conflict between parent and child
(2) To protect child's interest; for child's welfare; in interest of justice; if parent indifferent to child
(3) Custody affected
(4) No parent or guardian
(5) Abuse and neglect (usually in the Child Abuse and Neglect Reporting Statute)
(6) Upon request of minor or parent
(7) If termination is a potential disposition in a neglect proceeding
(8) If parent is a minor and/or incompetent

* Mandatory appointed counsel for child/parent
⊛ Discretionary appointed counsel for child/parent
** Mandatory appointment of counsel for child
⊛⊛ Discretionary appointment of counsel for child
*** Mandatory appointment of counsel for parent
⊛⊛⊛ Discretionary appointment of counsel for parent

P-G. Ad L Guardian ad litem appointed for parent under conditions specified

Appendix E. continued TABLE II. Provisions for Counsel in Termination Statutes

	No Mention of Counsel	Right to Counsel for Parent and Child	Right to Counsel for Parent and Child and *Discretionary* Separate Counsel for Child	
			No Conditions Specified	Conditions Specified
Alabama[11]		X*		
Alaska[11]				(2)[1]
Arizona		P-G. Ad L (8)[3]		
Arkansas		X		
California		X***	X	
Colorado[11]		X*		(2)
Connecticut		P-G. Ad L (8)[2]		
Delaware		P-G. Ad L (8)[2]		
District of Columbia		X*		
Florida[11]		X		
Georgia		X*		
Hawaii		P-G. Ad L (8)[2]		
Idaho		P-G. Ad L (8); P***[9]		
Illinois		P-G. Ad L[1,4] (8)		
Indiana		X		
Iowa		X*		
Kansas[11]		X*		
Kentucky		P***[9]		
Louisiana		X*		
Maine	X			

Right to Counsel for Parent and Child and *Discretionary* Guardian Ad Litem for Child		Right to Counsel for Parent and Child and *Mandatory* Separate Counsel for Child		Right to Counsel for Parent and Child and *Mandatory* Guardian Ad Litem for Child	
No Conditions Specified	Conditions Specified	No Conditions Specified	Conditions Specified	No Conditions Specified	Conditions Specified
			(1)(2)(8)		
	(2)[1]				
		X			
	(5)				
			(1)(4)		(1)(2)(4)
	(2)[2]				
X[9]					
		X[4]			
					(1)(4)
		X			
		X			

	No Mention of Counsel	Right to Counsel for Parent and Child	Right to Counsel for Parent and Child and *Discretionary* Separate Counsel for Child	
			No Conditions Specified	Conditions Specified
Maryland	X			
Massachusetts	X			
Michigan[11]		X ☻		(6)
Minnesota		X*		
Mississippi				
Missouri		P***9. P-G. Ad L (8)		
Montana[11]		X⊛		
Nebraska		P-G. Ad L (8)[2]		
Nevada		[5]	X[5]	
New Hampshire		P***4 P-G. Ad L (8)		
New Jersey	X			
New Mexico		X		
New York		X*		
North Carolina	X			
North Dakota		X*		
Ohio [6,11]		X*		
Oklahoma[11]		X*		
Oregon		X*	X	
Pennsylvania	X			
Rhode Island		P-G. Ad L (8)[2]		

Right to Counsel for Parent and Child and *Discretionary* Guardian Ad Litem for Child		Right to Counsel for Parent and Child and *Mandatory* Separate Counsel for Child		Right to Counsel for Parent and Child and *Mandatory* Guardian Ad Litem for Child	
No Conditions Specified	Conditions Specified	No Conditions Specified	Conditions Specified	No Conditions Specified	Conditions Specified
				X^{10}	
X^2					
X^9					
X					
X^2					
				X^9	
		X			
			(1)(4)		(1)(4)
			(1)(4)		
			(2)		

205

	No Mention of Counsel	Right to Counsel for Parent and Child	Right to Counsel for Parent and Child and *Discretionary* Separate Counsel for Child	
			No Conditions Specified	Conditions Specified
South Carolina	X			
South Dakota[11]		X*		
Tennessee				
Texas		P-G. Ad L (8)[2]		
Utah		X		
Vermont	X			
Virginia		X*		
Washington		X*		
West Virginia[11]		X*		
Wisconsin		P-G. Ad L (8)[2]		
Wyoming		P-G. Ad L (8)[2]		

---

[1] No mention of right to counsel for parents was located.
[2] No mention of general right to counsel for parent and child was located.
[3] Court may also provide guardian ad litem as necessary for any party. Further provides that upon request of the court, agency, or county attorney's own motion, the county attorney may represent the child in termination proceedings.
[4] Guardian ad litem, who must be an attorney, must be appointed for child in any adoption proceeding. The Adoption Act is the statute under which termination of parental rights may occur.
[5] Only statutory reference is to court's discretion to appoint counsel for the child or petitioner.
[6] The Ohio statute refers to an award of permanent custody in which the natural or adoptive parents are divested of all legal rights and obligations due from them to the child or from the child to them.

[7] Statute allows exceptions when child is petitioner, attorney ad litem is appointed, or the court determines that the interests of the child will be represented by another party to the suit. A federal court, in a case currently before the U.S. Supreme Court, has found the guardian ad litem provision to be unconstitutional and stated that the court is required to appoint counsel to represent the interests of the child in any proceeding where termination of parental rights is sought. See, *Sims* v. *State Department of Public Welfare of State of Texas,* 438 F. Supp. 1179 (D. Texas 1977).
[8] Statute allows waiver of counsel if court approves and finds interests of child and parent or other party are not adverse.
[9] No mention of right to counsel for child was located.
[10] Guardian ad litem requirement can be waived if counsel has been appointed or retained to represent the child.
[11] Termination is a disposition in neglect; assumed counsel provisions in neglect apply.

Right to Counsel for Parent and Child and *Discretionary* Guardian Ad Litem for Child		Right to Counsel for Parent and Child and *Mandatory* Separate Counsel for Child		Right to Counsel for Parent and Child and *Mandatory* Guardian Ad Litem for Child	
No Conditions Specified	Conditions Specified	No Conditions Specified	Conditions Specified	No Conditions Specified	Conditions Specified
					(1) (2) (4) (5)[2]
				X[7]	
		X[8]			
X					
		X			

Legend

(1) If conflict between parent and child
(2) To protect child's interest; for child's welfare; in interest of justice; if parent indifferent to child
(3) Custody affected
(4) No parent or guardian
(5) Abuse and neglect (usually in the Child Abuse and and Neglect Reporting Statute)
(6) Upon request of minor or parent

(7) If termination is a potential disposition in a neglect proceeding
(8) If parent is a minor and/or incompetent

* Mandatory appointed counsel for child/parent
⊛ Discretionary appointed counsel for child/parent
** Mandatory appointment of counsel for child
⊛⊛ Discretionary appointment of counsel for child
*** Mandatory appointment of counsel for parent
⊛⊛⊛ Discretionary appointment of counsel for parent

P-G. Ad L Guardian ad litem appointed for parent under conditions specified

P Right to counsel specified only for parent

Appendix E. continued   **TABLE III. Statutory References to Counsel**

	Neglect Proceedings	Termination Proceedings
Alabama	Ala Code tit. 12, §15-63	tit. 12, §15-63
Alaska	Alaska Stat. §§9.65.130; 47.10.030; 47.10.050	§§9.65.130; 47.10.050
Arizona	Ariz. Rev. Stat. §8-225	§8-535
Arkansas	Ark. Stat. Ann. §§42-817; 45-413, 428:	§56-220
California	Cal. Welf. & Inst. Code §317; 318; 326 (West)	Cal. Civil Code §237.5 (West)
Colorado	Colo. Rev. Stat. §§19-1-106; 19-3-105	§19-4-101; 19-1-106
Connecticut	Conn. Gen. Stat. Ann. §§17-38a; §17-66b and c (West)	§45-61e (West)
Delaware	Del. Fam. Ct. R. 360	Del. Fam. Ct. R. 360; Del. Code Ann. §13‍1103
District of Columbia	D.C. Code Encycl. §16-2304 as amended by Act 2-53§402	§16-2304 as amended by Act 2-53§402
Florida	Fla. Stat. Ann. §§27.07; §39.09 (West)	§39.09
Georgia	Ga. Code Ann. §§24A-2001; 24A-3301	§§24A-2001; 24A-3301
Hawaii	Haw. Rev. Stat. §571-24	§571-62
Idaho	Idaho Code §§16-1606, 1608, 1618	§§16-2007; 2009
Illinois	Ill. Ann. Stat. ch. 37 §§704-5; §701-20 (Smith-Hurd)	ch. 4. §9.1-13
Indiana	Ind. Code Ann. §12-3-3-2 (Burns)	§31-3-1-7
Iowa	Iowa Code Ann. §§232.11, 232.28 (West)	§§232.28; 600A.6; 600A.7
Kansas	Kan. Stat. §§38-817; 821	§§38-817; 820; 821
Kentucky	Ky. Rev. Stat. §208.060	§199.600
Louisiana	La. Civ. Code Ann. art. 13:1575; 1579; 14:403 (West)	art. 13:1602
Maine	Me. Rev. Stat. tit. 22 §3858	
Maryland	Md. Ann. Code §§3-821; 834	
Massachusetts	Mass. Gen. Laws Ann. ch. 119, §29 (West)	
Michigan	Mich. Comp. Laws Ann. §§712A.17; 722.630	§712A.17
Minnesota	Minn. Stat. Ann. §260.155 (West)	§§260.231; 260.155
Mississippi	Miss. Code Ann. §§43-21-17; 43-23-15	§93-15-5

	Neglect Proceedings	Termination Proceedings
Missouri	Mo. Ann. Stat. §210.160 (Vernon)	§211.471
Montana	Mont. Rev. Codes Ann. §10-1310(12)	§10-1310(12)
Nebraska	Neb. Rev. Stat. §43-205.06	§43-209
Nevada	Nev. Rev. Stat. §§62.045; 62.085	§128.100
New Hampshire	N.H. Rev. Stat. Ann. 604-A:1a	§§170-C:8; 170-C:10
New Jersey	N.J. Stat. Ann. §§9:6-8:23; 9:6-8:43	
New Mexico	N.M. Stat. Ann. §§13-14-18; 13-14-25	§22-2-23
New York	N.Y. Fam. Ct. Act. §§249; 262; N.Y. Soc. Serv. Law §384-a	N.Y. Fam. Ct. Act §§249; 262; 611; N.Y. Soc. Serv. Law. §384-b
North Carolina	N.C. Gen. Stat. §§7A-283, 285	
North Dakota	N.D. Cent. Code §§27-20-26; 20-48	§§27-20-26; 20-48
Ohio	Ohio Rev. Code Ann. §2151.281; 2151.352	§2151.281; 2151.352
Oklahoma	Okla. Stat. Ann. tit. 10 §1109; 21 §846	tit. 10 §1109
Oregon	Or. Rev. Stat. §419.498	§419.498
Pennsylvania	Pa. Stat. Ann. tit. 11 §50-317 (Purdon)	
Rhode Island	R.I. Gen. Laws §§40-11-14; 14-1-30, 31	§15-7-10
South Carolina	S.C. Code §20-10-180	
South Dakota	S.D. Comp. Laws. Ann. §§26-8-22.1; 26-8-22.2; 26-10-12.1	§§26-8-22.1; 26-8-22.2
Tennessee	Tenn. Code Ann. §37-248	§37-248
Texas	Tex. Code Ann. tit. 2 §11.10	tit. 2 §11.10
Utah	Utah Code Ann. §§55-16-7; 78-3a-35	§78-3a-48
Vermont	Vt. Stat. Ann. tit. 33, §§647, 653	
Virginia	Va. Code §16.1-266	§16.1-266
Washington	Wash. Rev. Code Ann. §§13.34.090; 13.34.100; 26.44.053	§§13.34.090: 13.34.100
West Virginia	W. Va. Code §49-6-2	§49-6-2
Wisconsin	Wis. Stat. Ann. §48.25 (West)	§48.42
Wyoming	Wyo. Stat. Ann. §§14-8-117; 14-8-123; §14-28.12:1	§14-6-101

Appendix F.
CITATIONS TO STATE ADOPTION SUBSIDY STATUTES

State	Statutory Reference	State	Statutory Reference
Alaska	Alaska Stat. §§20.15.190 through 20.15.240	New Jersey	N.J. Stat. Ann. §§30-4C-46 through 30-4C-49
Arizona	Ariz. Rev. Stat. §§8-141 through 8-145	New Mexico	N.M. Stat. Ann. §§22-2-42 through 22-2-46
California	Cal. Welf. & Inst. Code §16120.1	New York	N.Y. Soc. Serv. Law T.9, §§450-458 (McKinneys)
Colorado	Colo. Rev. Stat. §§26-7-101 through 26-7-108	North Carolina	N.C. Gen. Stat. §§48-39.1 and .2
Connecticut	Conn. Gen. Stat. Ann. §§17-44a through 17-44d	North Dakota	N.D. Cent. Code §§50-09-01 through 50-09-20.1
Delaware	Del. Code Ann. tit. 31, §§304-305 (1977)	Ohio	Ohio Rev. Code Ann. §5153.16 (Baldwin)
District of Columbia	D.C. Code Encycl. §§3-114 through 3-119	Oklahoma	Okla. Stat. Ann. tit. 10, §60-13a (West)
Florida	Fla. Stat. Ann. §409.166	Oregon	Or. Rev. Stat. §§418.330 through 418.340
Georgia	Ga. Code Ann. §99-211(g)(6)	Pennsylvania	Pa. Stat. Ann. tit. 62, §§771-774 (Purdon)
Idaho	Idaho Code §§56-801 through 56-806	Rhode Island	R.I. Gen. Laws §15-7-25
Illinois	Ill. Ann. Stat. §23-5005(4)	South Carolina	S.C. Code §§15-45-310 through 15-45-380
Indiana	Ind. Code Ann. §§31-3-3-1 and 31-3-3-2 (Burns)	South Dakota	S.D. Comp. Laws Ann. §§28-7-3.1 through 28-7-3.2
Iowa	Iowa Code Ann. §§600.17 through 600.21 (West)	Tennessee	Tenn. Code Ann. §§36-102(8) 14-105(0)
Kansas	Kan. Stat. §§38-320 through 38-328	Texas	Tex. Ann. Civ. Stat. art. 46-2 (Vernon)
Kentucky	Ky. Rev. Stat. §199.555	Utah	Utah Code Ann. §55-15(b)-3
Maine	Me. Rev. Stat. tit. 19, §§541-544	Vermont	Vt. Stat. Ann. tit. 33, §2801
Maryland	Md. Ann. Code art. 16, §88A-88H	Virginia	Va. Code §§63.1-238.1 through 63.1-238.5
Massachusetts	Ch. 963 of the Acts and Resolves of Mass., 1971, as amended by Ch. 576, 1972	Washington	Wash. Rev. Code Ann. §§74.13.100, 103, 106, 109 through 136 and 26.32.115
Michigan	Mich. Comp. Laws Ann. §710.48	West Virginia	W. Va. Code §49-2-17
Minnesota	Minn. Stat. Ann. §393.07 (1a)(West)	Wisconsin	Wis. Stat. Ann. §48.48(12) (West)
Missouri	Mo. Ann. Stat. §§453.073 and 453.065 (Vernon)		
Montana	Mont. Rev. Codes Ann. §71-1516		
Nebraska	Neb. Rev. Stat. §§43-117 and 43-118		
Nevada	Nev. Rev. Stat. §127.186		
New Hampshire	N.H. Rev. Stat. Ann. §170-F		

[1] As of this writing, six states: Alabama, Arkansas, Hawaii, Louisiana, Mississippi, and Wyoming, had no adoption subsidy statutes. In the jurisdictions with statutes, there is great variation in the extent to which adoption subsidy programs are operational.

Appendix G.
ADOPTION EXCHANGES
TABLE I. National, Regional and Private Adoption Exchanges.

Exchange	Geographic Area Served
Adoption Resource Exchange of North America (ARENA) 67 Irving Place New York, New York 10003 (212) 254-7410	**All of North America**
Adoption Coordinating Project—Adoption Listing Service (ALS) 749 South Grand Avenue West Springfield, Illinois 62704 (217) 528-4409	**Illinois**
Adoption Listing Service of Ohio (ALSO) 4477 Georgette Avenue North Olmsted, Ohio 44070 (216) 779-8399	**Ohio**
Aid to Adoption of Special Kids (AASK) 3530 Grand Avenue Oakland, California 94610 (415) 451-1748	**California, western states**
Children's Adoption Resource Exchange (CARE) 3711 Macomb Street, N.W. Washington, D.C. 20016 (202) 686-1888	**Washington, D.C., Virginia, Maryland**
The CAP Book 33 South Washington Street Rochester, New York 14608 (716) 232-5110	**Eastern Region of the United States**
Delaware Valley Adoption Resource Exchange (DARE) 1501 Cherry Street Philadelphia, Pennsylvania 19102 (215) 568-5033	**Delaware, New Jersey, Pennsylvania**
Northwest Adoption Exchange P.O. Box 2526 Boise, Idaho 83701 (208) 345-6880	**Alaska, Idaho, Montana, Oregon, Utah, Washington**

Exchange	Geographic Area Served
Rocky Mountain Adoption Exchange P.O. Box 2692 Colorado Springs, Colorado 80901 (303) 471-5991	**Colorado, New Mexico, Wyoming**
Services to Unmarried Mothers and Adoption (SUMA) Community Chest Building 2400 Reading Road Cincinnati, Ohio 45202 (513) 621-8687	**Southwestern Ohio, Northern Kentucky**
Southeast Regional Adoption Exchange 970 Martin Luther King Jr. Drive, S.W. Suite 205 Atlanta, Georgia 30314 (404) 522-4373	**Alabama, Florida, Georgia, Kentucky, Mississippi, North Carolina, South Carolina, Tennessee**
Canadian Department of Health and Welfare Social Services Division Adoption Coordinator Brooke Claxton Building Tunney's Pasture Ottawa, Ontario, Canada K1A 1B5 (613) 992-4203	**All of Canada**

Source: Compiled by the North American Center on Adoption, November 1977. Address and phone numbers verified as of July 31, 1978. Note: Exchanges will often accept referrals from beyond the specific geographic areas served.

Appendix G. continued   TABLE II. State Adoption Exchanges

Alaska
Adoption Consultant
Division of Social Services
130 Seward Street, Room 315
Juneau, Alaska 99801
(907) 586-1862

Arizona
Adoption Consultant
Arizona Department of Economic Security
Social Services Bureau
Box 6123
Phoenix, Arizona 85005
(602) 271-3347

California
Adoption Section
California Department of Social Services
714/744 P Street
M.S. 19-31
Sacramento, California 95814
(916) 445-7964

Colorado
Adoption Consultant
Colorado Department of Social Services
Division of Children and Youth
456 Bannock Street
Denver, Colorado 80204
(303) 778-6363

Connecticut
Connecticut Adoption Resource Exchange
Division of Children and Youth Services
354 Woodland
Hartford, Connecticut 06112
(203) 566-7235

Georgia
Georgia State Department of Human Resources
State Office Building
618 Ponce de Leon Avenue, N.E.
Atlanta, Georgia 30308
(404) 894-4452

Idaho
State Adoption Coordinator
Idaho Department of Health and Welfare
c/o State House
Boise, Idaho 83720
(208) 384-3340

Illinois
Social Services Specialist
Department of Children and Family Services
One Old State Capitol Plaza
Springfield, Illinois 62706
(217) 785-2598

Indiana
Indiana Department of Public Welfare
141 South Maridian Street
Indianapolis, Indiana 46225
(317) 633-4521

Iowa
Adoption Specialist
Iowa State Department of Social Services
State Office Building
Des Moines, Iowa 50319
(515) 281-5874

Kansas
Adoption Specialist
Division of Children and Youth
Smith-Wilson Building
2700 West Sixth Street
Topeka, Kansas 66606
(913) 296-3283

Kentucky
Adoption Specialist
Kentucky Department for Human Resources
Bureau of Social Services
275 East Main Street
Frankfort, Kentucky 40601
(502) 564-6936

Louisiana
Louisiana Department of Public Welfare
P.O. Box 44065
Baton Rouge, Louisiana 70804
(504) 342-4008

Maine
State of Maine
Department of Human Services
State House
Augusta, Maine 04333
(207) 289-3456

Maryland
Social Services Administration
Maryland Resource Exchange
11 South Street
Baltimore, Maryland 21202
(301) 383-3609

Massachusetts
Massachusetts Adoption Resource Exchange (MARE)
600 Washington Street, 7th Floor
Boston, Massachusetts 02111
(617) 727-6180

Michigan
Michigan Adoption Resource Exchange (MARE)
P.O. Box 30037
300 South Capital Avenue
Lansing, Michigan 48909
(517) 373-3513

Minnesota
Adoption Unit
Minnesota Department of Public Welfare
Centennial Office Building
St. Paul, Minnesota 55155
(612) 296-3740

Missouri
Adoption Coordinator
Missouri Division of Welfare
Broadway State Office Building
Box 88
Jefferson City, Missouri 65103
(314) 751-4836

Nevada
Adoption and Licensing Specialist
Nevada State Welfare Division
251 Jenell Drive
Carson City, Nevada 89710
(702) 885-4771

New Hampshire
Director of Social Services
Child and Family Services of New Hampshire
99 Hanover Street
Manchester, New Hampshire 03105
(603) 668-1920

New Jersey
New Jersey State Exchange
P.O. Box 510
Trenton, New Jersey 08625
(609) 292-5268

New Mexico
Adoption Consultant
New Mexico Health and Social Services Department
P.O. Box 23
Santa Fe, New Mexico 87501
(505) 827-2285

New York
New York State Department of Social Services
State Adoption Service
Two World Trade Center
Room 3363
New York, New York 10047
(212) 488-5290

North Carolina
Supervisor of Adoptions
North Carolina Department of Human Resources
Family and Children's Services Branch
325 North Salisbury Street
Raleigh, North Carolina 27611
(919) 733-3801

Ohio
Placement Services for Children
Ohio Department of Public Welfare
30 East Broad Street, 32nd floor
Columbus, Ohio 43215
(614) 466-8446

Pennsylvania
Department of Public Welfare
P.O. Box 2675
Room 425
Health and Welfare Building
Harrisburg, Pennsylvania 17120
(717) 787-4882

South Dakota
South Dakota State Department of Social Services
Youth and Family Services
Illinois Street
Pierre, South Dakota 57501
(605) 773-3227

Tennessee
Adoption Specialist
Tennessee Department of Public Welfare
309 State Office Building
Nashville, Tennessee 37219
(615) 741-1666

Texas
Adoption Resource Exchange Consultant
Texas Department of Human Resources
J.H. Winters Building
300 East Riverside
Austin, Texas 78705
(512) 475-6713

Vermont
Vermont Department of Social and Rehabilitation Services
State Office Building
Montpelier, Vermont 05602
(802) 244-5181

Virginia
Child Welfare Supervisor
Virginia Department of Welfare
Division of Social Services
8007 Discovery Drive
Richmond, Virginia 23288
(804) 786-8863

Washington
Department of State Health Services
OB 41 C
Olympia, Washington 98504
(206) 753-7018

West Virginia
Adoption and Foster Family Services
West Virginia Department of Welfare
Division of Social Services
Building 6 - Room 850
1900 Washington Street, East
Charleston, West Virginia 25305
(304) 348-2400

Wisconsin
Agency Services Supervisor
Wisconsin Department of Health and Social Services
One West Wilson Street, Room 570
Madison, Wisconsin 53702
(608) 266-0690

Wyoming
Adoption Consultant
Wyoming Department of Health and Social Services
Hathaway Building
Cheyenne, Wyoming 82002
(307) 777-7561

Source: Compiled by the North American Center on Adoption, November 1977. Addresses and phone numbers verified as of July 31, 1978. State exchanges had not been established in 15 jurisdictions, Alabama, Arkansas, Delaware, District of Columbia, Florida, Hawaii, Mississippi, Montana, Nebraska, North Dakota, Oklahoma, Oregon, Rhode Island, South Carolina and Utah. For information on adoption services in those jurisdictions, contact the state adoption specialists. Note: There is significant variation in the type and quality of services provided by exchanges in individual states.

Appendix H.
INTERSTATE PLACEMENTS
TABLE I. Reported Interstate Placements by State and Service System, April 1976.

State	Service System	Means of Data Collection	Member Interstate Compact[2]	Number of Children Reported Out-of-State	Reported Number of Out-of-State Children In State
Alabama	Child Welfare	telephone[1]	No	NA	NA
	Mental Health	letter	Yes	CW/JJ	NA
	Juvenile Justice	letter	Yes	1	0
Alaska	Child Welfare	letter	No	19	NA
	Mental Health	letter	Yes	0	NA
	Juvenile Justice	letter	Yes	19	0
Arizona	Child Welfare	interview	No	2	NA
	Mental Health	interview	No	0	NA
	Juvenile Justice	interview	Yes	Unknown	38[3]
Arkansas	Child Welfare	telephone	No	2	Unknown
	Mental Health	letter	Yes	0	NA
	Juvenile Justice	no response	Yes	NA	NA
California	Child Welfare	telephone	Yes	Unknown	Unknown
	Mental Health	interview	No	Unknown	Unknown
	Juvenile Justice	interview	Yes	Unknown	Unknown
Colorado	Child Welfare	telephone	Yes	42	Unknown
	Mental Health	no response	Yes	NA	NA
	Juvenile Justice	no response	Yes	NA	NA
Connecticut	Child Welfare	telephone	Yes	130	Unknown
	Mental Health	no response	Yes	NA	NA
	Juvenile Justice	letter	Yes	58	Unknown
Delaware	Child Welfare	telephone	Yes	4	0
	Mental Health	letter	Yes	Unknown	1
	Juvenile Justice	no response	Yes	NA	NA
District of Columbia	Child Welfare	telephone	No	Unknown	Unknown
	Mental Health	no response	Yes	NA	NA
	Juvenile Justice	no response	Yes	NA	NA
Florida	Child Welfare	telephone	Yes	Unknown	287
	Mental Health	letter	Yes	2	CW
	Juvenile Justice	letter	Yes	0	0
Georgia	Child Welfare	telephone	No	Unknown	Uknown
	Mental Health	letter	Yes	1	NA
	Juvenile Justice	no response	Yes	NA	NA
Hawaii	Child Welfare	no response	No	NA	NA
	Mental Health	no response	Yes	NA	NA
	Juvenile Justice	no response	Yes	NA	NA
Idaho	Child Welfare	telephone	No	44[4]	65[4]
	Mental Health	letter	Yes	CW	CW
	Juvenile Justice	letter	Yes	0	0
Illinois	Child Welfare	telephone	Yes	174	Unknown
	Mental Health	letter	Yes	CW	Unknown
	Juvenile Justice	no response	Yes	NA	NA

Indiana	Child Welfare	telephone	No	329	Unknown
	Mental Health	no response	Yes	NA	NA
	Juvenile Justice	no response	Yes	NA	NA
Iowa	Child Welfare	telephone	Yes	207	Unknown
	Mental Health	letter	Yes	NA[5]	NA
	Juvenile Justice	no response	Yes	NA	NA
Kansas	Child Welfare	telephone	No	178[6]	Unknown
	Mental Health	letter	Yes	CW	0
	Juvenile Justice	no response	Yes	NA	NA
Kentucky	Child Welfare	telephone	Yes	45	Unknown
	Mental Health	letter	Yes	CW	0
	Juvenile Justice	no response	Yes	NA	NA
Louisiana	Child Welfare	lawsuit	Yes	715	NA
	Mental Health	lawsuit	Yes	CW	NA
	Juvenile Justice	not contacted	Yes	NA	NA
Maine	Child Welfare	telephone	Yes	0	Unknown
	Mental Health	letter	Yes	6	Unknown
	Juvenile Justice	letter	Yes	0	0
Maryland	Child Welfare	telephone	Yes	191	0
	Mental Health	letter	Yes	0	0
	Juvenile Justice	letter	Yes	111	Unknown
Massachusetts	Child Welfare	interview	Yes	173	NA
	Mental Health	interview	Yes	Unknown	Unknown
	Juvenile Justice	interview	Yes	33	Unknown
Michigan	Child Welfare	telephone	No	14	Over 100
	Mental Health	no response	Yes	NA	NA
	Juvenile Justice	letter	Yes	12	1
Minnesota	Child Welfare	telephone	Yes	107	Unknown
	Mental Health	letter	Yes	CW	Unknown
	Juvenile Justice	no response	Yes	NA	NA
Mississippi	Child Welfare	no response	No	NA	Unknown
	Mental Health	no response	No	NA	NA
	Juvenile Justice	letter	Yes	0	0
Missouri	Child Welfare	telephone	Yes	Unknown	Unknown
	Mental Health	no response	Yes	NA	NA
	Juvenile Justice	letter	Yes	0	0
Nevada	Child Welfare	telephone	No	44	Unknown
	Mental Health	no response	No	NA	NA
	Juvenile Justice	letter	Yes	10	0
New Hampshire	Child Welfare	telephone	Yes	11	Unknown
	Mental Health	letter	Yes	0	0
	Juvenile Justice	letter	Yes	Unknown	NA
New Jersey	Child Welfare	interview	No	735	Unknown
	Mental Health	interview	Yes	0	0
	Juvenile Justice	no response	Yes	NA	NA
New Mexico	Child Welfare	telephone	No	23	Unknown
	Mental Health	no response	Yes	NA	NA
	Juvenile Justice	letter	Yes	0	2

New York	Child Welfare	telephone	Yes	197[1]	Unknown
	Mental Health	telephone	Yes	Unknown	Unknown
	Juvenile Justice	letter	Yes	0	0
North Carolina	Child Welfare	telephone	Yes	24	Unknown
	Mental Health	letter	Yes	0	0
	Juvenile Justice	letter	Yes	0	0
North Dakota	Child Welfare	no response	Yes	NA	NA
	Mental Health	no response	Yes	NA	NA
	Juvenile Justice	no response	No	NA	NA
Ohio	Child Welfare	interview	Yes	Unknown	Unknown
	Mental Health	interview	Yes	Unknown	Unknown
	Juvenile Justice	interview	Yes	Unknown	Unknown
Oklahoma	Child Welfare	telephone	Yes	0	2
	Mental Health	no response	Yes	NA	NA
	Juvenile Justice	letter	Yes	0	4
Oregon	Child Welfare	telephone	Yes	8	Unknown
	Mental Health	no response	Yes	NA	NA
	Juvenile Justice	letter	Yes	1	1
Pennsylvania	Child Welfare	telephone	Yes	Unknown[1]	3
	Mental Health	no response	Yes	NA	NA
	Juvenile Justice	no response	No	NA	NA
Rhode Island	Child Welfare	telephone	Yes	62	Unknown
	Mental Health	letter	Yes	95	22
	Juvenile Justice	no response	No	NA	NA
South Carolina	Child Welfare	telephone	No	6	Unknown
	Mental Health	interview	Yes	0	Unknown
	Juvenile Justice	interview	No	0	1
South Dakota	Child Welfare	telephone	Yes	35	Unknown
	Mental health	interview	Yes	CW	15
	Juvenile Justice	interview	No	1	3
Tennessee	Child Welfare	telephone	Yes	3	Unknown
	Mental Health	letter	Yes	30	20-30
	Juvenile Justice	letter	Yes	0	0
Texas	Child Welfare	telephone	Yes	0	15[2]
	Mental Health	letter	Yes	0	0
	Juvenile Justice	letter	Yes	0	0
Utah	Child Welfare	telephone	Yes	5	3
	Mental Health	no response	No	NA	NA
	Juvenile Justice	letter	Yes	0	15[1]
Vermont	Child Welfare	telephone	Yes	22	Unknown
	Mental Health	letter	Yes	0	0
	Juvenile Justice	letter	No	2	0
Virginia	Child Welfare	telephone	Yes	436	Unknown
	Mental Health	letter	No	0	0
	Juvenile Justice	letter	Yes	30	0
Washington	Child Welfare	telephone	Yes	2	Unknown
	Mental Health	letter	Yes	2	6
	Juvenile Justice	letter	Yes	Unknown	Unknown

West Virginia	Child Welfare	telephone	Yes	7	Unknown
	Mental Health	no response	Yes	NA	NA
	Juvenile Justice	no response	Yes	NA	NA
Wisconsin	Child Welfare	telephone	No	8	100-150
	Mental Health	no response	Yes	NA	NA
	Juvenile Justice	no response	Yes	NA	NA
Wyoming	Child Welfare	telephone	Yes	31	0
	Mental Health	no response	Yes	NA	NA
	Juvenile Justice	letter	Yes	1	2

[1] Respondent indicated the office dealt only with foster home placements. Institutional placements were done locally.

[2] Compact on Child Placement membership as of January 1, 1976. By December 1977, only nine states and the District of Columbia were not members. Mental Health Compact membership was as of October 1977.

[3] Official interviewed estimated that ten percent of the training school population was from out-of-state. As of January 5, 1976, the total training school population was 380.

[4] Includes placements made by all the child-placing systems.

[5] Letter provided information on facilities to which children were sent, but no numbers.

[6] 149 reported to be "just across the bridge" in Kansas City, Missouri.

[7] Figure reflects New York City figure of 193 and four reported by the state.

[8] Numbers kept on children in foster homes, but not on children placed in institutions. Respondent thought that in 1973 one child was placed out of state, but there was no record of where. To get data it would be necessary to contact each county.

[9] Texas reports 15 children coming into the state since 9/1/75. Prior to that time, an estimated 1200-1300 children were placed in Texas by other states.

[10] Represents youth who have committed federal crimes and been placed through a federal contract.

Appendix H. continued
TABLE II. Summary of Interstate Placements by Service System.

Child Welfare
- 2 states reported not sending any children out of state
- 8 states and the District of Columbia did not know
- 4 states did not respond (Hawaii, North Dakota, Alabama, Mississippi)
- 37 states reported 4049 children out of state

Mental Health
- 12 states reported not sending any children out of state
- 8 states referred all children to the child welfare or juvenile justice systems
- 5 states did not know
- 20 states and the District of Columbia did not respond
- 6 states reported 136 children out of state

Juvenile Justice
- 11 states reported not making any out of state placements under state juvenile justice auspices
- 5 states did not know
- 20 states and the District of Columbia did not respond
- 14 states reported 306 children out of state

Appendix I.
INTERSTATE PLACEMENT REPORTED BY CHILD WELFARE ADMINISTRATORS IN 1976

[Table: A matrix showing interstate placement of children, with sending states listed as rows and receiving states listed as columns. Dots (•) indicate placements from one state to another.]

[1] While the New Hampshire administrator reported 11 children out of state he did not know in which states they were.

221

Appendix J.
SELECTED DEMOGRAPHIC CHARACTERISTICS OF SEVEN STUDY STATES

	1975[1] Total Population (In Millions)	1976[2] Percent of Population Under 18	1975[3] Percent of Population Black	1975[3] Percent of Population Other Minority	1975[4] Percent of Low Income Children
Arizona	2.2	32.6	3.0	6.2	18.7
California	21.2	29.2	7.6	4.4	14.6
Massachusetts	5.8	28.8	3.6	Under 1	16.6
New Jersey	7.3	29.4	11.9	1.0	10.8
Ohio	10.7	30.8	9.6	Under 1	13.2
South Carolina	2.8	32.8	30.8	Under 1	23.9
South Dakota	0.7	31.5	Under 1	5.8	14.6
U.S.A.	213.0	30.3	11.5	1.6	15.3

[1] U.S. Bureau of the Census, *Statistical Abstract of the United States; 1977,* (98th Edition) (Washington, D.C.; Government Printing Office, 1977), Table No. 10, Population-State: 1960-1976.

[2] U.S. Bureau of the Census, *Statistical Abstract, 1977,* Table 29, Population By Age-States: 1976.,

[3] U.S. Bureau of the Census, *Statistical Abstract, 1977,* Table 35, Population By Race-States: 1960-1975.

[4] U.S. Bureau of the Census, *County and City Data Book* , 1972 (Washington, D.C.: Government Printing Office, 1973), Items 50-67.

1974[5] Per Capita Income Rank	Population[6] Density (Per Square Mile)	2/76[7] Number of AFDC Recipients	2/76[7] AFDC Monthly Payment Per Recipient	2/76[7] Number of AFDC Foster Care Recipients	2/76[7] Average AFDC Foster Care Payment Per Child
25	15.6	67,018 [50,303][8]	$40.78	60	$154.50
6	127.6	1,444,850 [993,341]	85.14	13,352	292.70
15	727.0	361,768 [251,123]	87.63	2,515	251.81
4	953.1	451,508 [322,622]	83.08	2,638	168.26
23	260.0	590,288 [404,461]	65.25	4,806	67.89
44	85.7	139,774 [102,685]	27.74	653	88.35
34	8.8	25,239 [18,563]	68.38	476	150.61
	57.5	11,449,033 [8,115,312]	71.01	114,049	257.15

[5] U.S. Bureau of the Census, *Statistical Abstract, 1977* Table 716, Median Family Income, 1959-1969, and Per Capita Money Income, 1959-1974-States, By Per Capita Rank in 1974.

[6] U.S. Bureau of the Census, *Statistical Abstract,* Table 11, Population Rank, Percent Change and Density-States and Puerto Rico, 1920-1970.

[7] U.S. Department of Health, Education and Welfare, Social and Rehabilitation Service, National Center for Social Statistics, *Public Assistance Statistics, February 1976* (Washington, D.C.; HEW, 1976).

[8] Bracketed figures refer to number of child recipients.

Appendix K.
NUMBER OF CHILDREN IN OUT-OF-HOME PLACEMENT

TABLE I. Number of Children in Out-of-Home Placement by Agency and Study State[1] 1975-1976

Agency Responsible	Arizona		California		Massachusetts	
	Number	Percent	Number	Percent	Number	Percent
Child Welfare [AFDC Foster Care Program][3]	3,955[2] [44]	77 [1]	28,716 [15,941]	73 [55]	8,416 [2,468]	65 [29]
Juvenile Justice State Training Schools State Other County	324 NA See [1]	6	4,433 NA NA	11	619	5
Mental Health State Hospitals Other	31[2]	1	592 156 }	2	213 313 }	4
Mental Retardation State Schools Other	822[4]	16	2,669 1,586 }	11	2,229	17
Special Education	NA		NA[6]		923[7]	7
Other BIA Nursing Homes	NA[5] NA		1,000	3	187	1
TOTAL	5,132	100	39,152	100	12,900	99

[1]Sources for Table I are set forth in Table II. This table does not reflect a completely accurate count. For example, children who were the responsibility of the Bureau of Indian Affairs (BIA) in Arizona are not included. In some states, it was necessary for us to select between discrepant figures supplied by various state officials. In New Jersey, we did not compute the percentage of children in out-of-home placement because we did not have figures for the juvenile justice system. We can say with certainty, however, that approximately 100,000 of the children in the seven study states were in out-of-home placement.

[2]This figure includes 2,945 children in foster homes (492 of whom were supervised by the juvenile courts but paid for by the Department of Economic Security (DES), and 173 of whom were Indian children paid for by the BIA, but supervised by DES); and 1,010 children in institutions (485 of whom were supervised by juvenile courts and paid for by DES). The count of children in institutional placements is based on October 1975 data. It was not included in the DES Fiscal Year 1975 annual report on foster care, but was reported to CDF by state officials.

[3]These figures refer to the numbers and percent of children for whom the state received federal reimbursement through the AFDC Foster Care Program for a one month period. See Chapter 5 for a description of the AFDC Foster Care Program.

[4]This figure includes 152 mentally retarded children in state psychiatric

New Jersey		Ohio		South Carolina		South Dakota	
Number	Percent	Number	Percent	Number	Percent	Number	Percent
12,641 [609]	[5]	15,866 [4,850]	75 [31]	2,282[8] [653]	65 [29]	1,114 [466]	60 [42]
NA NA		2,503 560 }	15	775	22	99 45 171 }	17
476 111		825	4	NA		14	Under 1
1,767		1,241	6	450[9]	13	75 136 }	11
NA		NA		NA		58	3
NA		NA		NA		151	8
14,995		20,995	100	3,507	100	1,863	99

hospitals.

[5]BIA officials could not provide a figure on the number of Indian children residing on Arizona reservations who were out of their homes. They estimated that Region 9, which includes Arizona, served approximately 60,000 Indians and had 700 Indian children in placement, half of whom were in foster care, and half in institutional placements. These figures do not include children in BIA boarding schools, over one-half of whom, an official estimated, are there for "social reasons."

[6]The California Department of Education provided us with a list of Approved Placements for Fiscal Year 1975-76, but these included all private facilities, not just residential schools.

[7]This figure reflects placements in private residential facilities. Forty percent of these children were in out-of-state placements, 20 percent in other New England states. The Special Education Division also reported 2,447 children in state schools, 233 children in state hospitals, and 202 children in DYS secure facilities. We did not include these in the special education total, as we suspected they had been counted by other systems.

[8]This figure includes 1,813 children in foster homes and 469 children in institutions.

[9]The South Carolina Department of Mental Retardation has the authority to purchase foster home care. The Department provides no separate statistics on children. This figure represents *some* institutional care placements, but none of the foster home placements.

Appendix K. continued   **TABLE II. Sources for Table I**

	Arizona	California	Massachusetts
Child Welfare	Arizona Dept. of Economic Security, Annual Report, Fiscal Year July 1, 1974 to June 30, 1975 for foster care. DES report of June 1975 on institutional placements.	California Dept. of Benefit Payments, Program Information Bureau, "Public Assistance Facts and Figures, Dec. 1975," dated Feb. 9, 1976.	Figures supplied by the Dept. of Public Welfare at CDF's request. We note that the *Boston Globe* at the same time reported 9,624 children in foster care. R. Levey, "They're Nobody's Kids and Easy to Betray," *Boston Globe* 7 May 1976, p. 31.
Juvenile Justice	January 5, 1976 count of children in training schools, Arizona Dept. of Corrections.	California Dept. of Youth Authority, *Characteristics of California Youth Authority Wards, Dec. 31, 1975* (Sacramento: Div. of Research, 1975).	Figures supplied by Div. of Youth Services.
Mental Health	CDF interview with staff member of Div. of Behavioral Health.	Statistics compiled at CDF request by Center for Health Statistics.	Figures supplied by Div. of Children's Services, Dept. of Mental Health.
Mental Retardation	CDF interview with staff member of Bureau of Mental Retardation.	Statistics compiled at CDF request by Div. of Community Services, Dept. of Health and Welfare.	Figures supplied by Div. of Children's Services, Dept. of Mental Health.
Special Education	Not requested by CDF staff.	Not requested by CDF staff.	Figures supplied by Dept. of Special Education.
Other	CDF staff interview with Director of Social Service Branch, BIA, Region 9.	Estimate by officials in the Dept. of Health.	CDF interview with Dept. of Public Health officials.
AFDC-FC	*Public Assistance Statistics (PAS) June, 1975.* DHEW Publication No. SRS 76-03-100 NCSS Report A-2.	PAS, Nov. 1975.	PAS, Nov. 1975.

New Jersey	Ohio	South Carolina	South Dakota
CDF interview with case review unit supervisor.	Ohio Dept. of Public Welfare, "Ohio Public Welfare Statistics," January-March, 1975.	Reported to CDF. Figures are for Dec. 31, 1975.	South Dakota Dept. of Social Services, "Foster Family Care, Recommendations for Change." Statistics as of June 1976.
Not requested by CDF.	CDF interview with Ohio Youth Commission staff members.	Based on a count of the population in the three training schools on March 23, 1976. Does not include group home figures (estimated to be between 40 and 80).	The State Training School and Youth Forestry Camp reported to CDF 144 children were in care. Youth Services Program Div. reported to the appropriations committee of the legislature 171 children in residence. There may be some overlap in the two counts.
Statistics compiled at CDF request by Div. of Mental Health.	Reported to CDF by the Ohio Office of the Attorney General (1975 statistics).	No separate statistics on children available.	CDF request to state institutions; and interview with Director, Div. of Mental Health and Mental Retardation.
Reported in 1975 survey conducted by the New Jersey Association of Retarded Citizens.	Reported to CDF by the Ohio Office of the Attorney General (1975 statistics).	CDF interview.	CDF request to state institutions; and interview with Director, Div. of Mental Health and Mental Retardation.
Not available.	Not requested by CDF staff.	Not requested by CDF staff.	Reported to CDF staff.
			CDF interview with staff of Aberdeen BIA.
PAS, June 1975.	Sept. 1975 figures reported by Ohio fiscal office.	Reported to CDF by South Carolina officials.	PAS, June 1976.

Appendix L.
DESCRIPTION OF STATUTORY PROVISIONS FOR FOSTER CARE REVIEWS

Tables I, II, and III describe the results of our analysis of statutory provisions for the review of foster care cases in the 50 states and the District of Columbia. An attempt was made to cover laws and amendments enacted through December 1977, and more current information was used when available. This analysis covers only statutory provisions for reviews. (Relevant citations are provided in Table IV.) Therefore, it does not address reviews which may be conducted pursuant to administrative regulations or guidelines. Nor does it cover efforts undertaken by individual courts to systematically review out-of-home placements, such as reviews instituted as part of the National Council of Juvenile and Family Court Judges' Children in Placement Project. Further, the analysis is based only on a reading of the statutes, and does not cover the extent to or manner in which such laws are, in fact, implemented.

Table I

Table I summarizes the nature of the statutory provisions for the review of foster care cases in the 50 states and the District of Columbia. As can be seen from the Tables, there is much variation among the states in the extent to which they address by statute the periodic review of children in foster care.

In nine states, we found no specific statutory provision for the review of children once they are placed in out-of-home care pursuant to neglect or dependency proceedings.

In 20 states, statutes provide for judicial review of dispositional orders which commit the child to the custody of an agency, department, or individual, but not at periodic intervals. Thirteen of these simply state that the court may reconsider the disposition in a neglect or dependency case if the court deems it necessary or if a petition for reconsideration is before the court. Seven of the 20 require a court hearing prior to extending a child's placement beyond a specific length of time (e.g. one year, two years, three years). Two additional states provide for a one-time court hearing subsequent to the entry of a disposition, but do not mention subsequent periodic reviews.

Statutes in three states, including one of those that also requires a court hearing to extend a placement, require administrative reviews by the agency responsible for the care of the children in placement on a periodic basis.

Statutes in three states, including one of those that also requires a court hearing to extend a placement, require administrative reviews by the agency responsible for the care of the children in placement on a periodic basis.

Table II

Table II describes for each of the states requiring some form of independent review of children in foster care: (1) the cases to whom the review requirement applies; (2) the roles of the agency, court, and where applicable, the review board; (3) the frequency of review; (4) the due process protections specified; and (5) other relevant provisions addressed in the statute. There is considerable variety among these states in the comprehensiveness of the reviews, the specificity of procedures and dispositional alternatives, and the protections afforded interested parties.

In 8 of the 20 states the review procedure applies to all children in the care and custody of the public agencies (some of these states require all children entering care to go through a court proceeding). In the other 12, it applies only to children placed in care pursuant to a court order, not to children placed voluntarily by their parents.

Reviews in 14 of the states are the sole responsibility of the court. The court reviews vary as to whether the court must hold a hearing and whether notice of the hearing must be provided to the parties. A hearing is mandatory in four states, optional in seven, and not specified in the remaining three. In four states the review procedure involves both citizen review boards and the courts. In three of these states the court routinely reviews the recommendations of the review boards. In the fourth the court conducts subsequent reviews when the review board so recommends. In Maryland and South Carolina the review is conducted by a citizen review board but court action may follow.

Six of the 20 states require reviews at least every six months by a review board or court. In six additional states there must be an initial review within six months of placement and annual reviews thereafter. In the remaining states, the review schedules vary. For instance, the statutory provisions for review in the District of Columbia vary with the age of the child and the length of time in care. Reviews are required at least every six months for all children under the age of six and for any child who has been in care less than two years. Cases of children who are six years of age or over and have been in care two years or more are reviewed annually.

Table III

Table III describes in detail the statutory provisions for administrative reviews of children in foster care in three states where we found statutory references to such reviews. In two of the three states the reviews are semi-annual, in one they are annual. Two of the states require that reports of the reviews must be made to or filed with the court. In one state, failure by the agency to evaluate a child enables a parent to petition the court for modification of an order. In another, a parent may formally request a review of the decision of the agency, and if necessary appeal to the court.

TABLE I.
Foster Care Review Mechanisms Specified by Statute in 50 States and the District of Columbia

No Review Mentioned	Reconsideration of Court Order Upon Petition to Court	Court Hearing Necessary to Extend Placement Beyond A Specified Period	One time Court Review Required	Periodic Administrative Review Required	Periodic Judicial or Citizen Review Required
Arkansas Delaware Montana Nebraska Oklahoma Oregon Pennsylvania South Dakota Wyoming	Alabama Connecticut Illinois Indiana Kansas Kentucky Louisiana[1] Maine Massachusetts New Mexico Rhode Island Texas Wisconsin	Alaska Colorado Georgia Hawaii Idaho Minnesota North Dakota	Colorado (6 months after placement) Utah (2 years after placement)	Connecticut Idaho Mississippi	Arizona California District of Columbia Florida Iowa Maryland Michigan Missouri Nevada New Hampshire New Jersey New York North Carolina Ohio South Carolina Tennessee Vermont Virginia Washington West Virginia

[1]The Louisiana termination statute further provides that whenever parental rights are not terminated but the child has been abused, the court must annually review the case to determine what progress has been made in rehabilitating the parents so that reunification may occur.

Appendix L. continued

TABLE II. Statutorily Mandated Periodic Judicial or Citizen Reviews of Children in Foster Care

State	For Whom	Agency Role	Review Board Role	Court Role
Arizona	Children adjudicated dependent and placed by court order.	Prepare a permanent placement plan; conduct an administrative review of the placement and progress every 6 months, and submit a copy to the court.	Review plan and subsequent progress reports prepared by the placing agency to determine efforts made to implement the plan. Submit findings and recommendations to the court within 30 days, and to the agency and other interested parties.	Appoint local foster care review boards. Assign cases to review boards and forward agency's plan and progress reports to review boards. Annually reaffirm or revise dispositional order giving priority first to reunification of the family, and then to the permanent placement of the child.
California	Children adjudicated dependent and placed by court order.[2]			Conduct status renewal hearing.
District of Columbia	Children adjudicated neglected and placed by court order.	10 days prior to review hearing, submit report to court including information on services provided to child and parent, amelioration of problems and evidence of new problems, cooperation of parent with agency, and evidence of visitation.		Determine if placement continues to be necessary to safeguard child's welfare. If not, may order the child be returned home and services provided or enter any other dispositional order authorized in neglect proceedings, including termination of parental rights for purposes of adoption.

[2] Children in foster care in two demonstration counties in California are subject to a more detailed review. However, because it is not applicable statewide it is not described here.

Role Of Others	Frequency	Notice and Other Due Process Rights Specified	Other Provisions
Foster parents and other interested parties may be involved in review process when appropriate.	Review of cases by local review boards at least every 6 months. Annual judicial review.	Written notice of annual court review and right to participate to agency, foster parents, natural parents or guardian, foster child, if over 12, and such other persons as court may deem necessary.	(1) Protections for ensuring confidentiality of records in possession of review boards. (2) Training required for review board members. (3) Establishes state foster care review board. (4) Duties of local boards include informing natural parents, foster parents and others of rights and responsibilities, encouraging the timely return of children to their natural parents when appropriate, attempting to maximize stability and family continuity for children in care, and making recommendations regarding foster care policies and procedures to state foster care review board.
Probation officer annually files report and recommendation for disposition.	Annually.	Written notice of hearing by probation officer to parties in original proceeding and counsel of record. Court required to advise parties at hearing of future hearing date and rights to participation and counsel.	
	Under age 6, every 6 months. Other ages, every 6 months until in care 2 years, then at least annually.	Notice of hearing to all parties and their attorneys.	

State	For Whom	Agency Role	Review Board Role	Court Role
Florida	Children placed by court order and voluntarily placed children.	Petition the court to review the status of a child in care 6 months or more and furnish court with written report, including recommendations.		Shall review status of child and *may* hold hearing to determine if child should continue in care, be returned home, or freed for adoption. May dispense with hearing with consent of parties and base decision upon reports and affidavits.
Iowa	Children placed by court order.			Review all orders. May on own motion or motion of interested parties modify disposition after hearing is held.
Maryland	All children in public or private placements under jurisdiction of the Department of Social Services for more than 6 months.		Review cases to determine efforts made to acquire permanent and stable placements and submit a written report to the juvenile court and the local Department of Social Services on the status of such efforts. May make specific recommendations as to whether return home, continued placement, or initiation of termination proceedings for purposes of adoption is in the child's best interest.	*May* on its own motion or motion of any party, hold a hearing to consider review board report.

Role Of Others	Frequency	Notice and Other Due Process Rights Specified	Other Provisions
	At least annually.	Notice of hearing and a copy of the agency petition (including statement of dispositional alternatives) served upon agency, foster parent, natural parents, and other persons at court's discretion.	
	At least annually.		Notice of hearing to parties if disposition is to be modified.
Governor appoints members of local review boards.	Every 6 months.		(1) Creates state Citizen Board for Review of Foster Care for Children to: coordinate local board activities; make recommendations to the General Assembly regarding foster care policies and procedures; submit an annual report on the status of foster care children; and provide training for local boards. (2) Requires cooperation of agencies and institutions in furnishing necessary information to local board. (3) Makes board members subject to the same standards of confidentiality as employees of the Department of Social Services. (4) Board members must have demonstrated an interest in children through activities such as community service or professional experience, or possess background in law, sociology, psychology, psychiatry, education, social work or medicine.

State	For Whom	Agency Role	Review Board Role	Court Role
Michigan	Children placed by court order.	Provide information to county juvenile agent regarding possibility of re-establishing home for the child.		Shall rehear case to determine whether child shall remain in foster care in the temporary custody of the court.
Missouri	Children placed by court order and children placed voluntarily.	Agency must petition court to review non-court placements and then present written report on child's status to the court. In court placements periodic written status reports must be filed.		Shall review report and *may* hold hearing. Purpose of hearing to determine whether termination proceedings for the purpose of adoption should be instituted.
Nevada	Children placed by the court in a home or institution.	May be required to submit written report to court on child's progress and recommendations for further supervision, treatment or rehabilitation.		Review placement for purpose of determining if continued placement is in the best interest of the child and public and the child is being treated fairly. May request report from child's worker, guardian or custodian.
New Hampshire	Children adjudicated neglected.			Review disposition.

Role Of Others	Frequency	Notice and Other Due Process Rights Specified	Other Provisions
At six months, parents required to appear and show efforts made to reestablish a home. At subsequent hearings, parents must show efforts to reestablish home and also show why parental ties should not be terminated. County juvenile agent must submit report at hearing regarding possibility of reestablishing home for the child.	Six months after entry of disposition, and then annually thereafter until child is placed in permanent custody of court.		
	Every 6 months for court-ordered placements; unspecified for children placed voluntarily after an initial 6 month review.		
	Semiannually.		
	At least once within first year after disposition and at least annually thereafter.		

235

State	For Whom	Agency Role	Review Board Role	Court Role
New Jersey	All children placed outside their homes by the Division of Youth and Family Services	File notice of placements within 72 hours of placement and notice of any change in subsequent status of the child with the court. Prepare and revise as necessary the placement plan for each child which includes statement of goals and responsibilities of all parties, including services to be provided.	Act on behalf of the court to review whether placement is in child's best interest. Criteria to be used are spelled out in statute and include evidence as to whether the child's wishes were considered; whether parents have been encouraged to visit; and appropriateness of services. The review, if all notified parties consent, may be based solely on written materials. The review board must submit a written report within 10 days of its review to the court and agency with a finding as to whether return home, continued placement, or initiation of termination proceedings for purposes of adoption would be in the child's best interest.	(1) Approve placement or order child returned home within 15 days of notice of initial placement by determining whether continuation of the child in his home would be contrary to his welfare. (2) Establish child placement review boards as an arm of the court. (3) Review the findings of local board and make dispositional order. *May* hold a hearing.
New York	Children placed voluntarily.	File petition in family court to review foster care status of child in care for 18 months.		Court shall review child's foster care status. May rely on written materials and dispense with hearing if all notified parties consent. Court shall specify dispositional order: return home; continued placement; direct agency to legally free child for adoption; or order a child's adoptive placement. Court may order agency to undertake specific plan to reunite family. If petition for termination ordered and is not initiated within 90 days by the agency, court shall permit foster parents to file petition, except

Role Of Others	Frequency	Notice and Other Due Process Rights Specified	Other Provisions
	Action by review board within 45 days of initial placement and at least annually thereafter. Children already in care should be reviewed within 12 months of enactment of statute.	For Board Review: Written notice 15 days ahead of review and right to appear to agency, child, parents, and others at board's discretion. For Court Hearing: Notice must include statement of dispositional alternatives and be given 30 days in advance along with right to participate to agency, review board, child, parents, and others at court's discretion.	(1) Establishes a State Child Placement Advisory Council to: review policies, procedures and practices of the review boards and of the agency regarding child placement; establish procedures for training board members; monitor the effectiveness of the "Child Placement Review Act;" make an annual report on its effectiveness to the Supreme Court, the Governor and the Legislature. (2) Board members shall have either training, experience, or interest in issues concerning child placement or child development.
Foster parent where child has resided may also petition court for review.	After a child is in care 18 months, and at least every 24 months thereafter if child continues in foster care.	Notice of hearing including a statement of dispositional alternatives of court, and of right to participate to agency, foster parents, natural parents, and others at the court's discretion.	

State	For Whom	Agency Role	Review Board Role	Court Role
New York (Cont'd)				in specified circumstances. If adoption is ordered and agency fails to comply before rehearing, court may transfer custody of child to another agency.
	Children placed by court order pursuant to a finding of abuse or neglect.	Submit report to court at end of initial period of placement and annually when placement is extended. May petition court for extension of hearing.		Hold hearing on need for extension of placement. In addition to or in lieu of extension order, court may order agency to undertake specific plan to reunite family; or order agency to institute legal proceedings to free a child for adoption. If such proceedings are not initiated within 90 days, court shall permit foster parents to initiate petition, except in specified circumstances.
North Carolina	Children whose custody removed from parents.	Comply with court order to present information and assist the court in review.		Conduct periodic reviews to determine if the needs of the child are met and placement is in the child's best interest. Order the Department of Social Services, the juvenile counselor, or any other public or private community agency to assist in the review. Enter an order continuing the placement, providing for a different placement, or making such other provision as is deemed in child's best interest.

Role Of Others	Frequency	Notice and Other Due Process Rights Specified	Other Provisions
Foster parents may petition for extension hearing.	After a child is in care 18 months, and then annually thereafter to extend order.	Notice of hearing and right to participate to agency, natural parents and foster parents.	
	Semiannually the first year, then annually.	10 days notice to parents of periodic review.	Applies only to court orders entered after January 1, 1978.

State	For Whom	Agency Role	Review Board Role	Court Role
Ohio	All children in placement.	File with the court an initial report of its review 4 months after placement and then annually. Such report must include information on the involvement of the child's parents, recommended future plans for the child, and services offered to the family to restore the home.	If appointed by the court, review boards may approve review procedures used by agencies in preparing annual reports. May also review annual reports within 90 days and accept or order revised.	(1) Examine and approve review procedures used by agencies in preparing reports to the court. (2) Review annual reports within 90 days and accept or order revised. *or* (3) Appoint review boards to carry out (1) and (2) above. (4) If the court determines the custody or care arrangement is not in the child's best interest it may terminate the agency custody and place custody elsewhere. (5) Send copy of annual review findings to Department of Public Welfare.
South Carolina	All children in public or private foster care.	Provide such records and information to review boards as may be necessary.	Review cases of children who have been in care more than 6 months to determine efforts made to acquire a permanent home for the child. Also required to: encourage return home or, when not appropriate, the adoption of children; advise foster parents of their rights to petition for termination and adoption; and report to state Department of Social Services or other agencies deficiencies in agency efforts to find permanent homes for children.	Hold hearing upon petition of any person or agency aggrieved by local review board decision. Boards meet in family court chambers.

Role Of Others	Frequency	Notice and Other Due Process Rights Specified	Other Provisions
	Within 4 months of placement, then annually. Children already in care should be reviewed within 4 months of effective date of Act Jan. 1, 1977.		(1) Requires the Department of Public Welfare to report annually on the outcomes of reviews to the General Assembly (2) One board member shall represent the general public and the remainder must be trained or experienced in the care or placement of children.
Governor appoints members of foster care review boards in each judicial circuit, upon recommendation of county legislative delegations.	Every 6 months.	Person or agency aggrieved by decision of local board may request and receive a hearing before board and has right to petition the court to show cause why decision should not be modified or set aside.	(1) Creates state Advisory Board for Review of Foster Care of Children to: make recommendations to the General Assembly regarding foster care policies procedures and deficiencies in agency practice, and set rules for local boards. (2) Requires agency and institution cooperation with review boards in furnishing of records and other information as a condition of licensure.

State	For Whom	Agency Role	Review Board Role	Court Role
Tennessee	All children in court ordered placement following declaration of dependency or neglect.	Prepare a plan for each child in its care specifying long-term goals; and including a signed statement of responsibilities of parent, agency and caseworker, which includes the statutory definition of an abandoned child, and the procedures for termination of parental rights. Agency must report on plan to court every 6 months during first year, and annually thereafter. Copies of all reports on the implementation of the plan (except the initial 6 month report) must also go to the foster care review board.	Review plans for children in care and agency report 6 months after initial court review, then annually. Shall submit findings to the court and agency involved only if board determines need for full court review. Assessments and reports are advisory.	(1) Appoint members of foster care review boards. (2) Conduct review of children in care 6 months (not later than 7) to assess compliance with plan for child. (3) *May* conduct subsequent judicial reviews when deemed necessary or when advisory board recommends such review. (4) Direct review boards to review the plan and agency report periodically and to report recommendations to court when full court review required.
Vermont	All children for whom court has transferred legal custody or guardianship.	File notice with court, state's attorney and other parties of biennial review. File with court and state's attorney a report and recommendations.		Upon petition or own motion court shall order a hearing to review the order of disposition. If no hearing, initial order considered reviewed and remains in force. In reviewing case, court charged to consider the child's best interest taking into account: relationship with natural parents; foster parents; siblings; child's adjustment; role of natural parent; and likelihood that natural parent will be able to resume parental duties within reasonable period.

Role Of Others	Frequency	Notice and Other Due Process Rights Specified	Other Provisions
	Court review within 6 months of initial placement, and subsequently if deemed necessary by court or review board. Board review 6 months after court review and annually thereafter. Plans for children already in care shall be submitted to the court at least by July 1, 1977 (12 months after effective date of provisions.)		(1) Each board may include pediatrician or other doctor, lawyer, member of human resource agency staff, member of local mental health agency, parent of minor child, and person 18-25. Member of county department of human services office will serve as ex officio member. (2) Statement of confidentiality of plans, reports and other materials prepared on behalf of children in foster care.
Person, if other than agency, having legal custody required to file notice of biennial review with court, state's attorney and other parties, and to file with court and state's attorney report and recommendations.	Every two years.	Notice of biennial review to be filed with court, state's attorney, and other parties.	Failure to give notice or to review order does not terminate original order.

State	For Whom	Agency Role	Review Board Role	Court Role
Virginia	All children under legal custody of local department of public welfare or social services, or child welfare agency for whom a foster care plan has been filed with the court. (Foster care plan must be filed for children placed voluntarily and by court order.)	Within 60 days of initial order, file foster care plan with court. Such plan must specify care and services to be provided, provisions for visitation, nature of placement, goals and rationale for plan (return home, adoptive placement or permanent foster care).[3] Within 12 months of filing initial plan, file a petition with the court reporting on child's placement and progress; parent-child contacts; services provided to child and family; compliance with initial plan; and recommended disposition, including foster care plan if continuation in care is recommended.		(1) Send copy of intial foster care plan to child's attorney, child's parents, and other interested parties, and a portion of plan (excluding plans for adoptive placement or permanent foster care) to foster parents. (2) Judge or court staff must review agency petition and judge *may* order hearing for review of foster care plan and enter any appropriate dispositional order consistent with alternatives available at original hearing.
Washington	All children found to be dependent.	Provide court with a specific plan as to child's placement, plans for reunification, and action to be taken to maintain parent-child ties. Statute requires that an agency place a child as close to home as possible, preferably in his own neighborhood, unless a more distant placement is necessary to promote the child's or parent's well-being.		Review status of children to determine whether court supervision should continue. Shall continue child in care only if no parent is available or willing to care for the child, the child is unwilling to reside in the parent's custody, or return would present manifest danger to the child. If child continues in care, court shall establish in writing: reunification services provided; extent of parental visiting; cooperation between agency and parent; additional services needed; and when return home can be expected. Court shall order additional services if needed. Further, court shall advise parent that a petition to seek termination may be ordered at the next review hearing.

[3] The Virginia statue requires that prior to court ordered placement and the transfer of legal custody, there must be a finding that there is no less drastic alternative.

[4] The Virginia statute provides for placement in "permanent foster care" if diligent efforts to return the child home or place him for adoption have been unsuccessful or adoption is not a reasonable alternative under the circumstances. Permanent foster care can be used if it is a requisite to providing funds for the care of the child in an approved educational treatment or training program. Once placed the child shall remain until the age of majority. (§63.1-206.1)

Role Of Others	Frequency	Notice and Other Due Process Rights Specified	Other Provisions
Any party receiving copy of plan may petition court for its review.	Annually as long as child is in temporary foster care. (Temporary foster care refers to child who is not in adoptive placement or permanent foster care.[4]) Court may review case whenever petitioned by parties to do so if good cause is shown.	If hearing, notice of hearing, copy of agency petition and right to participate to child if over 12, child's attorney, child's parents, foster parents, agency, and others at court's discretion.	
	At least semiannually.		When a child is returned home following a review hearing, casework supervision shall continue for 6 months, at which time there shall be a hearing on the need for continued intervention.

State	For Whom	Agency Role	Review Board Role	Court Role
West Virginia	All children in physical or legal custody of the state department of welfare who have not been placed in permanent foster care [5], an adoptive home, or returned home.	Agency must file petition with court reporting on child's situation and efforts to make permanent plans for the child 20 months after placement, and supplementary petitions every 18 months thereafter.		*May* hold hearing and enter disposition.

---

[5] "Permanent foster care" requires written agreement in which the state department of welfare places control of child with family until child's emancipation.

Role Of Others	Frequency	Notice and Other Due Process Rights Specified	Other Provisions
	20 months after initial placement and then at 18 month intervals.	If hearing, notice and right to be present to child if over 12, child's parents, foster parents and others at the court's discretion.	State department shall annually report to court current status of placements of children in permanent care and custody of state who have not been adopted.

Appendix L. continued

TABLE III. Statutorily Mandated Periodic Administrative Reviews of Children in Foster Care

State	For Whom	
Connecticut	Children under supervision of Commissioner of Children and Youth Services	
Idaho	All children in the custody or under supervision of the Department of Health and Welfare.	
Mississippi	Each child under custody of the State Department of Public Welfare.	

Agency Role	Frequency	Other Provisions
Prepare and maintain written plan for care and treatment which includes a diagnosis and proposed plan of treatment. Review the treatment plan and placement every six months to determine its appropriateness.	At least every six months.	Child or parent if aggrieved by treatment plan or review decision may request in writing a hearing before the Commissioner, and have the right of further appeal to the court.
Make periodic evaluations of children in custody or under supervision to determine whether existing orders and dispositions shall be modified or continued. Reports of evaluations must be made to the court which vested custody of child with the department.	At least every six months.	Failure to evaluate or reevaluate a child within six months enables child, parent, guardian or custodian, or counsel to petition court for revocation or modification of an order. No petitions may be filed within four months of a prior hearing.
Administer a system of individualized plans and annual reviews for each child. The reviews shall be conduced by the Department of Public Welfare staff or others appointed by the Commissioner. The reviews shall include, at a minimum, an evaluation of the child: based on the extent of the parents' care and support, and parent-child communication; compliance with the service plan; methods of achieving the goal; and the services offered and/or used to establish a permanent home. Must file the plan with the court which awarded custody and, upon approval of the court, make it available to natural or foster parents. Must also report to the legislature annually as to the number of children re-reviewed and their status.	During the anniversary month for the child's entry into foster care and annually thereafter.	(1) Department of Public Welfare must maintain a registry of children in its custody which classifies children: in temporary custody for evaluation (up to 3 months); temporary custody with plan for return home (up to one year); temporary custody with plan for adoption (up to 2 years); freed for adoption; 14 years of age and over who can't return home and have chosen not to be adopted; and institutionalized children for whom adoption is not feasible. (2) Includes punishment for violation of confidentiality requirement—fine of no more than $1,000 or imprisonment of six months or both.

Appendix L. continued
TABLE IV. Statutory References to Reviews

Alabama	Ala. Code tit. 12, §15-74	Minnesota	Minn. Stat. Ann. §260.191
Alaska	Alaska Stat. §47.10.080	Mississippi	Miss. Code Ann. §43-15-5
Arizona	Ariz. Rev. Stat. §§8-515, 516	Missouri	Mo. Ann. Stat. §§453.305; 453.310
California	Cal. Welf. and Inst. Code §366 (West)	Nevada	Nev. Rev. Stat. §62.225
Colorado	Colo. Rev. Stat. §19-3-115	New Hampshire	N.H. Rev. Stat. Ann. §169.31-a
Connecticut	Conn. Gen. Stat. Ann. §§17-62; 17-421 (West)	New Jersey	N.J. Stat. Ann. §30.4C-50 (West)
District of Columbia	D.C. Code Encycl. §16-2323 (West)	New Mexico	N.M. Stat. Ann. §13-14-35
		New York	N.Y. Soc. Serv. Law §392
Florida	Fla. Stat. Ann. §409.168 (West)		N.Y. Family Ct. Act §1055
Georgia	Ga. Code Ann. §24A-2701	North Carolina	N.C. Gen. Stat. §7A-286 (2)
Hawaii	Haw. Rev. Stat. §571-48	North Dakota	N.D. Cent. Code §27-20-36
Idaho	Idaho Code §§16-1610; 16-1611; 16-1623	Ohio	Ohio Rev. Code Ann. §5103.151 (Baldwin)
Illinois	Ill. Ann. Stat. ch. 37, §705-8 (Smith-Hurd)	Rhode Island	R.I. Gen. Laws §14-1-42
Indiana	Ind. Code Ann. §31-5-7-17 (Burns)	South Carolina	S.C. Code Ann. §§43-43-10-43-13-70
Iowa	Iowa Code Ann. §232.36 (West)	Tennessee	Tenn. Code Ann. §§37-1501-37-1510
Kansas	Kan. Stat. §38-826	Texas	V.T.C.A. Family Code §14.08
Kentucky	Ky. Rev. Stat. §28.205	Utah	Utah Code Ann. §78-3A-39 (19), 42, 42, 45 & 47
Louisiana	La. Civ. Code Ann. §§13:1571.10; 13:1603 (West)		
Maine	Me. Rev. Stat. tit. 22, §3793	Vermont	Vt. Stat. Ann. tit. 33, §§658 and 667
Maryland	Md. Ann. Code art. 88-A, §§111-117	Virginia	Va. Code §16.1-282
Massachusetts	Mass. Gen. Laws Ann. ch. 119, §26 (West)	Washington	Wash. Rev. Code Ann. §13.34.130
		West Virginia	W. Va. Code §49-6-8
Michigan	Mich. Comp. Laws Ann. §712A.19	Wisconsin	Wis. Stat. Ann. §48.35 (West)

Appendix M.
ADMINISTRATIVE STRUCTURE OF STATE AGENCIES RESPONSIBLE FOR CHILDREN IN OUT-OF-HOME CARE AS OF 1976 IN THE STUDY STATES.

Child Placing System	Arizona	California	Massachusetts
Child Welfare	Family & Child Welfare Services, Social Services Bureau, Dept. of Economic Security	Family & Children's Services, Dept. of Health & Welfare	Div. of Social Services, Dept. of Public Welfare, Executive Office of Human Services
Juvenile Justice	State Dept. of Corrections	California Youth Authority, Dept. of Health & Welfare	Div. of Youth Services, Executive Office of Human Services
Mental Health	Div. of Behavioral Health Services, Dept. of Health Services	Community Services, Dept. of Health & Welfare	Children's Services, Div. of Mental Health, Dept. of Mental Health, Executive Office of Human Services
Mental Retardation	Bureau of Mental Retardation, Dept. of Economic Security	Community Services, Dept. of Health & Welfare	Div. of Mental Retardation, Dept. of Mental Health, Executive Office of Human Services
Special Education	Div. of Special Education, Dept. of Education	Div. of Special Education, Dept. of Education	Div. of Special Education, Bureau of Inst. Schools, Dept. of Education
Other			Office for Children, Executive Office of Human Services

New Jersey	Ohio	South Carolina	South Dakota
Div. of Youth & Family Services, Dept. of Institutions & Agencies	Bureau of Services for Families & Children, Div. of Social Services, Dept. of Public Welfare	Individual & Family Service Div., Bureau of Human Services, Dept. of Social Services	Community Services, Div. of Social Welfare, Dept. of Social Services
Dept. of Corrections & Parole, Dept. of Institutions & Agencies	Ohio Youth Commission	Dept. of Youth Services	Office of Juvenile Services, Div. of Corrections, Dept. of Social Services Board of Charities & Corrections
Div. of Mental Health, Dept. of Institutions & Agencies	Office for Children, Div. of Mental Health, Dept. of Mental Health	Dept. of Mental Health	Office of Mental Health, Div. of Mental Health & Mental Retardation, Dept. of Social Services
Div. of Mental Retardation, Dept. of Institutions & Agencies	Div. of Mental Retardation, Dept. of Mental Retardation	Dept. of Mental Retardation	Office of Developmental Disabilities, Div. of Mental Health & Mental Retardation, Dept. of Social Services
Div. of Special Education, Dept. of Education	Div. of Special Education, Dept. of Education	Office of Programs for Handicapped, Dept. of Education	Div. of Special Education, Dept. of Education
		Office of Child Advocacy, Dept. of Social Services	Office on Children & Youth, Div. of Human Development, Dept. of Social Services

Appendix N.
ORGANIZATION OF CHILD WELFARE SERVICES IN THE STUDY STATES AS OF 1976

Arizona:
State Supervised and Administered

Family and Child Welfare Services was part of Social Services Bureau, Department of Economic Security. Head of FCWS accountable to Assistant Director for Program Services. Child welfare field staff in district offices of Department of Economic Security were accountable to Assistant Director for Field Services. All traditional child welfare responsibilities were within FCWS.

California:
State Supervised-County Administered

Family and Children's Services was in the Department of Health. It was in the Service Operations Unit which, along with Adoptions and Special Services for the Blind and Service Management, was part of the Community Services Unit in that Department. Fifty-eight county offices providing child welfare services were responsible to local boards of supervisors. The Adoptions Unit, which had higher organizational status than the FCS unit, was entirely state run. Licensing of children's facilities was handled by the state unit responsible for all licensing.

Massachusetts:
State Supervised and Administered

Child welfare services were handled in the Office of Social Services in the Department of Public Welfare. The delivery system was three-tiered: the local offices provided information and referral, preventive and foster home services; regional offices provided protective and adoption services; the state offices provided supervision of group homes. Licensing was carried out by the Office for Children.

New Jersey:
State Supervised and
Administered

The Division of Youth and Family Services in the Department of Institutions and Agencies provided child welfare services. The Division was organized into five major units: field services; fiscal and management; contract development and administration; regulatory; and legislative. The field services unit was comprised of the Bureau of Family Services, the Bureau of Residential Services, the Bureau of Resource Development (adoptions), and the Case Audit and Review Unit. The central field service unit was responsible for 21 district offices, four regional adoption centers, and several group homes run by the Division. Licensing functions were carried out within the field service unit.

Ohio:
State Supervised-County
Administered

The Division of Social Services included a Bureau of Services for Families and Children responsible for all child welfare functions except licensing; and a Licensing Bureau, responsible for standard setting and consultation to counties. In 42 counties, children's services boards were responsible only for children's services. In the remaining 46 counties, child welfare functions were carried out within the county Department of Public Welfare.

South Carolina:
State Supervised-County
Administered

The Department of Social Services was divided into four bureaus: support services, fiscal operations, public and medical assistance, and human services. The Individual and Family Service Division in the Bureau of Human Services was responsible for all traditional child welfare services. There were 46 county offices.

South Dakota:
State Supervised and
Administered

The Division of Social Welfare in the Department of Social Services included financial assistance and community services. Community services included all traditional child welfare functions except licensing. Licensing was carried out by the Office on Children and Youth.

Appendix O.
1975 - 1976 ADOPTION DATA FOR SEVEN STUDY STATES

	Arizona	California	Massachusetts
No. Terminations During Previous Year	121 (1975)	844[3]	No Response to CDF Questionnaire
No. Children Voluntarily Relinquished During Previous Year	NA	1,255	
No. Children Placed In Adoptive Homes During Previous Year	119 (1976)	2,735	
No. Children In Adoptive Homes Not Legally Adopted	NA	2,944 (1976)	
No. Adoptions Finalized During Previous Year	NA	2,407	
Race of Children Known	NA	Yes[4]	
No. With Special Needs	NA	[5]	
No. Subsidized Adoptions Finalized in Previous Year	NA	572[6]	
No. Children Adopted By Foster Parents	NA	502	
Total No. Subsidized Adoptions Ever Completed	25 (Estimate of No. approved in 1976)	3,000	
No. Children Freed For Adoption But Not In Adoptive Homes	83	1,649	
Race Known	Yes[2]	No	
No. With Special Needs	46	NA	
Does state have a special category of "long-term foster care?"	No	Yes	

[1]This table reflects total adoptions, not just adoptions of children in foster care. Unless otherwise noted, data were supplied by state adoption units in response to CDF questionnaire.

[2]Of the Arizona children awaiting adoption, 64 percent were white; 6 percent black; 7 percent American Indian; 9 percent Spanish-speaking; and 10 percent mixed.

[3]The California figure includes only children for whom parental rights were terminated and adoptive placements made.

[4]In 1975, 68 percent of the California children in adoptive placements were white; 7 percent black; 6 percent Spanish-speaking; 16 percent mixed, American Indian, or other; under 1 percent unknown.

[5]The California figure reported to us did not reflect an unduplicated count of children with special needs and therefore is not cited.

[6]Figure refers to the number of subsidized adoptive placements, rather than the number finalized.

New Jersey	Ohio	South Carolina	South Dakota
NA	NA	67	No Response to CDF Questionnaire[12]
NA	NA	153	
559	NA	174	
525	NA	208	
399 (1975)	7,588	126	
NA	Yes[8]	Yes[9]	
63	NA	24	
95	76	NA[10]	
NA	NA	18	
577	265	NA	
41	NA	128	
Yes[7]	NA	Yes[11]	
41	NA	57	
No	No	Yes	

[7] Of the children awaiting adoption in New Jersey, 49 percent were white and 51 percent black.

[8] Ohio reported racial information on approximately half of the children adopted. Of those, 92 percent were white, the remainder nonwhite.

[9] Of the children adopted in South Carolina, 71 percent were white, 25 percent black, and 4 percent mixed.

[10] The South Carolina adoption subsidy legislation was not enacted until Spring 1976.

[11] Of the South Carolina children awaiting adoption, 45 percent were white, 51 percent were black and 4 percent mixed.

[12] South Dakota did not respond to our survey request. However, in interviews with CDF staff they reported that as of January 1976, 149 children were freed and awaiting adoption, 8 percent of whom were over 15 years of age. They further reported 92 approved adoptive homes with 56 potential parents willing to take Indian children over eight. There was no information on the number of these potential adoptive parents who were themselves Indian.

Appendix P. FEDERAL PROGRAMS AFFECTING CHILDREN WITHOUT HOMES

Program	Authorizing Legislation (Regulations)	Administering Agency (Program Office)[1]	Purpose
Aid to Families with Dependent Children	Social Security Act, Title IV-A, 42 U.S.C. §601, et seq. (45 CFR 201, et seq.)	HEW/SSA (Office of Family Assistance)	To provide federal funds to states for cash assistance payments to needy children and their families.
AFDC Foster Care	Social Security Act, §408, 42 U.S.C. §608 (45 CFR §233.110)	HEW/SSA (Office of Family Assistance)	To provide reimbursement to states for maintenance costs for children in licensed or approved foster family homes and private non-profit child care institutions.
Child Welfare Services	Social Security Act, Title IV-B, 42 U.S.C. §§620-625 (45 CFR 220)	HEW/OHDS (Administration for Children, Youth, and Families, Children's Bureau)	To help state and local agencies provide preventive and protective services for children, including foster care.
Emergency Assistance	Social Security Act, Title IV-A, 42 U.S.C. §601, et seq. (45 CFR §233.120)	HEW/SSA (Office of Family Assistance)	To assist needy families in emergency or crisis situations to avoid destitution or provide living arrangements if the family is without available resources for reasons other than refusal to accept employment.
Indian Child Welfare Assistance	25 U.S.C. §13 (25 CFR 20)	DOI/BIA (Office of Indian Services)	To provide maintenance payments for foster home care and appropriate institutional or other group care for dependent, neglected and handicapped Indian children in need of such care, and for whom such services are not available from other state or local welfare agencies, as well as services to children in care.

[1] The following abbreviations for federal agencies and offices are used throughout this appendix: HEW (Department of Health, Education and Welfare); SSA (Social Security Administration); OHDS (Office of Human Development Services); DOJ (Department of Justice); LEAA (Law Enforcement Assistance Administration); DOI (Department of Interior); BIA (Bureau of Indian Affairs); DOD (Department of Defense); DOA (Department of Agriculture); OE (Office of Education).

Type of Aid	Children Eligible for Program	Authorizing Congressional Committees (Subcommittees)
Formula grants; states make money payments directly to eligible needy families with dependent children. (Entitlement program)	In 24 states payments are limited to needy families with dependent children where one parent is deceased or absent from the home. The remaining states and the District of Columbia also extend benefits to needy families with unemployed fathers.	(H) Ways and Means (Public Assistance and Unemployment Compensation) (S) Finance (Public Assistance)
Formula grants; $100 average maximum monthly payment or Federal Medicaid percentage. (Entitlement program)	AFDC eligible children removed from their homes as a result of a judicial determination that continuation in such setting would be contrary to their welfare.	(H) Ways and Means (Public Assistance and Unemployment Compensation) (S) Finance (Public Assistance)
Formula grants; each state receives $70,000 with the remainder allocated on the basis of population under 21 and per capita income.	All children in need of child welfare services without regard to financial need, legal residence, social status or religion.	(H) Ways and Means (Public Assistance and Unemployment Compensation) (S) Finance (Public Assistance)
Federal reimbursement to states having approved plans. Payments (cash, in-kind aid or vouchers) limited to 30 days per family in a 12-month period. (Entitlement program)	Families with children who are in emergency or crisis situations. Specific emergencies covered vary by state.	(H) Ways and Means (Public Assistance and Unemployment Compensation) (S) Finance (Public Assistance)
Direct payments for maintenance costs and services.	Indian children under 18, or under 22 if assistance initiated before 18, who reside on or near a reservation, who require placement in a foster home or specialized non-medical care facility in accordance with the State AFDC Foster Care payment standards or have need of special services not available under other assistance or child welfare programs.	(H) Interior and Insular Affairs (Indian Affairs and Public Lands) (S) Select Committee on Indian Affairs

Program	Authorizing Legislation (Regulations)	Administering Agency (Program Office)	Purpose
Child Abuse and Neglect Prevention and Treatment	Child Abuse Prevention and Treatment Act, 42 U.S.C. §5101, et seq. (45 CFR 1340)	HEW/OHDS (Administration for Children, Youth and Families, **Children's Bureau.** National Center on Child Abuse and Neglect)	To assist states and other bodies to strengthen their capacity to **develop** programs which will help in identification and prevention of abuse and neglect, and provision of ameliorative services.
Juvenile Justice and Delinquency Prevention	Juvenile Justice and Delinquency Prevention Act of 1974, 42 U.S.C. §5601, et seq. (See State Planning Agency Grants Guideline Manual, and 43 *Federal Register* 36402-36410, August 16, 1978.)	DOJ/LEAA (Office of Juvenile Justice and Delinquency Prevention)	To assist states in planning, establishing, **operating, coordinating** or evaluating juvenile justice projects. To provide funds for special projects for the improvement of and development of alternatives to the juvenile justice system.
Runaway Youth Program	Juvenile Justice and Delinquency Prevention Act of 1974, Title III, Runaway Youth Act, 42 U.S.C. §5701, et seq. (45 CFR 1351)	HEW/OHDS (Administration for Children, Youth and Families, Youth Development Bureau)	To assist public or nonprofit private agencies develop local facilities to deal primarily with the needs of runaway youth and other homeless youth in a manner which is outside the law enforcement structure and juvenile justice system. Also authorizes technical assistance and short-term training to staff of runaway facilities.

Type of Aid	Children Eligible for Program	Authorizing Congressional Committees (Subcommittees)
Formula grants to states which meet certain requirements and grants and contracts for research, training and demonstration projects.	Eligibility varies by project. Child abuse and neglect defined as harm or threatened harm to the health or welfare of a child under 18 by a person responsible for the child's health and welfare.	(H) Education and Labor (Select Education) (S) Human Resources (Child and Human Development)
Formula grants; states meeting certain requirements receive $200,000 plus an additional amount allocated on the basis of population under 18. Discretionary grants for special emphasis projects.	Not applicable. To receive funds a state must include a number of provisions in its state plan, including provisions to remove status offenders from correctional facilities and to ensure that juveniles will not be detained in facilities where they have regular contact with adults. Special emphasis grants may be made to public and private agencies, organizations, institutions, or individuals. At least 20% of funds must go to private, nonprofit agencies, organizations or institutions with experience in dealing with youth.	(H) Education and Labor (Economic Opportunity) (S) Judiciary (Subcommittee to Investigate Juvenile Delinquency)
Project grants and contracts.	Programs serve youths under 18 who absent themselves from their home or legal residence without permission of their parents or legal guardian.	(H) Education and Labor (Economic Opportunity) (S) Judiciary (Subcommittee to Investigate Juvenile Delinquency)

Program	Authorizing Legislation (Regulations)	Administering Agency (Program Office)	Purpose
Social Services	Social Security Act, Title XX, 42 U.S.C. §1397, et seq. (45 CFR 228)	HEW/OHDS (Administration for Public Services)	To furnish services directed at the goals of achieving or maintaining self-support and/or self-sufficiency, preventing or remedying neglect, abuse, or exploitation of children and adults unable to protect themselves; preserving, rehabilitating, or reuniting families; preventing or reducing inappropriate institutional care when appropriate and providing services to persons in institutions.
Indian Social Services Counseling Program	25 U.S.C. §13 (25 CFR 20)	DOI/BIA (Office of Indian Services)	To provide counseling services to recipients of general assistance, to children in the Indian Child Welfare Assistance Program, and to other Indian children and adults in need of social services.
Medicaid	Social Security Act, Title XIX, 42 U.S.C. §1396, et seq. (42 CFR 446-452)	HEW/Health Care Financing Administration (Medicaid Bureau)	To provide financial assistance for medical services to individuals and families certified as eligible by the states.

Type of Aid	Children Eligible for Program	Authorizing Congressional Committees (Subcommittees)
Formula grants; 90% federal match for family planning services, 75% for all other services. Fees may be required. (Capped entitlement program)	Determined by state but *may* include any children in families with a monthly gross income under 115% of the median income for a family of 4, adjusted for family size. 50% of state's funds must go to AFDC, SSI or Medicaid eligible persons. Includes services to children in foster care as well as emergency shelter for children in need of protective services.	(H) Ways and Means (Public Assistance and Unemployment Compensation) (S) Finance (Public Assistance)
Provision of services by BIA staff.	Indian children who reside on or near a reservation who request or on whose behalf family and community services are requested.	(H) Interior and Insular Affairs (Indian Affairs and Public Lands) (S) Select Committee on Indian Affairs
Formula grants; state expenditures are matched by federal Medicaid percentage. (Entitlement program)	Child must be certified eligible by the state welfare or Medicaid agency. All states but Arizona have Medicaid programs. Eligibility varies by state, but in all states children are eligible if they receive AFDC or SSI payments or are under 21 and would be eligible for AFDC except for federal or state age or school attendance requirements. States have the option of extending coverage to the medically needy, to children under 21 who are financially needy but do not qualify for AFDC, and to SSI-eligible children. Financially eligible children under 21 in foster care and certain types of child care institutions are also often eligible, as are children adopted with subsidies in some states.	(H) Interstate and Foreign Commerce (Health and the Environment) (S) Finance (Health)

Program	Authorizing Legislation (Regulations)	Administering Agency (Program Office)	Purpose
Early Periodic Screening, Diagnosis and Treatment (EPSDT) Program	Social Security Act, Title XIX, 42 U.S.C. §1396, et seq. (45 CFR §205.146; 42 CFR §449.10)	HEW/Health Care Financing Administration (Medicaid Bureau)	To provide preventive health care to Medicaid eligible children by identifying, diagnosing and treating medical, dental and developmental problems.
Supplemental Security Income (SSI)	Social Security Act, Title XVI, 42 U.S.C. §1381, et seq. (20 CFR 416)	HEW/SSA (Office of Program Operations, Bureau of Supplemental Security Income)	To provide supplemental income, through federal financial assistance, to persons in financial need who are age 65 or older and to persons who are blind or disabled, including children.
SSI Disabled Children's Program	Social Security Act, Title XVI, 42 U.S.C. §1382d (42 CFR §§51a.301-321, (Interim Rule. December 16, 1977)	HEW/Public Health Service (Health Services Administration. Bureau of Community Health Services Office for Maternal and Child Health)	To ensure that children who receive SSI are referred to the state's crippled children's agency or other appropriate agency to determine their need for medical, education and social services. Children six or under or children who have never attended school must be provided services and children over six referred for services which will help them benefit from subsequent education or training or otherwise enhance their opportunities for self-sufficiency or self-support as adults.
Civilian Health and Medical Program of the Uniformed Services (CHAMPUS)	10 U.S.C. §1071, et seq. (32 CFR 199)	DOD/Asst. Sec. of Defense-Health Affairs (Office for the Civilian Health and Medical Program of the Uniformed Services)	To provide financial assistance for medical care by civilian sources to dependents of active, retired and deceased members of the uniformed services; in addition to basic medical care, assistance is available for certain services for handicapped dependents.

Type of Aid	Children Eligible for Program	Authorizing Congressional Committees (Subcommittees)
Formula grants; state expenditures are matched by the federal Medicaid percentage. (Entitlement program)	Children under 21 who are Medicaid-eligible, including children in out-of-home care.	(H) Interstate and Foreign Commerce (Health and the Environment) (S) Finance (Health)
Direct payments with unrestricted use. In some states federal benefit is supplemented by state payment. (Entitlement program)	Children who meet the federal eligibility criteria for blindness or disability and have access to less than the specified levels of income and resources. Children in foster care and certain types of institutions may be eligible. Coverage also extends to children in group facilities serving 16 or fewer persons.	(H) Ways and Means (Public Assistance and Unemployment Compensation) (S) Finance (Public Assistance)
Formula grants to the states.	All children who receive SSI.	(H) Ways and Means (Public Assistance and Unemployment Compensation) (S) Finance (Public Assistance)
DOD reimburses CHAMPUS contractors at a fixed rate set forth in contracts.	Children of active duty members of the uniformed services or of retired or deceased members who are under 21, or students and under 23, or older and dependent for support because of a physical or mental incapacity; only children of active duty members or certain deceased members are eligible for the handicapped programs.	(H) Armed Services (Military Personnel) (S) Armed Services (Manpower and Personnel)

Program	Authorizing Legislation (Regulations)	Administering Agency (Program Office)	Purpose
Crippled Children's Services	Social Security Act, Title V, 42 U.S.C. §701, et seq. (42 CFR 51a)	HEW/Public Health Service (Health Services Administration, Bureau of Community Health Services, Office for Maternal and Child Health)	To assist states, especially in rural areas and areas suffering from economic distress, in locating children with crippling conditions or suffering from conditions leading to crippling and providing a full range of diagnostic and corrective services, including hospitalization and other institutional care and aftercare.
Community Mental Health Centers	Community Mental Health Centers Amendment of 1975, 42 U.S.C. §2689, et seq. (42 CFR 54)	HEW/Public Health Service (Alcohol, Drug **Abuse and Mental** Health Administration, National Institute of Mental Health, Division of Mental Health Service Programs	To continue and expand community mental health services.
Special Supplemental Food Program for Women, Infants and Children (WIC)	National School Lunch Act of 1966, as amended, 42 U.S.C. §1786 (7 CFR 246)	DOA/Food and Nutrition Service	To provide special nutritious food supplements to pregnant and lactating women and to children under age 5 at nutritional risk because of inadequate income and nutritional need.
Title I Program for Handicapped Children in State-administered or State-supported Schools	Title I, Elementary & Secondary Education Act of 1965, as amended, 20 U.S.C. §241c-1 (45 CFR 116, 116b)	HEW/OE (Bureau of Education for the **Handicapped** [programmatic responsibility] and Bureau of Elementary and Secondary Education/Div. of Education for the **Disadvantaged** [fiscal responsibility])	To provide funds to state agencies to supplement and strengthen educational programs for handicapped children in state **operated** and state-supported schools.

Type of Aid	Children Eligible for Program	Authorizing Congressional Committees (Subcommittes)
Federal/state matched formula grants and special project grants.	All children below the age of 21 who have an organic disease, defect or condition which may hinder the achievement of normal growth or development, as defined by the state, are eligible for diagnostic services. Flexible income standards are applied for treatment services.	(H) Interstate and Foreign Commerce (Health and the Environment) (S) Finance (Health)
Federal grants to public or non-profit organizations or agencies.	Anyone residing in the catchment area of a center is theoretically eligible for its services. To be eligible for federal funds, a center must provide, in addition to other services, specialized services for **children and screening, follow-up care and transitional halfway house services for persons discharged from mental health facilities.**	(H) Interstate and Foreign Commerce (Health and the Environment) (S) Human Resources (Health and Scientific Research)
Federal grants to states.	Children under five years of age determined to be at nutritional risk because of inadequate income and nutritional need. States may establish their own income standards.	(H) Education and Labor (Elementary, Secondary and Vocational Education) (S) Agriculture. Nutrition and Forestry (Nutrition)
Formula grants; funds allocated on the basis of average daily attendance in the schools and a percentage of the average per pupil expenditure in the state or in the U.S.; funds distributed to facilities on a grant basis.	Handicapped children under 21 who are in need of special services and are in state supported schools, including facilities with which the state contracts for special educational services.	(H) Education and Labor (Elementary, Secondary and Vocational Education) (S) Human Resources (Education, Arts and Humanities)

Program	Authorizing Legislation (Regulations)	Administering Agency (Program Office)	Purpose
Title I Program for Children in State-administered Institutions Serving Neglected or Delinquent Children	Title I, Elementary and Secondary Education Act of 1965, as amended, 20 U.S.C. 241c-3 (45 CFR 116, 116c)	HEW/OE (Bureau of Elementary and Secondary Education/Div. of Education for the Disadvantaged)	To provide funds to state agencies for programs and projects designed to meet the special educational needs of children in state institutions for neglected or delinquent children.
Title I Program for Children in Local Institutions Serving Neglected or Delinquent Children	Title I. Elementary and Secondary Education Act of 1965, as amended, 20 U.S.C. §241a, et seq.(45 CFR 116, 116a)	HEW/OE Bureau of Elementary and Secondary Education/Div. of Education for the Disadvantaged)	To provide funds to local educational agencies for programs and projects designed to meet the special educational needs of educationally deprived children in school attendance areas with high concentrations of low income families and for children in local institutions for neglected or delinquent children.
BIA Boarding School Program	25 U.S.C. §13 (BIA Manual)	DOI/BIA (Office of Indian Education Programs)	To operate federal boarding schools for Indian children living on Indian owned or restricted trust lands where other facilities are not available and to maintain federal dormitories for children attending public schools.
School Lunch Program in Residential Institutions	National School Lunch Act, Sec. 17 as amended by PL 94-105, 42 U.S.C. §1751, et seq. (7 CFR 210)	DOA/Food and Nutrition Service	To make children's residential institutions eligible for the school lunch program.

Type of Aid	Children Eligible for Program	Authorizing Congressional Committees (Subcommittees)
Formula grants to state agencies; funds allocated on the basis of the ADA in the institutions and a percentage of the average per pupil expenditure in the state or in the U.S.	Educationally disadvantaged children under age 21 who are in institutions for delinquent or neglected children for which the state agency is responsible for providing free public education. These include public or private nonprofit residential facilities for children adjudged delinquent, adult correctional facilities, and public or private nonprofit residential facilities for at least 10 neglected children for whom the facility has been granted custodial responsibility.	(H) Education and Labor (Elementary, Secondary and Vocational Education) (S) Human Resources (Education, Arts and Humanities)
Formula grants to local educational agencies. State allocation based in part on count of children 5 to 17 in school district residing (for at least 30 days) in local institutions for neglected or delinquent children. The local educational agencies are to provide programs in the institutions.	Educationally disadvantaged children ages 5-17 who reside in local institutions for delinquent children (public or private residential facilities, including adult correctional institutions) or for neglected children (public or private residential facilities operated for the care of at least 10 children committed or placed voluntarily).	(H) Education and Labor (Elementary, Secondary and Vocational Education) (S) Human Resources (Education, Arts and Humanities)
Direct operation of the boarding schools.	Children of one fourth or more degree of Indian blood who are members of a federally recognized tribe and reside on or near a reservation are given priority.	(H) Education and Labor (Elementary, Secondary and Vocational Education) (S) Select Committee on Indian Affairs
Formula grants on a performance funding basis.	Financially eligible children under 21 in public or licensed private nonprofit residential child care institutions which operate principally for the care of children, including homes for the mentally retarded, emotionally disturbed, physically handicapped and unmarried mothers; group homes, halfway houses, orphanages, temporary shelters, long term care facilities for chronically ill children and juvenile detention centers.	(H) Education and Labor (Elementary, Secondary and Vocational Education) (S) Agriculture, Nutrition and Forestry (Nutrition)

Program	Authorizing Legislation (Regulations)	Administering Agency (Program Office)	Purpose
Food Donation Program-Commodity Distribution to Institutions Portion	7 U.S.C. §612c (7 CFR 250)	DOA/Food and Nutrition Service	To make surplus commodities available for distribution to qualifying households, individuals, schools, charitable institutions, nutrition programs for the elderly and summer camps.
Foster Grandparent Program	Domestic Volunteer Services Act of 1973, 42 U.S.C. §5002, et seq. (45 CFR 1208)	ACTION (Older Americans Volunteer Programs)	To provide volunteer opportunities to low income persons age 60 and over by having them render supportive services, for which they receive a stipend, to children with special needs in health, education, welfare or related settings, both institutional and non-institutional.
Retired Senior Volunteer Program (RSVP)	Domestic Volunteer Services Act of 1973, 42 U.S.C. §5001, et seq. (45 CFR 1209)	ACTION (Older Americans Volunteer Programs)	To develop a recognized role in the community for adults age 60 and over through significant volunteer service. No compensation for service is provided.
Assistance to States for the Education of Handicapped Children	Education for All Handicapped Children Act, 20 U.S.C. §1401, et seq. (45 CFR 121a)	HEW/OE (Bureau of Education for the Handicapped)	To establish necessary rights to insure that all handicapped children receive the free appropriate public education to which they are entitled. Grants are provided to the states to assist them in providing for the education of all handicapped children, with priority given to handicapped children receiving no education and children who are severely handicapped.

Type of Aid	Children Eligible for Program	Authorizing Congressional Committees (Subcommittees)
Donated foods to qualifying facilities.	Children in eligible institutions which include non-penal non-educational public facilities and nonprofit private facilities organized for charitable or public welfare purposes, nonprofit private hospitals, and state correctional institutions for minors.	(H) Education and Labor (Elementary, Secondary and Vocational Education) (S) Agriculture, Nutrition and Forestry (Nutrition)
Grants or contracts for up to 90% of the cost of the project; 100% funding in special circumstances.	Generally children with special needs who are 17 or under, with preference to younger children. However, a child may continue with a volunteer through age 20 if improvement is expected and there is a written plan for an alternative relationship for the person after age 20. Children with special needs include physically handicapped, delinquent, emotionally disturbed, mentally retarded or dependent and neglected children who are in hospitals, correctional facilities and other residential institutions; in schools, day care establishments or in private residences. The child care facilities must be licensed or certified.	(H) Education and Labor (Select Education) (S) Human Resources (Unemployment and Poverty)
Grants to state agencies on aging and other public and nonprofit private agencies and organizations for up to 90% of the cost for the development of and/or operation of volunteer projects. The required local share increases 10% each year the grant is continued.	Children being served at RSVP volunteer stations which include but are not limited to schools, courts, day care centers, hospitals, welfare agencies, nursing homes and institutions.	(H) Education and Labor (Select Education) (S) Human Resources (Unemployment and Poverty)
Formula grants to states distributed on the basis of the number of children 3-21 who are receiving special education and related services multiplied by an annually increasing percentage of the state's average per pupil expenditure.	Children who have been evaluated as mentally retarded, hard of hearing, deaf, speech impaired, visually handicapped, seriously emotionally disturbed, orthopedically impaired, deaf-blind, multi-handicapped, or having specific learning disabilities, and because of those conditions need special education and related services. To receive funds a state must include a number of provisions in its annual state plan, including an assurance to provide full education opportunities to all handicapped children, due process safeguards and placement in the least restrictive environment.	(H) Education and Labor (Select Education) (S) Human Resources (Handicapped)

Program	Authorizing Legislation (Regulations)	Administering Agency (Program Office)	Purpose
Civil Rights Act for Handicapped Persons	Rehabilitation Act of 1973, Section 504, 29 U.S.C. §794 (45 CFR 84)	HEW serves as the coordinator of all 504 enforcement programs throughout the government. The Office for Civil Rights is responsible for compliance in HEW programs.	To prohibit any recipient of federal funds from operating programs in a manner that discriminates in any way against beneficiaries who are handicapped, believed to be handicapped, or have a record of handicaps.
Developmental Disabilities Program	Mental Retardation Facilities and Community Mental Health Centers Construction Act of 1963, as amended by PL 91-517 and PL 94-103, the Developmentally Disabled Assistance and Bill of Rights Acts, 42 U.S.C. §6001, et seq. (45 CFR 1385, 1386, 1387)	HEW/OHDS (Administration for Handicapped Individuals, Developmental Disabilities Office)	To provide financial assistance to states for planning, administration, services and construction of facilities for the developmentally disabled. At least 30% of a state's allotment in FY 77 and thereafter must be used for developing and implementing plans designed to eliminate inappropriate placement in institutions of persons with developmental disabilities. Funds are also available for special projects and for the establishment of demonstration facilities and training programs in university affiliated facilities.
Child Welfare Research and Demonstration Program	42 U.S.C. §626 (42 CFR 205; 45 CFR 16)	HEW/OHDS (Administration for Children, Youth and Families, Children's Bureau)	To provide funds for special research or demonstration projects to improve the quality of child welfare programs and demonstrate new service approaches.

Type of Aid	Children Eligible for Program	Authorizing Congressional Committees (Subcommittees)
Civil rights act.	All handicapped persons are protected by Section 504. It applies to all recipients of federal funds and to all programs and activities that benefit from such assistance.	(H) Education and Labor (Select Education) (S) Human Resources (Handicapped)
Formula grants; allotted on the basis of population, need for services and facilities for the developmentally disabled and per capita income. Grants to **public or nonprofit entities** (for up to 90% of the cost of the project) are also available for special projects, as are project grants to university affiliated programs.	Children participating in or affected by projects must have a developmental disability that is a disability which is attributable: 1) to mental retardation, cerebral palsy, epilepsy, or autism, 2) to any other condition found to be closely related to mental retardation (in terms of intellectual and adaptive problems or required treatment, or 3) to dyslexia resulting from one of the above. The disability must further have originated before age 18, be expected to continue indefinitely and constitute a substantial handicap. A child with a developmental disability may receive services in his own home, a foster home, or an institution.	(H) Interstate and Foreign Commerce (Health and the Environment) (S) Human Resources (Handicapped)
Grants and contracts to public or private nonprofit institutions of higher learning and public or nonprofit agencies or organizations engaged in research or child welfare activities.	Eligibility varies with each demonstration project, but generally any child in need of child welfare services.	(H) Ways and Means (Public Assistance and Unemployment Compensation) (S) Finance (Public Assistance)

Program	Authorizing Legislation (Regulations)	Administering Agency (Program Office)	Purpose
Social Services Research and Demonstration Program	42 U.S.C. §§626, 1310, 1315 (42 CFR 205; 45 CFR 16, 63, 204)	HEW/OHDS (Administration for Public Services)	To provide funds for research or demonstration projects to improve social services program management and develop improved social service delivery; including child welfare services.
Juvenile Justice and Delinquency Prevention, National Institute for Juvenile Justice and Delinquency Prevention	Juvenile Justice and Delinquency Prevention Act of 1974, 42 U.S.C. §§5651-5661	DOJ/LEAA (Office of Juvenile Justice and Delinquency Prevention, National Institute for Juvenile Justice and Delinquency Prevention)	To conduct and coordinate research and evaluation of juvenile justice and delinquency prevention activities, serve as a national clearinghouse and information center on juvenile delinquency, and provide training for persons dealing with juveniles.
Child Welfare Services Training Grants	42 U.S.C. §626 (42 CFR 205; 45 CFR 16)	HEW/OHDS (Administration for Children, Youth and Families)	To train personnel for work in the field of child welfare.
Social Services Training Grants	42 U.S.C. §1397 et seq. (45 CFR §§228.80-85)	HEW/OHDS (Administration for Public Services)	To provide training directly related to the provision of social services for staff of the Title XX agency, service delivery personnel of provider agencies, and students committed to employment in the Title XX agency.

Type of Aid	Children Eligible for Program	Authorizing Congressional Committees (Subcommittees)
Grants and contracts. Grants to state agencies and nonprofit private organizations; contracts with profit or nonprofit organizations.	Not applicable. These are primarily research, rather than direct service projects, a portion of which concern protective services for children and youth.	(H) Ways and Means (Public Assistance and Unemployment Compensation) (S) Finance (Public Assistance)
Project grants, contracts and technical assistance to public or private agencies, organizations or individuals.	Not applicable. Most of these are research and evaluation projects.	(H) Education and Labor (Economic Opportunity) (S) Judiciary (Subcommittee to Investigate Juvenile Delinquency)
Grants to accredited public or nonprofit institutions of higher learning which may be any of three types: teaching grants, traineeship grants, or short-term in-service training grants.	Not applicable. Short-term training can be provided to foster parents, institutional personnel, homemakers, day care staff and personnel.	(H) Ways and Means (Public Assistance and Unemployment Compensation) (S) Finance (Public Assistance)
Formula grants; state agency may then provide training through grants to accredited educational institutions, financial assistance to students, or in-service training.	Not applicable. In-service and short- and long-term training in educational facilities may be provided to foster parents caring for Title XX children, and foster parents contracting with the agency to provide special services, as well as other agency staff, provider agencies, or individuals with whom the agency has purchase-of-service contracts.	(H) Ways and Means (Public Assistance and Unemployment Compensation) (S) Finance (Public Assistance)

Appendix Q.
AFDC FOSTER CARE PROGRAM EXPENDITURES FOR FISCAL YEAR 1976, AND JUNE 1976 PROGRAM RECIPIENTS

State	Federal Expenditures[1]	Recipients of AFDC-FC-June 1976[2]		
		Number of Children	Number in Foster Homes	Number in Institutions
Alabama	1,152,001	1,491	1,393	98
Alaska	514,716	206	153	53
Arizona	36,233	73	66	7
Arkansas	426,621	538	513	25
California	24,319,090	13,412	10,957	2,455
Colorado	1,082,164	761	560	201
Connecticut	2,209,578	1,963	1,589	374
Delaware	449,120	541	435	106
District of Columbia	537,750	317	176	141
Florida	74,173	118	118	0
Georgia	1,635,383	2,181	1,903	278
Guam	9,406	28	28	0
Hawaii	36,876	46	46	0
Idaho	582,217	473	451	22
Illinois	5,815,500[3]	4,139	NA	NA
Indiana	1,673,100	3,569	NA	NA
Iowa	1,000,150	769	621	148
Kansas	2,809,313	1,705	1,284	421
Kentucky	1,670,043	1,847	NA	NA
Louisiana	2,126,871	1,769	1,694	75
Maine	1,663,177	1,206	NA	NA
Maryland	3,364,392	3,778	3,400	378
Massachusetts	3,797,511	2,515	2,164	351
Michigan	7,396,440	4,368	3,786	582
Minnesota	5,662,933	2,757	2,408	349
Mississippi	975,694	1,010	1,010	0
Missouri	1,027,216	1,808	1,652	156
Montana	499,468	407	407	0
Nebraska	509,744	630	578	52
Nevada	228,652	205	196	9
New Hampshire	397,011	621	501	120
New Jersey	1,279,694	2,575	1,957	618
New Mexico	119,856	149	123	26
New York	73,474,009	25,255	12,021	13,234
North Carolina	718,135	2,617	2,106	511
North Dakota	476,713	470	404	66
Ohio	2,369,420	4,921	4,611	310
Oklahoma	537,112	646	646	0
Oregon	3,118,539	2,046	1,781	265
Pennsylvania	5,985,629	6,556	NA	NA
Rhode Island	233,135	200	184	16
South Carolina	463,956	667	667	0
South Dakota	558,076	466	420	46
Tennessee	1,418,455	1,747	1,552	195
Texas	1,028,780	3,420	3,200	220
Utah	519,657	402	NA	NA
Vermont	497,797	484	388	96
Virginia	3,708,964	3,419	3,232	187
Washington	2,139,670	1,755	1,573	182
West Virginia	537,269	532	448	84
Wisconsin	3,777,019	3,281	2,667	614
Wyoming	85,681	59	NA	NA
Total	$176,730,109[4]			

[1]Source: U.S. Department of Health, Education and Welfare, Social and Rehabilitation Service, Division of Finance, Office of Financial Management, *State Expenditures for Public Assistance Programs Approved Under Titles I, IV-A, X, XIV, XVI, XIX, XX of the Social Security Act, Fiscal Year 1976* (Washington, D.C.: HEW, 1977), p. 11, as adjusted for Illinois.

[2]Source: U.S. Department of Health, Education and Welfare, Social and Rehabilitation Service, National Center for Social Statistics, *Public Assistance Statistics - June 1976* (Washington, D.C.: HEW, 1976), Table 7.

[3]Data not supplied by the state. Figure compiled from monthly estimates of expenditures.

[4]Total adjusted to include expenditures for Illinois.

Appendix R.
MEDICAID ELIGIBILITY COVERAGE OF FINANCIALLY NEEDY CHILDREN UNDER 21 AS OF DECEMBER 1977

State	All Financially Needy Children Under 21	All Financially Needy Children in Foster Care[1]	All Financially Needy Children In Psychiatric Hospitals[2]	All Financially Needy Children In Intermediate Care Facilities[3]	All Financially Needy Children In Subsidized Adoptions[4]
Alabama		•			
Alaska		•		[12]	
Arizona	No Medicaid Program				
Arkansas	•				
California	•				
Colorado		•	•	•	
Connecticut	•				
Delaware		•			
District of Columbia	•				
Florida		•			
Georgia		•			
Hawaii[13]		•		•	•
Idaho		•		•	
Illinois		•			
Indiana			•		
Iowa		•			•
Kansas[14]		•	•	•	•
Kentucky[15]		•[5]	•		
Louisiana		•	•	•	
Maine	•				
Maryland	•				
Massachusetts	•				
Michigan	•				
Minnesota	•				
Mississippi		•			
Missouri		•[6]			•
Montana		•	•	•	
Nebraska[16]		•			
Nevada		•			•
New Hampshire		•			
New Jersey	•				
New Mexico		•		•	
New York	•				
North Carolina		•[7]			
North Dakota		•[8]	•	•	•
Ohio	No Reasonable Classifications Covered				
Oklahoma	•				
Oregon[17]		•[9]	•	•	
Pennsylvania	•				
Rhode Island		•[5]			
South Carolina		•			
South Dakota		•[10]			
Tennessee		•[5]	•		•
Texas		•[11]			
Utah	•				
Vermont	•				
Virginia		•		•	
Washington	•				
West Virginia		•			
Wisconsin	•				
Wyoming	No Reasonable Classifications Covered				
TOTALS	17	30	9	11	7

Source: Compiled from data obtained from the Eligibility Policy Branch, Division of Policy and Standards, Medicaid Bureau, Health Care Financing Administration, HEW, December 1977.

[1] Refers to children under age 21 in foster homes or private institutions for whom public agencies are assuming some financial responsibility, unless otherwise noted.

[2] Refers to children under age 21 receiving active treatment in Medicaid-certified psychiatric hospitals.

[3] Refers to children under age 21 in Medicaid-certified intermediate care facilities, unless otherwise noted.

[4] Refers to children under age 21 in subsidized adoptions for whom public agencies are assuming some financial responsibility.

[5] Also covers children placed in foster homes or private institutions by private nonprofit agencies.

[6] Covers only children in foster homes.

[7] Also covers children for whom county departments of social services have custody and/or placement responsibility and who are not in corrective institutions.

[8] Also covers children placed in foster homes by private nonprofit agencies.

[9] Also covers children in independent living situations with all or part of their maintenance cost paid by Children's Services Division.

[10] Limited to foster children for whom the Department of Social Services is assuming full or partial responsibility.

[11] Limited to children for whom the Department of Public Welfare assumes financial responsibility who are in foster family homes or private nonprofit child-care institutions licensed or certified by that Department, or in foster family homes licensed or certified and supervised by licensed public or private nonprofit child placing agencies.

[12] Covers children under 21 in Medicaid-certified intermediate care facilities for the mentally retarded.

[13] Also covers individuals under 21 in Medicaid-certified skilled nursing facilities.

[14] Also covers individuals under 21 who are members of an AFDC or General Assistance family.

[15] Also covers children of unemployed fathers (but not the specified relative or second parent) meeting the state's broader definition of unemployment.

[16] Also covers children under 21 who are considered "essential persons" by SSI.

[17] Also covers children under 21 deprived of parental support or care for any reason specified in the Act, and living with a relative specified in Section 406(A) of the Act.

Appendix S.
CONTACTS CONCERNING INNOVATIVE EFFORTS DISCUSSED IN CHAPTER 6

Direct Service Programs

Comprehensive Emergency Services Program
The National Center for Comprehensive Emergency Services
The Urban Observatory
700 Second Avenue South
Nashville, Tennessee 37210

The Door
James J. Turanski, M.D.
Program Director
The Door — A Center of Alternatives
618 Avenue of the Americas
New York, New York 10011

Family Reception Center
David Martin, DSW
Project Director
The Family Reception Center
441 Fourth Avenue
Brooklyn, New York 11215

Homebuilders Program
Jill Kinney, Ph.D.
Homebuilders Program
Catholic Children's Services of Tacoma
5410 North Forty-fourth Street
Tacoma, Washington 98407

Mother and Child Residence
Florence Kreech, Director
Louise Wise Services
6 East Ninety-third Street
New York, New York 10028

Project Ku-nak-we-sha
Maxine Robbins
Acting Director
Project Ku-nak-we-sha
Yakima Tribal Family and Children Services
P.O. Box 344
Toppenish, Washington 98948

San Antonio Children's Center
Dr. Carl Pfeifer
Director
San Antonio Children's Center
2939 W. Woodlawn Avenue
San Antonio, Texas 78228

Administrative and Judicial Efforts to Protect Children and Families

Concern for Children In Placement Project
D. Jene Whitecotton, Esq.
Project Director
National Council of Juvenile Court Judges
P.O. Box 8978
Reno, Nevada 89507

Freeing Children for Permanent Placement
Victor A. Pike
Permanent Planning Project
Children's Services Division
P.O. Box 17407
Portland, Oregon 97217
(for information about administration and intervention techniques)

David L. Slader
Metropolitan Public Defender
514 S.W. Sixth Avenue
Portland, Oregon 97204
(for discussion of legal issues)

Parents Rights Unit, Special Services for Children
Linda Greenman, Director
Natural Parents Unit
Special Services for Children
New York City Department of Social Services
Human Resources Administration
80 Lafayette Street
New York, New York 10013

South Carolina Foster Care Review Boards and the Office for Child Advocacy
Barbara Chappell, Director
Office of Child Advocacy
Division of Health and Social Development
1800 St. Julian Place
Columbia, South Carolina 29204

Advocacy Groups

Association for Children of New Jersey
(Formerly Citizen's Committee for Children of New Jersey)

Linda J. Wood, Acting Administrator
744 Broad Street, Suite 1220
Newark, New Jersey 07102

California Children's Lobby
Elizabeth Berger
California Children's Lobby
P.O. Box 448
Sacramento, California 95802

Citizen's Committee for Ohio Children's Services
Virginia Colson
3592 Delamere Avenue
Columbus, Ohio 43220

FLOC
Fred Taylor, Director
For Love of Children
2025 Massachusetts Avenue, N.W.
Washington, D.C. 20036

Mary Ann Stein, Director
Child Advocacy Center
1025 Fifteenth Street, N.W.
Washington, D.C. 20005

Illinois Foster Children's Association
Lewis and Clark College
P.O. Box 306
Godfrey, Illinois 62035

Institute for Child Advocacy
James Lardie, Director
Institute for Child Advocacy
2800 Euclid Avenue
Cleveland, Ohio 44115

Junior League
Jewel Dean J. Londa
Executive Director
The National Association of Junior Leagues, Inc.
825 Third Avenue
New York, New York 10022

National Action for Foster Children
Raymond S. McClelland
Executive Director
National Action for Foster Children Committee, Inc.
611 East Wells Street
Milwaukee, Wisconsin 53202

National Commission for Children In Need of Parents
Victor Weingarten
Executive Director
National Commission for Children In Need of Parents
801 Second Avenue
New York, New York 10017

National Foster Parents Association
Harley Mackie
President
808 West Commercial
Broken Arrow, Oklahoma 74012

North American Council on Adoptable Children
250 East Blaine
Riverside, California 92507

Children's Defense Fund

The Children's Defense Fund (CDF) is a national, nonprofit public charity created to provide long-range and systematic advocacy on behalf of the nation's children. Through research, public education, litigation, community organizing and monitoring federal administrative and legislative policies and programs, CDF seeks to change policies and practices resulting in the neglect or mistreatment of millions of children. Our goal is to place the needs of children and their families higher on the public policy agenda.

CDF is supported primarily by foundations. We have no chapters and are not a membership organization, but work closely with other groups to help individuals, parents, advocacy groups and national networks work on behalf of children.

CDF is now beginning a major effort to diversify and ensure its immediate and long-term funding base through solicitation of individual and group contributions. We hope we can attract a core of regular CDF sponsors who will make us one of their annual charities in any amount they can afford.

As important as financial help is the increased interest and involvement of individuals and groups on behalf of children. We hope all taking the time to read this book will begin to:

- Become informed about the needs of children nationally and in your own area.
- Talk to other parents, individuals and groups in your community to gain strength from numbers to pursue local change for children.
- Speak up to unresponsive policymakers and political officials who fail to protect children's interests or provide them with needed services.
- Write letters on selected children's issues to your Representative, Senator, state legislator or local city council people, and let CDF know if you or others are willing to do so on behalf of any of our issues. Request a copy of our *National Legislative Agenda for Children* if you do not know how to begin.
- Give good local child advocacy groups your financial support in any amount you can afford. One of CDF's goals is to help ensure that in a few years all 50 states will have effective local groups working actively to achieve specific goals for children. All of us need your help in building an effective national and local network for children.

CDF Board of Directors

Lisle C. Carter, Jr. (Chairman)
President, University of the District of Columbia
(Former HEW Assistant Secretary for Individual and Family Services)
Washington, D.C.

Julius L. Chambers, Esq.
Chambers, Stein, Ferguson & Becton
President, NAACP Legal Defense and Educational Fund
Charlotte, North Carolina

Marian Wright Edelman
Director, Children's Defense Fund
Washington, D.C.

Winifred Green
Director, Southeastern Public Education Program of the American Friends Service Committee
Jackson, Mississippi

Hubert E. Jones
Dean, School of Social Work, Boston University
Chairman, Massachusetts Advocacy Center
Boston, Massachusetts

Vernon E. Jordan, Jr.
President, National Urban League
New York, New York

Ruby G. Martin, Esq.
General Counsel, U.S. House of Representatives Committee on the District of Columbia
Washington, D.C.

Joseph L. Rauh, Jr., Esq.
Rauh, Silard & Lichtman
Washington, D.C.

Hillary Rodham, Esq.
Rose, Nash, Williamson, Carroll, Clay & Giroir
President, Arkansas Advocates for Children and Families
Little Rock, Arkansas

Gilbert Y. Steiner
Senior Fellow, The Brookings Institution
Washington, D.C.

Rachel B. Tompkins
Director, Citizens' Council for Ohio Schools
Cleveland, Ohio

Thomas A. Troyer, Esq.
Partner, Caplin & Drysdale
Washington, D,C.

Nan Waterman
Chairwoman, Common Cause
Washington, D.C.

Andrew Young*
U.S. Permanent Representative to the United Nations
New York, New York

* On leave

Other CDF Publications

Books

Children Out of School in America

School Suspensions: Are They Helping Children?

The Elementary and Secondary School Civil Rights Survey: An Analysis

Doctors and Dollars Are Not Enough

EPSDT: Does It Spell Health Care for Poor Children?

Children in Adult Jails

Who Needs Child Care? Policy Options for the '80s

Handbooks

94-142 and 504: Numbers That Add Up to Educational Rights for Handicapped Children

How Special Education Advocacy Can Work: A Mississippi Case Study

Your School Records

Misclassification: The Resegregation of Black Children in Public Schools

Health Care for Children: Policies and Principles for Child Advocates

A Brief Guide to Children Without Homes

Federal Programs Affecting Children Without Homes

For the Welfare of Children

It's Time to Stand Up for Your Children

Where Do You Look? Whom Do You Ask? How Do You Know? Resources for Child Advocates

Title XX: Social Services in Your State

The Child Care Handbook

National Legislative Agenda for Children

What is CDF?

CDF Annual Report

Special for International Year of the Child

A Portrait of Inequality: Black and White Children in America

America's Children and Families: A Profile

Children and the Federal Budget: What the President Proposes

A Child Advocate's Guide to Capitol Hill and Federal Agencies

Building a House on the Hill for Our Children

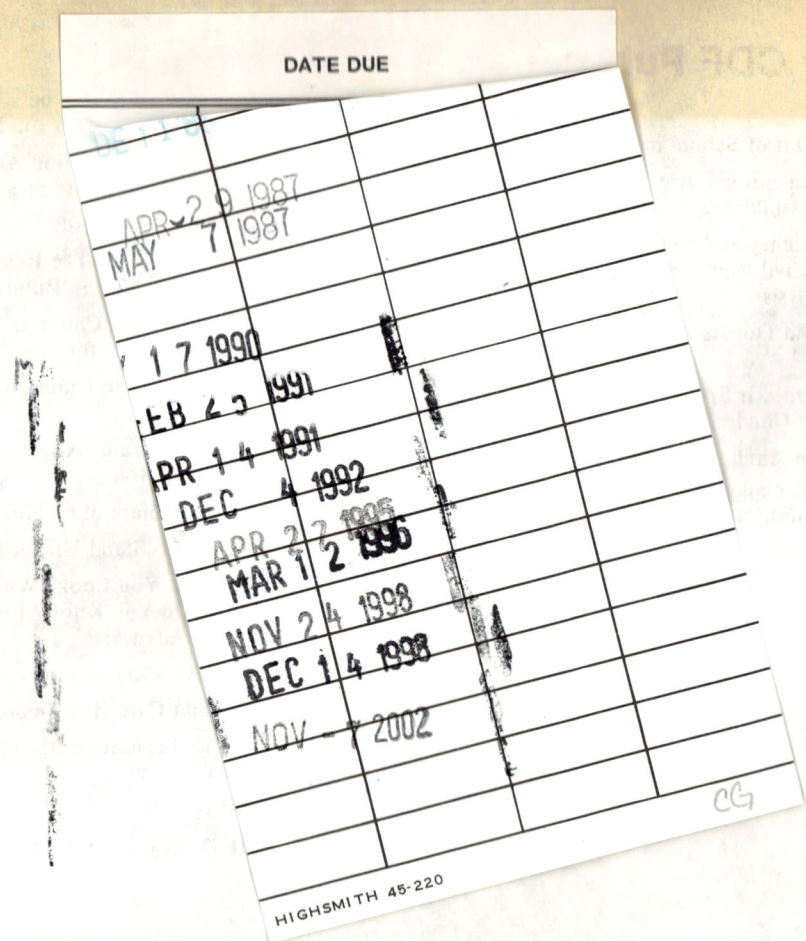